second edition

SUCCESSFUL COMMUNICATION *with* PERSONS *with* ALZHEIMER'S DISEASE

An In-Service Manual

Mary Jo Santo Pietro, PhD, CCC-SLP
Associate Professor of Speech Language Pathology;
Director, Speech and Hearing Clinic,
Kean University
Union, New Jersey

Elizabeth Ostuni, MA, CCC-SLP
Director, Accent on Communication,
Sparta, New Jersey

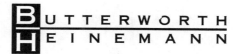

BUTTERWORTH
HEINEMANN

An Imprint of Elsevier

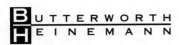

An Imprint of Elsevier

11830 Westline Industrial Drive
St. Louis, Missouri 63146

Previous edition copyrighted 1997

Acquisitions Editor: Kellie White
Associate Developmental Editor: Jennifer L. Watrous
Publishing Services Manager: Pat Joiner
Project Manager: Karen M. Rehwinkel
Senior Designer: Mark A. Oberkrom
Publishing Director: Linda Duncan

Printed in the United States of America

Last digit is the print number: 9   8   7   6   5   4   3   2

second edition

SUCCESSFUL
COMMUNICATION
with PERSONS *with*
ALZHEIMER'S DISEASE
An In-Service Manual

To all the caregivers who came to our workshops and taught us so much.

A LIVING WILL

When they say I cannot
hear you, sing me lullabies
and folk songs, the ones
I sang to you. I will hear them
as an unborn child can hear
its mother's music through
the waters of the womb.

When they say I can feel
nothing, press your face
against my forehead, rest your
hand against my cheek. I
will feel them as the woman
at the window feels the wind
outside the glass.

When they say I'm past
all caring, brush my hair
and braid in ribbons. I will
know it as the seashells
on my table know the
rhythms of the sea.

When they tell you
to go home, stay with me
if you can. Deep
inside I will be
weeping.

Naomi Halperin Spigle

From Martz SH (editor): I am becoming the woman I've wanted, Watsonville, Calif, 1995,
Papier-Mache Press, p. 216.

Notes to the Instructor

THE LEARNING OBJECTIVES OF THIS TEXT

1. To make the job of professionals working directly with persons who have Alzheimer's disease easier, more efficient, and more pleasant.
2. To provide the highest quality of life available for the nursing home resident who has Alzheimer's disease.
3. To furnish all nursing home employees with basic information about communication processes, problems, and strengths of people who have Alzheimer's disease.
4. To instruct caregivers in specific techniques shown to be effective in improving communication with patients with Alzheimer's disease.
5. To promote discussion and problem-solving related to sensitive communication issues.
6. To encourage administrators and managers to design policies, programs, and procedures that support facility-wide use of effective communication.

Human beings use more than words to communicate. Our tone of voice, gestures, the clothes we wear, and the way we decorate our homes also send messages about what we think and how we feel. Even with all these avenues of expression available, we often struggle to find the right words or to understand what someone means when they speak. The challenge is far greater when we try to communicate with persons who have Alzheimer's disease, an illness characterized by major communication problems. Still, better communication with our patients and with our co-workers is a worthwhile goal. It is also an achievable one.

As speech-language pathologists, we have spent many years working directly with Alzheimer's disease patients at home, in adult daycare centers, and in long-term care facilities, and from early to late stages. We have conducted countless practical workshops with nursing home personnel. Caregivers' stories have enlivened and energized our audiences; their questions and insights have brought personal wisdom and experience to the learning process. But still we hear questions like these from seasoned staff as well as new employees:

- "Why does she keep asking me the same question?"
- "What does he mean he wants his mother? I've told him over and over, she's dead."
- "Why can't I talk her into taking her bath?"
- "What do I say when he accuses me of taking his wallet?"
- "How can I get her to stop yelling all the time?"

The volume of these questions has convinced us that there is an essential component of information and skills that most formal education programs neglect: the basic "how-tos" of communicating with residents who have Alzheimer's disease. It is also increasingly evident that time and money are inter-dependent resources as nursing facilities struggle to balance quality care within severe budget limitations. Both assets are protected when intelligent communication practices are at the center of every procedure and every care-giving technique.[1,2] We have culled the literature for solid suggestions and proven techniques for improving communication with persons who have Alzheimer's disease.

The result is this book, *Successful Communication with Persons with Alzheimer's Disease*. The book is comprised of a series of 12 self-contained in-service sessions, each in-service focusing on a specific aspect of communication that is crucial in the care of these residents. The intended audience is the direct care staff in nursing facilities who cope daily with frail and cognitively confused elders. But nursing homes that routinely "walk the extra mile" toward excellence will build components of these in-services into continuing education programs for support staff as well. Administration and management, buildings and grounds maintenance teams, housekeeping, food services, volunteers, and contract businesses—in short anyone and everyone who has even occasional contact with residents who have Alzheimer's disease has need of the communication skills described in this book.

Successful Communication with Persons with Alzheimer's Disease is also a solid resource for employees in other settings in which elderly persons with cognitive deficits spend their time: private homes, group homes, adult daycare centers, and rehabilitation hospitals. Because of its practical approach, this text is an ideal choice for nursing aide certification programs and college classes in gerontology, in which care-giving practices and ethics are shaped.

OVERVIEW OF THE SECOND EDITION

This textbook provides instructors and in-service participants with a ready-to-go format.

Outline of User-Friendly Text

Our intent in writing *Successful Communication with Persons with Alzheimer's Disease* has been to develop materials that are easy to understand, whether the learner has the support of a course instructor or is using the text for independent study. Each of the 12 in-services include these convenient features:

- Chapter outline
- An introductory premise
- Learning objectives
- Definitions of important terms
- Quick Tip Summaries of key information
- Real-life examples, case studies, and scripts from actual encounters with persons who have Alzheimer's disease
- Self-study questionnaires, checklists, and quizzes
- Activities for team or group discussions, role-plays, and on-the-job practice
  Lecture-ready overheads of all Quick Tip Summaries can be found in Appendix 2.

Successful Communication with Persons with Alzheimer's Disease is divided into four main parts. Part I, which includes the Introduction and In-services 1 and 2, focuses on communication deficits that are specific to Alzheimer's disease, as well as those resulting from the other medical and psychological problems that persons face because they are growing older.

Part II consists of In-Services 3 and 4, and acquaints the reader with the concepts of communication-impaired environments and the ways in which surroundings either support or interfere with a resident's attempts to communicate. We have collected new resources on physical and psychosocial environments that can truly make the resident feel "at home."

In Part III, professional caregivers are encouraged to examine their own communication strengths, weaknesses, and attitudes. In-Services 5, 6, 7, and 8 bring caregivers "face to face" with the sensitive issues of diversity, (verbal) abuse in the nursing home setting, and interactions with families. New material presents information on how nursing facilities are addressing these challenging realities.

Part IV is devoted to specific communication techniques and programs. In-

Services 9, 10, and 11 present reliable programs reported in the past, and several recent well-researched models that are transforming the way we communicate with persons who have Alzheimer's disease. All have been selected on the basis of ease of implementation and minimal expense. In-Service 12, "Last Things: When a Person with Alzheimer's Disease is Dying," is all new. This in-service offers suggestions to families and direct care staff for maintaining communication with terminally ill, cognitively-impaired residents when traditional interventions are no longer helpful.

Each of the 12 in-services in *Successful Communication with Persons with Alzheimer's Disease* is designed as an independent lesson, that is, each in-service is "topic specific." The in-service training schedule can follow the exact sequence of the book, or the instructor may prefer to select specific in-services based on particular needs of certain residents, direct care staff, or setting. Instructors will soon see, however, that the information presented in Part I (Introduction, In-Services 1 and 2) is basic to the student's understanding of all subsequent material. If instructors choose to begin with any of the later in-services in the book, students should first be required to read these three introductory sections and to pass the quizzes on In-Services 1 and 2 to ensure that this important content has been mastered.

An alternative mode of study is also available to those who cannot attend classes. Shortly after the publication of the first edition, the authors recorded a set of audiocassette tapes entitled, like the first book, *Successful Communication with Alzheimer's Disease Patients*. The taped program was based on the content of that book. The program is approved for nursing continuing education credits for several health care professions and is available, with permission of Elsevier Science, through the Center for Health Care Education.[3]

Suggestions for Selecting a Qualified Instructor

A major presenting symptom of Alzheimer's disease is a decline in communication skills. Because of the close relationship between the disease process, communication skills, and the behavior management of these residents, the ideal choice for instructor, consultant, or co-planner for the in-services in this book is a speech-language pathologist.

Speech-language pathologists who work in nursing homes, home health care settings, and adult daycare centers specialize in the gerontologic aspects of communication. They are experienced in providing in-service programs. Their national professional organization, The American Speech-Language-Hearing Association is a resource for additional materials on communication problems associated with aging and dementia.

The in-services in the second edition of *Successful Communication with Persons with Alzheimer's Disease* can also be conducted effectively by other health care professionals. However, the instructor should have a thorough understanding of the complex changes in language that occur in residents with Alzheimer's disease, what those changes signal, and how to respond most skillfully to them. Whatever your background, we encourage you to read the following suggestions before proceeding.

Suggestions for Creating Meaningful Learning Experiences

The teaching goals for *Successful Communication with Persons with Alzheimer's Disease* are twofold: (1) to deepen the participants' knowledge about the communication skills and deficits of residents who are aging and in cognitive decline; and (2) to improve their own communication with those residents, as well as with each other and the residents' families. One way to meet both goals is to develop a variety of opportunities for students to experience the content of the text. Several of the 14 suggestions for promoting course participation that follow encourage participants to use or to re-create the classroom material in some way. Additional activities and discussions form part of each in-service. Many Good Practice activities center on a role play of communication situations that arise from the participants' own experiences and observations. Below are some guidelines for conducting successful role plays, adapted from Koury and Lubinsky's chapter in *Dementia and Communication*[4]:

1. For students new to role-playing, the instructor should first model how role-play is done by playing one of the roles.
2. Students should be encouraged to "think on their feet."
3. Stop the action if a player becomes too anxious or runs out of ideas. Redirect the action with a question, or allow someone else to give it a try. Then encourage the first student to try again. The idea is to build a successful repertoire of responses, not be made to feel humiliated and inadequate by the practice.
4. Ask the audience to make suggestions to help the players.
5. Replay a less-than-inspired role-play to give players a second chance to learn appropriate responses. Or encourage more than one pair to enact a particular role-play and ask the audience to reflect on the effectiveness of different communication styles and dynamics between the two pairs.
6. Coach more experienced players with emotionally charged statements such as "You're frustrated, even angry now. She actually *slapped* you!"
7. Summarize strategies for communication repair frequently. Ask the group to judge which strategies would be most effective with particular residents with whom they now work.
8. Videotape (or tape record) the role play to capture fine teaching points and illustrate good use of technique—but only after students have had some practice and experience with role play. It takes a skilled instructor to turn this form of self-confrontation into a positive learning experience, but the effort is worthwhile.

Suggestions for Promoting Course Participation

Instructors and training departments will have a higher rate of attendance and gain stronger administrative support if they emphasize the benefits and services of the program. Here are 14 ideas for getting started.

1. Establish an in-house (or corporate) certification program for employees who complete all 12 in-services.
2. Link the certificate or completion of all of the in-services to a pay raise.
3. Arrange with the state or corporate office for attendees to received continuing education (CE) credits. This book contains ample learning activities, quizzes, and Quick Tip Summaries in ready-to-go formats to provide evidence to reviewers that the course merits CE credits.
4. Create a title such as "Communication Specialist" for those who have completed all 12 in-services. These persons could assist with additional in-service training sessions. Write articles for the in-house newsletter or community publication, or conduct short-term studies based on questions and issues that arise during the classes on communication.
5. Develop incentives that motivate participants to seek certification and at the same time make behavioral changes: Offer a prize to the participant who makes frequent use of one of the conversational strategies; who spots an especially obvious or bothersome physical barrier to communication in his or her setting; or who writes a well-detailed description of a resident's communication skills or deficits.
6. Recognize and reward participants who complete half the units (e.g., a "half-way certificate") with items such as 2 hours compensatory time; an empty frame for the anticipated certificate of completion; a bookmark inscribed with an inspirational quotation; mention of the student's name in the in-house newsletter; 1 day's parking privilege in the CEO's parking place; a letter to the attendee's supervisor with copies for the personnel file; or a flower or special ribbon to be worn for the rest of the week. Each time someone comments on

the flower or asks "why the ribbon?", the communication in-service program becomes more visible and more positive in the eyes of the rest of the staff.

7. Keep participants' interested by arranging a visit to the local university's speech and hearing clinic, contracting with an audiologist to screen each student's hearing or to speak about the effects of hearing loss on job performance, inviting a lawyer to explain state laws and regulations regarding elder abuse and the "whistle-blower" protection clauses, or asking a foreign-born staff member or volunteer to talk about cultural differences in communication that he or she has experienced since moving to the United States.

8. Stress the commitment of management to improvement of the communication climate; arrange for a top administrator to drop in and meet each student personally, or to introduce the first program in a series.

9. Extend the in-service *learning experience* by assigning pairs of students to give 15-minute mini-sessions and demonstrations in their work settings. Then ask them to review their *teaching experience* during the next communication in-service that they attend.

10. Give a prize or perk to the student who recruits the most attendees for the next in-service or set of in-services on communication.

11. Invite a local newspaper (hopefully with photographer) to attend the graduation of those participants who complete all 12 in-services successfully. Have the press release ready with the names and hometowns of all participants.

12. Include the opportunity for special training in communication skills in all staff recruitment literature.

13. Advertise the program to the Volunteer Department, or require that a certain number of communication classes be a routine part of new volunteer orientation.

14. Cut costs by co-sponsoring the program with a nearby nursing facility, home health agency, Certified Nursing Assistant training program, Office on Aging, or junior college.

A FINAL WORD

Of course, not all problems in a nursing home can be solved by improving communication skills of staff or residents. Nevertheless, it is our hope that mastery of the concepts and skills in *Successful Communication with Persons with Alzheimer's Disease* will help caregivers and support staff discover more situations that can be managed better and with less effort than they might ever have imagined. Good luck!

MJSP & EJO

REFERENCES

1. McCallion P, Toseland R, Lacey D, Bands S: Educating nursing assistants to communicate more effectively with nursing home residents with dementia, *The Gerontologist*, 39:5, 546-558, 1999.

2. Schirm V, Albanese T, Garland T, Gipson G, Blackmon D: Caregiving in nursing homes, *Clinical Nursing Research*, 9:3, 280-297, 2000.

3. Santo Pietro MJ, Ostuni E: *Successful communication with Alzheimer's disease patients.* Audiocassette program for nursing home personnel, available through Center for Health Care Education, P.O. Box 6844, Monroe Township, NJ 08831. 1998.

4. Koury LN, Lubinsky R: Effective in-service training for staff working with communication impaired patients. In Lubinsky R, editor: *Dementia and communication*, Philadelphia, 1991, BC Decker, p. 279.

Acknowledgments

Once again we would like to thank Lilly Miller at the Center for Health Care Education who gave us so many opportunities to meet with nursing home personnel at every level throughout the state of New Jersey. In essence, over the years they trained us in what they needed to communicate successfully with their Alzheimer's patients.

Thanks also to Faerella Boczko, MA, CCC-slp at the Jewish Home and Hospital for Aged in the Bronx, NY. Her expertise and dedication to the improved communication for her Alzheimer's patients was an education and inspiration. Thanks to everyone on the Saul Unit who made the Breakfast Club and so many other programs work.

Many thanks to the staff and residents of the Sussex County Homestead Nursing Home, Mary Lou Schnurr, CNHA, Director, for their generous support of the Healing Touch research projects and for their role in providing several of the conversations and case illustrations in this manual.

A sincere thank you to all the speech-language pathologists who have become interested in the treatment of persons with Alzheimer's disease over the last decade. Thanks for all the techniques you've developed, all the wisdom you've shared, and all the care you've given. We do have a role to play here.

And finally, thanks so much to Karen Rehwinkel and Jennifer Watrous, patient and inspired editors at Elsevier/Butterworth-Heinneman. It's been a joy to work with you.

Communication in the Nursing Home

PREMISE   We depend on communication to accomplish most of life's tasks. The better we communicate, the more likely we are to be understood and to get what we need from other people. When people do not communicate effectively, misunderstandings develop and mistakes are made. In the nursing home, effective communication not only ensures accurate decision making and efficiency, but also promotes understanding and a sense of well-being in both residents and staff.

LEARNING OBJECTIVES
- Discuss the concept of communication as defined in this text.
- Give examples of verbal and nonverbal communication.
- Provide at least three reasons why human beings communicate.
- Describe the seven basic requirements for engaging in effective communication with others.
- List at least five reasons why effective communication in a nursing home is so important.

DEFINITIONS   **Communication**   Communication occurs when we send or receive messages, and when we assign meaning to another person's signals. Every communication takes place in a specific *environment* that has both *physical* and *psychosocial* aspects. Each person involved in communication is both a *source* (speaker) and a *receiver* (listener).

Our *spoken words* provide only 7% of any message communicated between two people. *Expression*, or how one says the words (sadly, sarcastically), accounts for 35% of any message communicated, and *body language* accounts for approximately 58% of any message.[1] This means that more than 90% of our messages are communicated nonverbally.

All human beings communicate. In fact, when two people are in the same room, it is impossible *not* to communicate. Because communication is largely body language, messages are sent even when no words are said. Lovers, enemies, competitors, casual acquaintances, and complete strangers convey volumes to one another without ever saying a word. We may not communicate with great success, but we are always communicating *something* to one another.

Effective communication   You have communicated effectively when the message you intend is accurately understood by another who then responds appropriately.

Communication competence   Your ability to communicate effectively is your communication competence. Simply stated, the greater your knowledge of communication, the greater your communication competence. The more ways you have to express yourself, the greater the likelihood you will communicate effectively in any situation.

Verbal communication   The actual words we speak comprise our verbal communication. In general, verbal communication constitutes less than 10% of the total messages we convey. (See "Speech", "Language", "Voice", In-Service 2.)

Nonverbal Communication   Nonverbal signals constitute as much as 93% of any message. Culture, personality, and emotions contribute to an individual's style of nonverbal communication. These nonverbal signals include the following:
- *Expression:* The rate of speaking and the pitch, volume, and intonation of the voice

- *Body position:* Proximity to listener; at eye level, above, or below the listener
- *Body orientation:* Positioning toward or away from the listener
- *Gesture:* The presence, frequency, and expressiveness of hand movements
- *Touch:* The presence, meaningfulness, and gentleness of touch
- *Facial expression and eye contact:* The ability to show interest, emotion, and empathy
- *Personal appearance:* The condition of clothes, hair style, cosmetics, and scents
- *Personal environment:* Choices of living quarters, music, companions

Nonverbal communication serves many purposes. It can emphasize or restate what you have said verbally. It can substitute for verbal communication, such as when you shrug your shoulders rather than say, "I don't know." Nonverbal communication can regulate verbal communication. If you lower your voice at the end of a sentence, you are letting your conversational partner know that it is his turn to speak. When you turn away from someone, you are rejecting further conversation. Sometimes nonverbal communication contradicts verbal communication, such as when a person with a red face and bulging veins yells *"Angry? No, I'm not angry!"*

Nonverbal styles vary from person to person. Some people use nonverbal signals to generously enhance their communication. Others rarely use gestures and facial expression. Sometimes we send unintentional messages because we are not aware of the nonverbal signals we use. Remember, we cannot *not* communicate.

ILLUSTRATION OF NONVERBAL COMMUNICATION

The story is told about a script writer who complained to movie producer Sam Goldwyn, *"I'm telling you a sensational story. All I'm asking for is your opinion, and you fall asleep!"*

Mr. Goldwyn responded, *"Isn't sleeping an opinion?"*

WHY WE COMMUNICATE

The primary purpose of communication is the exchange of information between people. An equally important reason we communicate is to meet our individual needs. We communicate those wants and needs to people that can help us obtain necessities such as food, shelter, and clothing. Communication helps us secure our safety and protection from danger, whether calling the police or reading the "slippery when wet" sign.

Communication is also essential to the fulfillment of our most basic social and emotional needs. Others can only show love, acceptance, and concern for us through communication. When we do not receive expressions of love and acceptance, we are at risk for major health problems—depression, failure-to-thrive syndrome, heart disease, and cancer—to name just a few.

Communication meets our need for self-actualization. By communicating we let other people know who we are, what we are doing, and the principles on which we stand. Without communication we would have no professional, political, or educational expression.

Another reason we communicate is to exert power or control over other people. Communication is our chief means of managing others, of trying to get others to do what we want. Finally, we use communication to meet the needs of others—to provide them with information, praise, and support, and to express our affection for them. We care for others through our words and gestures. Communication is a powerful therapeutic tool. Through communication, we help restore psychological well-being to others and to ourselves.

▶ **QUICK TIP SUMMARY**

Why We Communicate[2]

We communicate:

1. To give and gain information.
2. To meet our need for food, shelter and clothing, security, and safety.
3. To meet our need for social and emotional health.
4. To engage in self-actualization and self-disclosure.
5. To control, exert power, manage.
6. To meet the needs of others.
7. To use as a therapeutic tool.

WHY EFFECTIVE COMMUNICATION IS SO IMPORTANT

When people communicate effectively, they achieve more of their goals and have more life satisfaction. In a nursing home, effective communication is especially important. Effective communication saves time. If people understand our messages the first time, we do not have to waste time repeating them. Effective communication prevents mistakes. If people understand our instructions, they are less likely to make mistakes that have to be remedied later.

Effective communication has a beneficial effect on residents and caregivers alike. It reduces power struggles, calms patients, and prevents catastrophic behaviors. In return, caregivers experience less stress, and there is less potential for abusive incidents. Effective communication provides the caregiver with critical information about the patient. If you know more about a patient's capabilities, you can allow him to do more and thereby prevent the buildup of learned helplessness (see definition, In-Service 1).

Effective communication reduces the isolation and depersonalization of both resident and caregiver. Sharing each other's accomplishments, problems, backgrounds, likes and dislikes builds self-esteem and promotes personal bonding between caregiver and resident. From an administrative viewpoint, effective communication can clearly reduce the level of worker stress and reduce the rate of worker burnout. The bottom line is that effective communication in the nursing home can and does save the facility money.

▶ **QUICK TIP SUMMARY**

The Importance of Effective Communication in the Nursing Home

Effective communication:

1. Saves time.
2. Prevents mistakes, saves work later on.
3. Calms the residents, calms the caregivers.
4. Defuses power struggles, prevents catastrophic behaviors, reduces the potential for abusive incidents.
5. Prevents residents from learning helplessness.
6. Reduces isolation and depersonalization of both residents and caregivers.
7. Promotes personal bonding between residents and caregivers.
8. Promotes self-esteem in residents and caregivers.
9. Cuts down on worker stress, reduces high rates of caregiver burnout.
10. Saves money for the facility.

REQUIREMENTS FOR EFFECTIVE COMMUNICATION

Think of the last time you had a real heart-to-heart conversation with a close friend or loved one. A heart-to-heart conversation is one of the best illustrations of effective communication. What does it take to make a heart-to-heart conversation work? What conditions are necessary?

1. *A place:* You need a place that is *quiet* and free of distractions; a place that is *private* and *comfortable*. Quiet, private, comfortable places are difficult to find in many nursing homes.

2. *A shared language:* To have a heart-to-heart conversation, you and your friend must speak the same language. The less language you share, the tougher it is to communicate. Not only words, but the body language of nods, gestures, and eye gaze can have different meanings in different languages. Even persons who speak different dialects of the same language can have different vocabularies and different cultures. Gender and generation gaps within each language also create communication breakdowns between people of different genders and ages. Seldom do residents and caregivers in a nursing home share a totally common language. They must often overcome regional, cultural, gender, and age-related differences to make communication work.

3. *A common frame of reference:* Every individual has a personal frame of reference, a personal set of experiences, interests, values, and beliefs. Your frame of reference grows out of personal preference and experience, socioeconomic and cultural factors, and historical events. Persons who did not live during the Great Depression might not put as much value on job security as those who did. Persons who have never experienced persecution or prejudice may not be sensitive to the pain that some words cause to holocaust or civil rights survivors. The people with whom you communicate best, with whom you like to have heart-to-heart conversations, generally share your frame of reference. Few workers in nursing home settings truly share common frames of reference with the residents for whom they care, and vice versa.

4. *A certain set of mental abilities:* Certain basic mental abilities are required for effective communication. They include the following:

a. *Perception:* To understand and respond to someone's message, two people must be able to see and hear each other. When having a heart-to-heart conversation, you tend to watch your partner's face and listen carefully. Many elderly nursing home residents have deficits in hearing and vision that interfere with their perception. Many caregivers, busy with their chores, do not look at residents while talking to them; do not listen to what they say. Important messages often go unnoticed.

b. *Attention:* To communicate well, the speaker and the listener must be able to pay attention to each other. You do not feel like sharing your innermost feelings unless you have someone's close attention. One symptom of Alzheimer's disease and other dementias is difficulty in maintaining attention. Medications and anxieties also interfere with the ability to attend. Nursing home personnel are frequently too busy or distracted to pay close attention to residents' attempts at communication. Both partners miss messages from lack of attention.

c. *Intellectual understanding:* To communicate effectively, two people must be able to understand each other's ideas. You are unlikely to bother explaining your thoughts to persons who cannot grasp them. Alzheimer's disease, by definition, robs people of the intellectual ability to understand. Caregivers, in turn, make fewer efforts to share information. The less intellectual stimulation the patients receive, the less practice they get in processing it. The inevitable decline in intellectual functioning is hastened by the lack of effective communication. An ongoing spiral of deterioration is set in motion.

d. *Memory:* To stay on topic and to add details to a story, a speaker must have an intact memory. *Long-term memory* is needed to remember who you are talking to, and what you are talking about. *Short-term memory* is needed to remember your partner's questions and remarks long enough to form responses. Alzheimer's disease is characterized by the loss of memory. Caregivers, too, find that they cannot remember all the details in the lives and medical histories of all the residents in their care. Limitations in the memories of both residents and caregivers not only reduce the effectiveness of communication, but also stifle the desire of either one to communicate.

5. *Openness:* Openness is a willingness to listen to and honestly appraise your partner's message even if you think you will not agree. If your partner is not open to your message, you are apt to withhold your ideas and opinions; you do not speak up if you believe your words will "fall on deaf ears." Persons with Alzheimer's disease often appear self-absorbed and uninterested in the messages of others. Equally damaging to the communication process, however, are staff members who show little openness to the messages of residents. Many caregivers admit they have little desire to hear them.

6. *Expectation of response:* When you speak earnestly to someone, you expect a response—at least a nonverbal acknowledgment, preferably a carefully worded answer! If your heart-to-heart partner were to sit silently after hearing your important announcement, you would probably say, "Well? Say something!" Research shows that persons with Alzheimer's disease continue to expect responses too, until quite late in the illness. Their expectations often go unmet. Conversely, staff members seldom expect responses from these residents. They hurry on without realizing that low expectations beget low returns.

7. *Respect and trust:* The final requirements for good communication are respect and trust. The person with whom you had your last heart-to-heart conversation was undoubtedly someone you respected and trusted. Otherwise you would not have told your secrets, shared your opinions, or bared your soul. You would not have felt safe. New residents with Alzheimer's disease might find it hard to trust people in the unfamiliar new setting of a nursing home. In homes in which the staff turnover rate is high, the formation of trusting relationships is especially difficult. Residents with Alzheimer's disease are often deeply suspicious of those who care for them. For their part, some caregivers appear not to respect the integrity of demented residents. They take for granted their right to enter a resident's room, search through belongings, and forcibly direct the resident's life. Some of these actions may be necessary, but their abrupt execution does not convey a sense of respect and trust; it engenders suspicion and defensiveness.

► **QUICK TIP SUMMARY**   **What is Required for Effective Communication?**

1. A place
2. A shared language
3. A common frame of reference
4. A certain set of mental abilities
   a. Perception
   b. Attention
   c. Intellectual understanding
   d. Memory
5. Openness
6. Expectation of response
7. Respect and trust

SOME FINAL NOTES ON COMMUNICATION

1. Effective communication is possible without one or more of the requirements discussed here. Lovers become engaged in a crowded subway, blind and deafened individuals manage businesses, and people from different cultures develop close friendships. However, the fewer requirements that can be met, the greater the effort communication partners must make to compensate. Learning to communicate effectively under less than optimal conditions is the greatest challenge faced by caregivers of persons with Alzheimer's disease.

2. We tend to understand others based on our personal points of view and cultural biases. Everyone does.

3. Effective communication does not guarantee agreement. A good fight can be good communication.

4. Our attitudes, or what we say to ourselves inside our heads, eventually find expression in how we behave and talk to others. A caregiver who thinks, "If he does that one more time, I'll. . ." is more likely to speak with open irritation to that resident than the caregiver who thinks, "I'm going to stay calm when Joe starts insulting me again."

5. The only people we can control are ourselves. No one else can make us say anything we don't want to say. No one else can make us lose control over our actions if we know clearly what we are supposed to do.

6. We *can* change the ways we communicate. We *can* change our attitudes. With practice and experience, we *can* develop effective communication skills even though our residents with Alzheimer's disease are losing theirs. This book is dedicated to the proposition that our work with Alzheimer's patients can be improved tremendously by changing the ways we communicate.

GOOD PRACTICE I-1

Benefits of Good Communication

Directions: Match the number from the "Importance of Effective Communication in the Nursing Home" list in the "Quick Tip Summary" that corresponds to the examples below. If this activity is done as a group, discuss your answers together. Opinions may differ.

1. ___ We don't have to cover for each other's absences on our unit now like we used to. I'm feeling less stressed and more like I can do my job as it should be done.

2. ___ Last week we spent a total of one-half employee hour in social contact with one of our most combative residents (5-minute segments throughout the day and evening). His catastrophic reactions have dropped from two per day to three per week.

3. ___ Two of the residents with Alzheimer's disease on our unit are starting to feed themselves.

4. ___ We have a new chart on our bulletin board. We select one resident with Alzheimer's disease each week. The staff member who can elicit the highest number of responses from that resident (either verbal or nonverbal) wins a lottery ticket.

5. ___ Our supervisor provided us with 10 hours of communication training last year. It was useful at home and on the job. I wasn't surprised to learn that our unit has the lowest rate of staff turnover in the facility.

GOOD PRACTICE I-2

Benefits of Good Communication

Directions: In a team discussion, describe your own real-life experiences related to the following benefits of good communication. In the spaces below, write the best example of each.

1. Saves time: _____

2. Prevents mistakes and accidents: _____

3. Calms the resident; calms the caregiver: _____

4. Reduces isolation of the caregiver and resident; promotes personal bonding:
_____

5. Saves facility time and money: _____

Discussion Point: In what ways could these ideas be adapted to your setting?

GOOD PRACTICE I-3

Tuning in to Verbal and Nonverbal Communication: A Television-Based Exercise

Directions: Tune in to a popular TV soap opera or dramatic presentation. Set the kitchen timer for 1 minute. Close your eyes. Listen, then write down the different emotions you heard when the actors spoke.

A. Verbal Communication: Expression.

1. Which emotions did you recognize? _____

2. What changes in the actor's voice let you know that different emotions were being expressed:

       ___ Spoke faster ___ Voice was high ___ Speech was louder

       ___ Spoke slower ___ Voice was low ___ Speech was softer

What else did you notice about listening to the conversation with your eyes closed?

_____

_____

B. Nonverbal Communication: Body Language

Now for 1 minute, open your eyes but turn off the TV sound. Watch the actors' body language and facial expressions. If an actor used any of the gestures and postures listed below, write a word in the blank that names the emotion you think the actor was trying to show:

Head shake _____	Head nod _____
Head droop _____	Chin up _____
Shoulders droop _____	Shoulders hunched _____
Shoulders "squared" _____	Hands clenched _____
Hands "fiddling" _____	Body forward _____
Body relaxed, "open" _____	Arms or legs crossed _____
Wide, rapid stride _____	Slow stride _____

GOOD PRACTICE I-4
Experiencing Effective Communication: A Personal Exercise

Directions: Think of the last time you had a true heart-to-heart communication with another person. Identify the place and language of the communication and answer yes (Y) or no (N) to the 20 questions. Add up the number of "yes" responses and multiply by five to get a percentage score. If your communication was effective, your score should be 80% or better.

Place where heart-to-heart occurred: _____

Language spoken in the conversation: _____

1. Was the place quiet? ( )
2. Was the place private? ( )
3. Was the place comfortable? ( )
4. Was the conversation in your native language? ( )
5. Was the conversation in your communication partner's native language? ( )
6. Did you and your communication partner share a common cultural background? ( )
7. Did you and your communication partner have a similar frame of reference? ( )
8. Could your partner hear what you said? ( )
9. Did your partner pay attention to your message? ( )
10. Did he or she understand your message? ( )
11. Could he or she remember what you said? ( )
12. Could you understand the meaning of your partner's message? ( )
13. Was your partner "open" to your message? ( )
14. Were you open to your partner's message? ( )
15. Did your partner respond to your message? ( )
16. Did you respond to your partner's message? ( )
17. Did you trust your partner? ( )
18. Did your partner appear to trust you? ( )
19. Did you respect your partner? ( )
20. Did your partner respect your ideas? ( )

Number of yes (Y) responses ___ × 5 = ___%
(% overall communication effectiveness)

Discussion Point: In contrast, think of the last time you attempted to have a conversation with a person with Alzheimer's disease. Score that conversation on the above scale. How does it compare to the score on your heart-to-heart?

REFERENCES   1. DeVito JA: *Essentials of human communication*, New York, 1993, Harper Collins, pp 6-7.
2. Lubinski R: *Dementia and communication*, Philadelphia, 1991, BC Decker, Inc, pp 142-151.

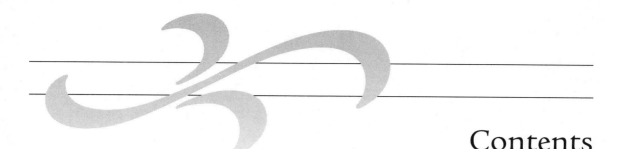

Contents

second edition

SUCCESSFUL
COMMUNICATION
with PERSONS *with*
ALZHEIMER'S DISEASE
An In-Service Manual

Characteristics of Communication in Persons with Alzheimer's Disease and Related Disorders

Communication Problems and Strengths of Patients with Alzheimer's Disease and Related Disorders

PREMISE

Alzheimer's disease causes a person's communication skills to deteriorate along a predictable course. Deterioration of memory, understanding, speech, language, and social skills takes a toll on a resident's ability to communicate effectively. While some skills are lost, other abilities undergo characteristic changes. In addition, persons with Alzheimer's disease experience communication breakdowns as part of aging. To better understand the communication behaviors of persons with Alzheimer's disease, caregivers must think not only about what is lost and what is changed but also about what is preserved.

LEARNING OBJECTIVES

- Identify and describe characteristic communication losses and changes in persons with Alzheimer's disease who are in the participants' care.
- Identify the communication breakdowns in elderly residents that are primarily due to aging.
- Recognize and describe the communication abilities preserved until the later stages in Alzheimer's disease patients with whom the participants work.

DEFINITIONS   **Communication disorder**   A communication disorder is a condition that interferes with a person's ability to be understood or to understand the communication of others. Speech that deviates so far from the speech of others that it calls attention to itself or causes distress for the listener or the speaker also is considered a communication disorder.[1]

Communication breakdown   Communication breakdown occurs when a listener does not understand the words or the intent of the speaker's message. Breakdowns in communication occur for many reasons. They happen every day to everyone and they are not always the result of a communication disorder.

Learned helplessness   "Learned helplessness arises when persons learn through repeated experiences that their actions have little effect on the outcome of the situation—especially in the 'restricted' environment of a nursing home."[2]

COMMUNICATION BREAKDOWNS CAUSED BY ALZHEIMER'S DISEASE

As a patient goes from the early to the middle and late stages of Alzheimer's disease, the number of lost abilities increases, and the changes become more marked.

Communication Losses Characteristic of Alzheimer's Disease   In Table 1-1, communication abilities are divided into four categories: *memory, understanding, speech and language skills,* and *social skills.* The table explains which abilities persons with Alzheimer's disease lose as the disease progresses.

TABLE 1-1	Communication Losses Characteristic of Alzheimer's Dementia			
STAGE	MEMORY	UNDERSTANDING	SPEECH AND LANGUAGE SKILLS	SOCIAL SKILLS
Early	Loses time orientation Loses some long-term and short-term memory (not always apparent in conversation) Loses recently acquired information Cannot retain five-item lists or phone numbers	Loses ability to understand rapid speech, speech in noisy or distracting environment, complex or abstract conversation, sarcastic humor or innuendo	Loses ideas of what to talk about Loses ability to process language rapidly (apparent in pauses and hesitancies) Loses rapid naming ability Uses related words such as "salt" for "sugar" (ability to self-correct retained)	Loses ability to stay on topic Loses control over anger and argumentativeness Loses "conversational bridges," making speech seem blunt and rude Loses ability to pay attention to speaker for more than a few minutes
Middle	Loses time and place orientation (not person) Loses additional long-term and short-term memory (apparent in conversation) Loses abstract vocabulary and concepts, names of less-familiar people Cannot remember three-item lists or three-step commands Cannot retain information soon after it is presented	Loses ability to understand ordinary, prolonged conversation Loses ability to focus and maintain attention in presence of distraction or noise Loses ability to understand what is read, although mechanics of reading are preserved Loses some ability to read facial cues, although perception of emotional meaning is retained	Loses naming abilities, especially of abstract or specific words Loses fluency (more pauses, revisions, sentence fragments) Loses ability to self-correct Loses loudness of voice and vocal expression in conversation Loses creative, "propositional" use of language	Cannot see things from another's point of view (becomes more egocentric) Asks fewer questions Starts fewer conversations Makes less eye contact Seldom comments or self-corrects Withdraws from social situations Loses "niceness" in conversation

Continued

TABLE 1-1	**Communication Losses Characteristic of Alzheimer's Dementia — cont'd**			
STAGE	MEMORY	UNDERSTANDING	SPEECH AND LANGUAGE SKILLS	SOCIAL SKILLS
Late	Loses orientation to time, place, and person Loses ability to form new memories Loses ability to recognize family members	Loses ability to understand most word meanings Loses overall awareness Doesn't seem to know when being spoken to	Loses ability to finish sentences Loses grammar and diction (speaks in jargon) May lose speech altogether, may become mute	Loses awareness of social interaction or expectations Loses apparent desire to communicate

Modified from Ostuni E, Santo Pietro MJ: *Getting through: communicating when someone you care for has Alzheimer's disease*, Vero Beach, FL: Speech Bin, 1991.

Communication Changes Characteristic of Alzheimer's Disease

Professional caregivers will quickly recognize characteristic changes that appear in the communication of Alzheimer's patients.

1. *Stereotypic language.* Persons with Alzheimer's disease use more stereotypic language in their everyday exchanges. They are apt to make remarks such as "You got me!" or "Can't say as I do." or "Easier said than done!" over and over again.

2. *Empty speech.* Persons with Alzheimer's disease tend to talk in generalizations or empty speech. Specific words that tell the listener "who," "what," or "where" are replaced by more vague or general terms. Instead of saying, "Please warm up my coffee in the microwave on the counter," a person with Alzheimer's disease might say, "Here, put this in that thing over there."

3. *Paraphasias.* Persons with Alzheimer's disease frequently confuse words that are related. Sometimes they say the opposite of what they mean; sometimes they say a word that is wrong but comes from the same category (e.g., "hot" instead of "cold" or "salt" instead of "sugar"). These errors are called paraphasias.

4. *Violations of conversational rules.* Violations of conversational rules are statements or comments that break the unwritten rules of normal human conversation. They are responses that are inappropriate, egocentric, blunt, or rude. Crying, walking away, swearing, and making a totally unrelated statement are typical violations of conversational rules.

5. *Windows of lucidity.* A window of lucidity is a moment or two in time when a person with Alzheimer's disease suddenly remembers things or talks clearly about ideas that appeared to be long forgotten (Box 1-1). All Alzheimer's disease patients seem to experience occasional windows of lucidity.

BOX 1-1 Window of Lucidity

In addition to Alzheimer's disease, poor health was taking a toll on Grandma K. She was dying of pneumonia. She had not spoken in more than 6 months and did not appear to recognize anyone. Her daughter, Harriet, called all the grandchildren to the nursing home because Grandma K was not expected to live through the night. The last to arrive was the youngest, John, who was in his late twenties. John raced down the hall, found Grandma K's room, and stood panting in the doorway. The entire family was gathered around the old woman's bed. Grandma K opened one eye, looked directly at her grandson and said, "John, did you ever get married?"

COMMUNICATION BREAKDOWNS CAUSED BY AGING

Most people with Alzheimer's disease are elders. Part of growing old is coming face to face with many losses, and these losses directly affect the ways in which people communicate. The communication disabilities of Alzheimer's disease patients are compounded by the losses they experience because of aging.

1. *Loss of independence.* Most elderly nursing home residents lose their physical and financial independence. The entire dynamic of their communication with others therefore changes. Their energy becomes consumed with getting through another day. Much of their conversation revolves around their physical ailments and the possessions they once had.

Some caregivers find it difficult to treat as an equal a person who is no longer physically independent. These caregivers talk down to and treat dependent elderly residents as if they were children. Elderly residents, including those with Alzheimer's disease, typically respond to this "parent-child" attitude in one of two ways: either they settle comfortably into the dependent role and develop a crippling *learned helplessness* ("I can't do anything unless you help me."), or they react angrily and defensively (Box 1-2). Either way, communication based on a caregiver's parent-child attitude causes problems.

Financial dependence also generates communication problems for nursing home residents. Many patients do not have the resources to obtain essentials or simple pleasures. Long distance telephone calls, bottles of cologne, or hearing-aid batteries must be handled or purchased by relatives or caregivers. Residents can only hope others will remember their personal needs and preferences.

2. *Loss of livelihood and social role.* Most of us define ourselves by what we do for a living and by our place in the family and the community. How we talk to others is determined by the roles we play in jobs, families, and society. When we no longer have those roles, we lose our usual communication places and partners. Our role-related vocabulary is no longer useful. For this reason, some elderly persons feel isolated even though they live with their age peers in the nursing home. They feel that they have little in common with other residents and, literally, that they are not who they once were. Helping residents know "who they used to be" is an important part of the role of the professional caregiver (see In-Service 11 for activities related to a resident's personal history).

3. *Loss of physical attractiveness and grooming skills.* Loss of physical attractiveness presents a very real barrier to communication. Research has shown that people are more likely to choose "attractive" rather than "unattractive" persons for communication partners. Dry wrinkled skin, cloudy eyes, yellow toenails, and other changes to an aging body are not on most people's lists of "beautiful features." Senior citizens are no different from most people. They, too, shun what they perceive as "unattractive" (Box 1-3).

BOX 1-2   **Parent-Child Power Struggle**

Marya was having a tough day. "Come on, sweetie," she cajoled Mr. Miller, "time to get dressed for breakfast. Gotta look nice for all the ladies!" Mr. Miller made no response. "Manny, did you hear me?" Still he made no response. Marya's patience ran short. "Hey, come on. This is the third time I've asked you this morning. Now you do what I say, Mister, or you'll be sorry!" [This was the same thing she had said to her 9-year-old that morning.] Suddenly Mr. Miller exploded, "Who do you think you are, telling me when to get dressed? I'll get dressed when I damn well please! Now get out of my room!"

Loss of physical attractiveness is made worse by the effects of the deteriorating grooming skills of persons with Alzheimer's disease. Unkempt hair, body odor, the smell of urine or halitosis, unshaven stubble, all these discourage potential communication partners. Furthermore, people who feel disheveled often do not feel like socializing. It is especially crucial to keep residents with Alzheimer's disease looking and smelling good. They become progressively less aware of their grooming as they become more impaired in their communication. The grooming process itself is an excellent opportunity for communication between patient and caregiver. There are good memories associated with being pampered and made beautiful. A resident with Alzheimer's disease who senses that he or she is well groomed may feel more like seeking companionship or at least like accepting the approach of others more readily.

4. *Loss of energy.* When energy levels are low, people feel less like making an effort to talk. All elderly people experience some loss of vigor as a normal part of aging. Institutionalized elderly persons get little exercise, little time outdoors, and diminished intellectual and emotional stimulation, all of which result in a major loss of energy, even before medications and pureed diets are introduced. Activities, foods, and sensory stimulation that increase energy levels will have a direct effect on an Alzheimer's disease patient's motivation to communicate.

5. *Loss of family and friends.* It is a fact of life that as a person becomes older, more and more loved ones disappear. The people with whom the person has been communicating most intimately—parents, siblings, spouses, coworkers, and friends—die or move away or visit the nursing home less often. These losses are painful. Alzheimer's disease patients may not recall everyone they have lost, but they sense the losses nonetheless. They grieve for loved ones, including their former selves, whom they cannot remember.

Grieving makes it difficult for elderly residents to invest in new communication partners. Starting over requires more energy than most elderly persons can muster. Furthermore, staff turnover, shift changes, and the frequent relocation of the residents make losses a daily, even hourly, occurrence. An Alzheimer's disease patient with any awareness senses this constant change or "loss" as troubling and confusing (Box 1-4).

6. *Loss of familiar environments.* For nursing home residents, the ultimate symbol of helplessness and loss is the loss of their familiar living quarters. New residents are assailed by unidentifiable sights, sounds, smells, and textures. They are distressed by having roommates instead of spouses, call bells instead of telephones, and trays instead of dishes. Uniforms, mimeographed menus, and fluorescent lighting constantly remind them that they are no longer at home. And every few hours a new set of faces arrives. This explains why many Alzheimer's disease patients never become oriented to their new surroundings (Box 1-5).

7. *Loss of first-language partners.* Many elderly nursing home residents do not share a first language with their fellow residents or with the direct-care staff

---

BOX 1-3   Perception of Old as Unattractive

Martha, an 81-year-old retired pharmacist, spent most of her days alone in her room. The unit staff members were concerned because, although she was still capable, she was speaking less and less to others. One of the nurse's aides brought Martha the news that Mr. Simms, a long-time pharmacist from a local drugstore, had recently entered the home. Perhaps, the aide suggested enthusiastically, Martha and Mr. Simms would enjoy sitting together for lunch once in a while. "You could talk about your pharmacies," the aide offered. "What?" scoffed Martha, "That old man?"

BOX 1-4 Loss of Friends and Caregivers

Jim sat morosely in his wheelchair. His speech came in fragments and was interrupted by long pauses, but the message was clear enough: "Some nice young folks . . . ." [He meant the student nurses who rotated through the unit each spring term.] "One came over . . . came a lot." He paused. "Asked her where it was . . . Had to get it all ready . . . going to paint my room." Jim's hand trembled. "She said she'd help me. But they left . . . never came back." Later Jim said, "I can't get it ready by myself." Jim was experiencing the pain of trying to develop lasting relationships in a nursing home.

BOX 1-5 Loss of Familiar Environments

A group of nursing home residents with middle-stage Alzheimer's disease often huddled in their wheelchairs in a small circle. Two topics seldom failed to bring forth some response: their mother's names and memories of the first night they spent in the nursing home. "I heard a baby cry," said one frail lady. [She must have heard another resident crying from a nearby room.] "Had to sleep alone," added another. [The emotion was still keen.]

---

members. They may be immigrants for whom English is a second language, or they may be American born, but the staff is composed largely of persons who speak English as a second language. Regardless of the situation, persons who are old and unwell find it increasingly difficult to speak or understand their second language. They may resort to talking in their first language. They also have more trouble understanding any language that is spoken with a heavy accent. Caregivers who do not share the same first language with a patient face an extra challenge communicating when that person has Alzheimer's disease.

► **QUICK TIP SUMMARY**   **Communication Breakdowns Caused by Aging**

Aging brings with it a host of physical, psychosocial, and environmental changes and losses. The result is that nursing home residents experience a drastic depletion in topics, places, and people needed for communication.

- Loss of physical and financial independence
- Loss of livelihood and social role
- Loss of physical attractiveness and grooming skills
- Loss of energy
- Loss of family and friends
- Loss of familiar environments
- Loss of first-language partners

COMMUNICATION ABILITIES PRESERVED UNTIL LATER STAGES OF ALZHEIMER'S DISEASE

Despite language loss by patients with Alzheimer's disease, many skills that support communication are remarkably preserved and remain for a long time. When working with Alzheimer's disease patients, caregivers should keep in mind six abilities that are nearly always preserved:

1. *The use of procedural memories.* Persons with Alzheimer's disease begin to lose memory for words, information, and events quite rapidly. But procedural memory, or the knowledge of how to perform familiar tasks, remains relatively intact until the later stages of dementia. Some scientists believe this phenomenon occurs because procedural memory is the most elemental of human memory systems and is the only memory system capable of operating independently. This system sustains some very complex human activity, from walking and washing our hands to playing the piano and driving a car. Examples of procedural memory include social rituals, such as passing plates, pouring coffee, or setting the table, and recreational activities, such as playing the piano or dancing. Although persons with Alzheimer's disease can no longer plan a complete meal or master the subtlety of chess, they may still be able to mix batter and flip pancakes and to make the basic moves in checkers. Anderson[3] has explained that procedural memory is like a computer program, whereas other types of memory are like the data stored in the computer. Persons with Alzheimer's disease begin to lose data rapidly, but the program still functions. They forget where they are going, but they still know how to walk; they forget what they are saying, but they still know how to talk. During the early stages of Alzheimer's disease, some patients are even able to learn new procedural memories.

2. *The ability to access early life memories.* One phenomenon repeatedly mentioned by family caregivers is the ability of persons with Alzheimer's disease to recall childhood memories better than they recall information from more recent decades. Families are dismayed to note that although Dad cannot remember the name of his spouse of 45 years or those of any of his children, he easily recalls the name of his mother, who died when he was 12 years old. When asked to talk about his home, he describes not the house he built himself and in which he raised a family but the house in which he was raised.

Earliest memories appear to be so "hard-wired" that they resist deterioration for a very long time. Some families find this upsetting and engage in endless efforts to bring their loved one back to the present: "No, Dad, your mother died when you were 12! Don't you remember Addie? Your wife, Addie? Our mother?" If the children were to accept and enjoy the old memories their father summons, they would find greater satisfaction in their conversations.

3. *The ability to recite, read aloud, and sing with good pronunciation and grammar.* Speech-language pathologists and linguists who have studied the language of Alzheimer's disease patients have observed that although these patients have little to say, they say it with good grammar. They can still respond automatically to greetings, recite prayers, and sing old songs. This automatic singing and speaking ability often brings them comfort and joy.

4. *The ability to engage in social ritual.* Alzheimer's disease patients retain the ability to use social ritual: "Please pass the sugar." "How are you today?" "Fine, thank you." "Would you like some coffee?" "No, thanks." In several studies that looked at the dining abilities of patients with Alzheimer's disease, subjects carried out social rituals, such as offering one another candy and making small talk, surprisingly well. Alzheimer's disease patients can exchange greetings, ask the time, excuse themselves, and accept compliments. The skill of taking turns during conversation is also maintained well into the middle stages of the disease.

5. *The desire for interpersonal communication.* Sometimes residents with Alzheimer's disease drive the staff crazy with their constant complaining and asking for things they do not need. Their real need is for human contact. They may have learned that if they do not complain or demand, no one talks to them. Most patients with Alzheimer's disease retain a strong desire to communicate until the late stages of the disease. A conversation study showed that loss of the desire to communicate was a signal that the patient was passing into a more severe stage of the disease.[4]

6. *The desire for interpersonal respect.* The best evidence that Alzheimer's disease patients retain their desire for respect is how quickly they show resentment when treated with disdain by their caregivers. From the patients' point of view, lack of respect includes having caregivers talk to them or yell at them as if they were children, being ignored, being called by "pet" names when they have not granted permission to do so, being moved from place to place, and receiving medical treatment without explanation. Although their behavior may indeed be childlike and exasperating, Alzheimer's disease patients expect to be treated as adults, and they react more positively and perform better when addressed as adults.

GOOD PRACTICE 1-1

Communication Abilities Lost in Early, Middle, and Late Stages of Alzheimer's Disease

Directions: The emergence of each of the communication symptoms below may indicate that the resident has entered a particular stage of the disease. Refer to Table 1-1 to determine which stage of the disease each symptom indicates, and make a check in the correct column.

Symptom	Early	Middle	Late
1. Resident first appears confused about the time of day.			
2. Resident makes mistakes that he or she no longer corrects.			
3. Resident no longer starts a conversation.			
4. Resident speaks in jargon or is mute.			
5. Resident can read mechanically but does not understand what is read.			
6. Resident no longer recognizes close family members.			
7. Resident has difficulty seeing things from another's point of view.			
8. Resident has little control over anger and argumentativeness.			
9. Resident cannot retain recent information.			
10. Resident cannot form new memories.			

GOOD PRACTICE 1-2

Characteristic Changes in the Communication of Alzheimer's Disease Patients

Directions: Identify the underlined words in residents' quotes below as examples of empty speech, paraphasias, stereotypic phrases, or violations of conversational rules. (Hint: Some quotes might fit more than one category.)

	Empty Speech	Paraphasia	Stereotypic Phrase	Violation of Conversational Rules
1. "Oh no you don't. <u>I never was one for that kind of thing. No, I never went in for that kind of thing.</u>"				

Continued

GOOD PRACTICE 1-2

Characteristic Changes in the Communication of Alzheimer's Disease Patients — cont'd

	Empty Speech	Paraphasia	Stereotypic Phrase	Violation of Conversational Rules
2. "I used to like to do <u>that</u>. We used to, you know, do <u>stuff like that</u> all the time."				
3. "I'm dying of the <u>cold</u> in here! Open the window. Give us some cool air!"				
4. "Oh yes, I was always a big <u>foot-ball</u> fan. When I was little, my Dad took me to see Babe Ruth and the, you know, the Yankees."				
5. "<u>A mile a minute. A mile a minute.</u> Everybody nowadays goes a mile a minute."				

GOOD PRACTICE 1-3

Role Play of Communication Breakdowns Caused by Aging

Directions: For each scenario, select a participant to play the part of the resident and another participant to play the part of the staff member. Draw each participant aside individually and explain the type of character he or she is to act out and the circumstances of the situation. This allows each role player to know how his or her character will act but not what the other person is going to do. After each scenario, discuss these two questions:

1. How did you feel in this situation?
2. How would you have preferred the other person to behave or respond?

Resident's Role	Staff Member's Role
Scene 1	
Sadie is small, helpless, and whiny. She only talks about her ailments. She is confined to a wheelchair. She [thinks she] needs help with everything.	Susan has a strong personality and a large number of residents under her care. She is very efficient and wants to get Sadie to breakfast by 7:30 AM. It is now 7:25 AM.
Scene 2	
George is able to walk using his walker, but only slowly and with great care. He is very unsteady and needs to concentrate on each step.	Alana takes every opportunity to practice her English and she has a naturally friendly manner. She feels compelled to engage George in conversation on his long walk to the activity room.
Scene 3	
Hiram is feeling lonely and depressed. His familiar roommate has moved to another floor, he does not recognize his new aide, and his family has not come to visit in a long time. He doesn't want to do anything.	Barbara, the new aide, is kind and gentle. She has been told that Hiram needs to get out of his room more.

REFERENCES

1. Van Riper C, Emerick L: *Speech correction: an introduction to speech pathology and audiology*, Englewood Cliffs, NJ, 1990, Prentice-Hall, p. 34.
2. Foy S, Mitchell M: Factors contributing to learned helplessness in the institutionalized aged: a literature review, *Phys Occup Ther Geriatr* 9:1, 1990.
3. Anderson JR: *Language, memory, and thought*, Hillsdale, NJ, 1990, Lawrence Erlbaum Associates.
4. Santo Pietro MJ, and others: Conversations in Alzheimer's disease: implications of semantic and pragmatic breakdowns. Presented at the annual convention of the American Speech-Language-Hearing Association, Seattle, 1990.

Additional Communication Disorders Frequently Found in Older Residents with Alzheimer's Disease

IN-SERVICE OUTLINE	Premise
	Learning Objectives
	Definitions
	How to Recognize and Compensate for Additional Communication Disorders
	Sensory Impairments
	Speech and Language Disabilities
	Medical Problems
	▶ QUICK TIP SUMMARY: Communication Breakdowns Resulting From Sensory Impairments, Speech and Language Disabilities, or Medical Problems Not Related to Alzheimer's Disease
	Coping with Sudden Changes in Communication Patterns
	Sudden Changes in Speech
	Sudden Changes in Language
	Sudden Changes in Voice
	GOOD PRACTICE 2-1: Responding to Other Communication Problems or Sudden Changes in Communication Abilities
	GOOD PRACTICE 2-2: Case Study of a Communication-Impaired Resident

PREMISE

According to estimates, at least 50% of all nursing home residents have significant communication disorders unrelated to dementia, and Alzheimer's disease patients have these disorders at a higher rate than do other elderly persons.[1] In addition, many nursing home residents have medical disabilities that weaken their communication skills. The presence of Alzheimer's disease makes management of these other disorders more, rather than less, imperative. Additional handicaps should not be dismissed with the attitude, "Well, she has dementia. No sense worrying about that hearing problem." If a patient is doubly communication handicapped, he or she is doubly hard to reach.

LEARNING OBJECTIVES

- Differentiate the four aspects of communication: speech, language, voice, and hearing.
- List at least four recommendations for supporting effective communication in persons with Alzheimer's disease who have either conductive or sensorineural hearing loss.
- List at least three typical speech patterns that result from drug intake, and discuss caregiving measures that could either relieve symptoms or increase sensitivity to these changes.

- Identify and report sudden differences in speech, language, or voice patterns of residents that signal significant changes in medical status.

DEFINITIONS **Hearing** Hearing is a sensory process. Hearing depends on the proper functioning of all three parts of the ear: the outer ear and ear canal, which gather sound; the middle ear, which contains three tiny bones that transfer sound from the outer ear to the auditory nerve; and the inner ear, the nerve center that converts sound to electrochemical impulses that the brain interprets and to which it responds. Adequate hearing is essential to understanding the speech and communication of others. Adequate hearing also is important in the production of clearly articulated speech. Persons who cannot hear their own speech gradually lose precise articulation and may speak with voices too soft or too loud.

Speech Speech is the way the words sound when a person talks. Are they clearly spoken? Slurred? Misarticulated? Does the person say "sue" for "shoe" or "nursh" for "nurse"? Ordinarily, if residents with Alzheimer's disease do not have additional communication disorders, their speech does not deteriorate until the final stages of the disease.

Language Language is composed of vocabulary, grammar, and intention to communicate. Sentences are put together with words and grammar to express ideas and feelings. Language breakdown in Alzheimer's disease patients begins early and worsens as cognitive and memory skills decline.

Voice Voice is the sound produced by vibrations of the vocal cords within the larynx, or "voice box," in the throat. The sound of the voice indicates whether the speaker is a man, a woman, an older person, or a child. Voice reveals the health, emotion, and purpose of the speaker.

HOW TO RECOGNIZE AND COMPENSATE FOR ADDITIONAL COMMUNICATION DISORDERS

Additional communication disorders experienced by aging persons with Alzheimer's disease can be divided into three subsets: (1) sensory impairments, (2) medical problems, and (3) speech and language disabilities. Coping with the additional communication problems of patients with Alzheimer's disease is easier if the underlying causes are understood.

Sensory Impairments 1. *Hearing impairment.* Impaired hearing is a serious and common communication problem among persons with Alzheimer's disease. More than one half of all Americans older than 65 years have marked hearing impairment; however, the incidence of hearing loss among patients with Alzheimer's disease may be as much as 20% higher than the incidence among elderly persons without Alzheimer's disease.[2,3]

Even an otherwise healthy person who has a hearing loss may find the constant effort to understand others exhausting. Many persons become suspicious and depressed and withdraw from social contact when they have unaided hearing loss. When a resident with Alzheimer's disease has a significant hearing loss, communication with that person is difficult.

Conductive hearing loss results from malfunctions of the outer ear or middle ear. It can be caused by wax buildup in the ear canal, inflammation of the ear canal (swimmer's ear), buildup of fluid behind the ear drum caused by allergies or upper respiratory infection, or a buildup of bony material in the ear (otosclerosis). Conductive hearing loss leads to "fuzzy" hearing or a feeling of pressure or pain in the ear (Recommendation Box 2-1).

RECOMMENDATION BOX 2-1

Recommendations for Helping Persons with Alzheimer's Disease Who Have Conductive Hearing Loss

- Clean wax and hair from ears. Check for water trapped in the canal after the patient has shampooed or showered.
- Be alert to signs of fluid buildup in the middle ear, especially after an allergy attack or upper respiratory illness: redness of the ear canal, a painful reaction to touch around the ear, unusually "quiet" speech, and instances of increased misunderstanding or lack of response to the speech of others. These symptoms *should be reported* to the patient's physician.
- Establish eye contact with the patient before speaking. Speak more slowly, but do not exaggerate your lip movements. Speak more loudly, but lower the pitch of your voice. A lower-pitched voice is more easily understood by persons with hearing loss.

Sensorineural hearing loss, or "nerve deafness," results from a malfunction of the inner ear or auditory nerve. It can be caused by long exposure to loud noise (e.g., machinery, gunfire, or loud music), a high fever, certain medications, and old age itself (presbycusis). Persons with sensorineural hearing loss have trouble differentiating many of the consonant sounds that give speech its clarity. They hear the speaker talking but cannot understand the words. Often the louder the speech is, the more difficulty the person has discerning the consonants; this is called *rollover.* Persons with sensorineural hearing loss can seldom be treated medically, but they often can be helped with hearing aids properly fitted by an audiologist.

Many elderly persons who have nerve deafness experience recruitment. A person with recruitment might not hear soft speech at all, but shouting causes the auditory system to suddenly "kick in," and the person hears the shout at its true level of loudness, causing him or her to jump and complain.

A number of persons with nerve deafness also experience incessant ringing in the ears, or tinnitus. Tinnitus also is caused by medications, extreme tension of the temporomandibular joint (jaw hinge), or trauma to the cervical (back of neck) area, such as whiplash or herniated disks. (Herniated disks are a common result of osteoarthritis.) Tinnitus not only is extremely distracting but also interferes with the ability to hear what others are saying. Persons with tinnitus are very uncomfortable in noisy settings (e.g., television playing, people talking, or trays clattering) because both noise and stress increase tinnitus (Recommendation Box 2-2).

2. *Vision disorders and blindness.* Loss of vision constitutes a barrier to good communication. Clouding of vision by cataracts, glaucoma, macular degeneration, or loss of visual acuity increases the Alzheimer's disease patient's uncertainty about a speaker's identity. Clouded vision also can interfere with reading a speaker's facial expressions, and important information about a speaking partner's appearance and body language is lost.

As Alzheimer's disease progresses, many patients are able to read written words long after they have lost the ability to understand spoken language. If they have untreated visual impairment, however, or if they are not wearing their corrective lenses, these residents are unable to use written words as an aid to better functioning (Recommendation Box 2-3).

RECOMMENDATION BOX 2-2

Recommendations for Helping Persons with Alzheimer's Disease Who Have Sensorineural Hearing Loss

- Do not talk to the person against a noisy background. Close the door (if the nursing home allows) or leave it only slightly ajar; roll the wheelchair to a quieter area or turn down the radio.
- Establish eye contact with the person before speaking. Speak more slowly. Lower your pitch, but use a normal, not louder tone of voice. Never shout at a person who has sensorineural hearing loss.
- If the resident has a hearing aid, encourage him or her to wear it. Learn to fit the earpiece snugly into the ear canal, to find the best settings, and to check for dead batteries. Many persons with Alzheimer's disease tolerate hearing aids well throughout the progression of the disease.
- Learn how to maintain the hearing aid: clean the tubing, replace batteries, and check for air leaks, which cause the aid to whistle or squeak.

RECOMMENDATION BOX 2-3

Recommendations for Helping Persons with Alzheimer's Disease Overcome Visual Problems

- Visual problems sometimes account for a resident's apparent disorientation to place and time. Be sure that each patient's vision has been checked within the past 6 months.
- Be sure that printed material and signs are in large, bold print and are well lit (see In-Service 3).
- Check that eyeglasses fit well, are clean, and are worn by the patient. Many patients who have worn glasses for years tolerate them well throughout the course of the disease.

Speech and Language Disabilities

1. *Aphasia.* Aphasia is a language problem that generally results from a stroke or other injury to the left side of the brain. Aphasic patients have difficulty in understanding and expressing language. Some patients have difficulty in the auditory comprehension of language but are able to speak fluently (fluent or Wernicke's aphasia). Others struggle to say one word at a time but appear to understand language fairly well (nonfluent or Broca's aphasia). The most common type of aphasia affecting elderly persons is global aphasia, or the severe loss of the ability to receive and express language.[4]

Persons with aphasia often have weakness or paralysis on the right side of the body (hemiplegia), and a loss of vision in the right visual field of each eye (hemianopsia). Many stroke survivors are labile, crying or laughing at the slightest provocation. Persons with aphasia can be expected to react with anger out of frustration because they can no longer speak with ease.

When a person has a series of small strokes, or transient ischemic attacks (TIAs), the result may be not only mild aphasia but also multiinfarct dementia (MID). MID closely resembles Alzheimer's disease in everything except its progression. Alzheimer's disease follows a steady decline, whereas MID tends to plateau until the next series of small strokes.

The language problems of aphasia are different from those of Alzheimer's disease. Aphasia does not typically create problems with reasoning and remembering or cause disorientation or personality changes as does Alzheimer's disease. Aphasic patients often are acutely aware of their limitations. An Alzheimer's

---

RECOMMENDATION BOX 2-4

Recommendations for Communicating with an Alzheimer's Disease Patient Who Is Also Aphasic

- Position yourself in the patient's visual field, usually on patient's left side.
- Get the person's attention before speaking; for example, sit at eye level, hold the person's hands, and say the person's name.
- Speak slowly and clearly, and use short sentences. Allow the tone of your voice and manner of touch to convey emotional support.
- Give the patient time to respond. Respect any attempts to verbalize. Strongly reinforce the patient's nonverbal responses, such as hand squeezing, pointing, or directed gaze.
- Talk to the patient and provide plenty of opportunities for the patient to observe, if not to engage in, communication with others.

RECOMMENDATION BOX 2-5

Recommendations for Helping Alzheimer's Disease Patients Who Have Dysarthria

- Give the patient plenty of time to speak.
- Speak slowly and encourage the patient to do likewise. Many dysarthric persons sound clearer if they can control their rate of speaking.
- Provide the dysarthric patient with firm hip, trunk, and head support for improved clarity of speech and for safer eating. Patients speak best when they are sitting in an upright position.

---

disease patient who has moved beyond the early stages of the disease is not so aware. Most aphasic patients, no matter how old or how long after onset, respond well to direct, patient-centered communication intervention by a speech-language pathologist. The most effective communication intervention with Alzheimer's disease patients, however, must focus on improving the communication styles of caregivers and providing environmental support and activities to help maintain declining language skills as long as possible (Recommendation Box 2-4). Patients with both disorders present complex management issues.

2. *Dysarthria.* A speech problem caused by muscle weakness resulting from nerve damage is called *dysarthria.* Nerve damage can result from stroke, tumors, trauma, viral infection, toxic poisoning, or degenerative conditions, such as Parkinson's disease. Symptoms of dysarthria vary widely depending on which part of the nervous system is damaged. Some patients have slurred speech and a nasal voice quality, whereas others strain to produce any speech at all. Speech might sound uneven, sporadic, even drunk, or it might be breathy, rapid, monotonous, and barely audible (Recommendation Box 2-5). Table 2-1 identifies the six common dysarthric syndromes, their associated conditions, sites of lesion in the nervous system, and the symptoms that accompany them.

3. *Dysphagia.* Patients with muscle weaknesses of the face, mouth, or throat may also have trouble controlling saliva, chewing, or swallowing (dysphagia). Swallowing is a complex behavior that takes place in the four stages described in Table 2-2 and Figure 2-1.

TABLE 2-1 Six Types of Dysarthria and Associated Symptoms

TYPE OF DYSARTHRIA	ASSOCIATED CONDITIONS	SITE OF LESION	SPEECH SYMPTOMS
Flaccid dysarthria	Bulbar palsy, facial palsy, myasthenia gravis	Lower motor neurons	Hypernasality, imprecise consonants, breathiness, monotonous tone
Spastic dysarthria	Pseudobulbar palsy, multiple strokes, tumors, encephalitis, brain damage at birth	Large motor neurons on both sides of brain	Contracted but weak muscles, slow movement with limited range, hypernasality, "strain-struggle" or harsh voice with low pitch
Ataxic dysarthria	Multiple sclerosis, stroke, alcoholism, trauma to back of head	Cerebellum or cerebellar pathway	Slow rate, uneven rhythm of speech, articulation errors, sounds "intoxicated"
Hypokinetic dysarthria	Parkinson's disease, Shy-Drager syndrome, stroke	Basal ganglia deep in brain, associated structures	Rigidity, tremor at rest, limited range of movement, soft voice, imprecise articulation, monotone
Hyperkinetic dysarthria	Dystonia, athetosis or chorea associated with Huntington's disease, Meige's syndrome	Basal ganglia or other parts of brain	Twisting, writhing, or rapid movements or muscle spasms, sudden sighs, strained or no voice, distorted vowels, hypernasality
Mixed dysarthria	Amyotrophic lateral sclerosis, multiple sclerosis, Wilson's disease	Multiple neurologic systems	Varied symptoms combining both flaccid and spastic dysarthria

TABLE 2-2 Complex Behavior of the Swallowing Stages

STAGE	COMPLEX BEHAVIOR
Anticipatory phase	Saliva builds up and the lips shape to the size of the spoon, cup, etc. For persons with Alzheimer's disease, this phase may be affected by a lack of interest in food, reduced production of saliva, a poor sense of smell, or poor ability to physically position oneself upright.
Oral phase	Food or liquid is placed in the mouth; the tongue cups around it and holds it. The tongue and jaw mix food with saliva and move it toward the teeth for chewing. Food is chewed to form a bolus while the lips and the lower facial muscles provide an anterior seal to prevent leakage. When the bolus is ready to be swallowed, the base of the tongue elevates and retracts, and the hard palate squeezes the bolus back to the soft palate, which moves forward and upward. In persons with Alzheimer's disease, inadequate lip seal, impaired chewing due to low muscle tone, paralysis, or missing teeth can interfere with the oral phase.
Pharyngeal phase	When food reaches the throat, the larynx (voice box) elevates, tilts forward, and closes to prevent food from entering the trachea (wind pipe). The pharyngeal muscles contract, the esophagus opens, and the bolus descends. In Alzheimer's disease patients, failure in the pharyngeal swallow phase can cause the bolus to enter the lungs and cause aspiration pneumonia. If the soft palate does not work to block off the nasal passages, food and liquid can leak out the nose.
Esophageal phase	Peristalsis (rhythmic muscle contraction) moves the bolus down the esophagus. In Alzheimer's disease patients, if peristalsis is slow or absent, residue can remain on the esophageal walls and cause medical problems such as reflux (backup of food).

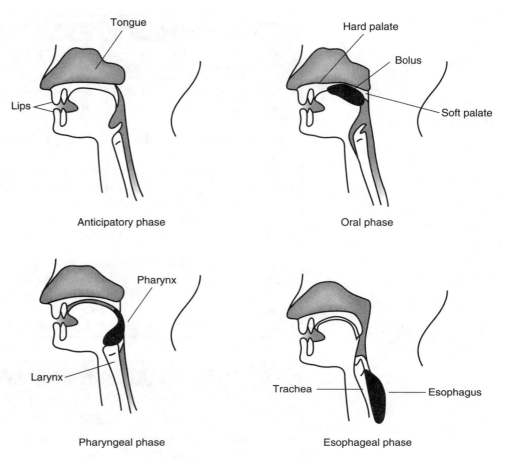

FIGURE 2-1   The four stages of swallowing.

Dysphagia is prevalent among the elderly because neuromuscular function deteriorates somewhat in both strength and speed among healthy elderly persons. Elderly persons are prone to an array of pathologic conditions associated with dysphagia, including stroke, arthritis, diverticulitis, head injury, and progressive neuromuscular disorders. Swallowing also is affected by social, psychological, and environmental factors, such as depression, loss of appetite, reduction in activity level, stressful environments, and malnutrition.

You should be alert to the following symptoms of dysphagia:
- Choking on food or drink
- A wet, gurgly voice
- An extended period of chewing followed by difficulty triggering a swallow
- Chronic drooling or facial droop
- Low-grade fever signaling aspiration pneumonia

Persons with dysarthria and dysphagia, like those with aphasia, can be helped by speech-language pathologists who teach muscle strengthening exercises and compensatory ways to communicate and swallow effectively (Recommendation Box 2-6).

RECOMMENDATION BOX 2-6

Recommendations for Working with Alzheimer's Disease Patients Who Have Dysphagia

- Monitor residents carefully for signs of difficulty with swallowing. Any choking or changes in eating behavior should be reported immediately to the physician.
- Make sure the resident is sitting upright, is well-supported, and is fully alert when eating.
- Note carefully feeding instructions and record observed swallowing problems.
- Remind residents to close their lips and to chew.
- Check to see that the patient's mouth is clean before offering another bite. Encourage independent eaters to eat slowly.
- Encourage patients at risk to "swallow again" when food may have collected in the mouth. If still in doubt whether swallow was complete, tell patient to "tuck the chin" or softly stroke the throat until swallowing occurs.
- Encourage frequent sips of liquid to help clear pocketed food.
- Require patients to remain in an upright position for 30 minutes after every meal.
- Swab around teeth and under tongue before allowing the person to lie down.

RECOMMENDATION BOX 2-7

Recommendations for Supporting Alzheimer's Disease Patients Who Have Voice Problems

- Provide good upright trunk and head support when the resident is preparing to speak. Persons who are slumped sideways in their chairs or beds have a more difficult time getting enough breath and muscle support for strong voicing.
- Eliminate background noise and interruptions in places and at times conversation among residents is likely to occur. Do not force residents to compete with noise such as a television or clattering dishes.
- Use simple positive reinforcement and reminders for speaking louder and more clearly: "Ah, Mabel, you are in good voice today!" "Charlie, please speak up. Sara wants to hear about your daughter's visit."
- Listen to residents' voices after meals to make sure their throats are free of bits of food that make the voice sound "wet." Instruct the patient to swallow or clear the throat.

---

4. *Voice problems.* The most underreported communication disorders in nursing homes are voice problems.[5] General frailty, neurologic deterioration, injury, or weakness can make an older person's voice so soft it cannot be heard. Years of smoking, drinking, or using medical or recreational drugs; chronic upper respiratory disease; or prolonged screaming or crying can leave a resident's voice hoarse and difficult to understand. The voices of elderly persons also can be monotonous, shaky, or intermittent.

Because a large percentage of elderly persons do not hear well, those who cannot speak loudly enough to be heard by the other residents are at an enormous disadvantage during conversation. Of greater importance, if a patient calls for help and cannot be heard, that resident's life can be at risk. Some voice problems can be managed successfully by a physician or a speech-language pathologist. Others can be relieved with a portable microphone and amplifier (Recommendation Box 2-7).

RECOMMENDATION BOX 2-8

Recommendations for Making Communication Easier for the Residents with Alzheimer's Disease Who Have a Tracheostomy

- Eliminate background noise so that the patient can be more easily heard.
- Use simple verbal reminders and perhaps physical cues to help the patient remember to cover the stoma before speaking: "George, use your finger. Cover your stoma."
- Use your own gloved finger to cover the stoma if the patient is unable to do so. Cue the patient to inhale, and then apply gentle pressure while he or she speaks a few words.
- Keep a "magic slate" or pad and pen available at bedside.

RECOMMENDATION BOX 2-9

Recommendations for Communicating with Alzheimer's Disease Patients with Chronic Illnesses

- Adjust expectations to the patient's level of energy and illness.
- Schedule important moments of communication for times when the patient is most alert and comfortable.

---

5. *Tracheostomy.* Patients who breathe through tracheostomy tubes have a special type of speech-voice disorder. The air they breathe is not exhaled through the vocal cords and out of the mouth. They cannot produce voice unless the opening, or stoma, is completely covered by a finger or two or unless they have had a valve (e.g., Passy-Muir) implanted. A resident with a "trach" needs special medical care and special help with communication. First, these patients have great difficulty producing audible voices under the best of circumstances. Second, they may need help to activate what little voice they do have. Many elderly patients do not have the dexterity to adequately cover the stoma themselves. Most Alzheimer's disease patients must be reminded to do so (Recommendation Box 2-8).

Medical Problems

1. *Chronic illness.* Persons newly admitted to nursing homes have an average of four concurrent illnesses. The most frequent are diabetes, arthritis, heart disease, atherosclerosis, osteoporosis, emphysema, cancer, and Parkinson's disease. Persons with Alzheimer's disease also have these medical conditions. Beyond the stress of dementia, such illnesses drain a resident's energy and receptiveness and increase the difficulty of communication. Knowing the effects of an individual resident's medical problems can help you estimate the extent to which illness interferes with communication (Recommendation Box 2-9).

2. *Drug and medication problems.* One of the most common impairments in communication among the elderly is caused by medication. When assessing a resident's communication impairment, the direct effects and the side effects of medications must be taken into account. Elderly patients with chronic conditions are highly vulnerable to the long-term effects of drugs. Because they have multiple medical conditions, these residents are susceptible to toxic drug interactions. They are also more likely than younger persons to have atypical reactions to drugs. Sometimes the effects of medications masquerade as primary illnesses, such as depression, anemia, confusion, and dementia (Recommendation Box 2-10).

3. *Problems with oral hygiene and nutrition.* Tooth decay, poorly fitting or absent dentures, dry mouth (xerostomia), or sores in the mouth affect how much a person feels like talking and how clearly he or she talks. Someone fighting the problems of

---

RECOMMENDATION BOX 2-10

Recommendations for Recognizing the Effects of Medication on Communication[6]

If the patient is taking:	Look for:
Antihistamines, antiseizure medications, antidepressants	Painfully dry mouth, sores and bleeding gums, agitation
Steroids, tranquilizers	Slurred speech
Cardiac medications, pain killers	Drowsiness
Aspirin, chemotherapeutic agents	Ringing in ears (tinnitus), hearing loss
Psychotropic drugs	Nervous tics, involuntary movements, difficulty opening jaw to eat or speak
Sleeping pills, tranquilizers, pain killers	Disorientation, intermittent memory loss

---

RECOMMENDATION BOX 2-11

Recommendations for Preventing Communication Problems Due to Poor Oral Hygiene and Nutrition

- Strongly encourage good oral hygiene and advocate for regular dental consultations.
- Know where the resident's dentures are kept. Make sure they are placed in the mouth correctly and comfortably.
- Immediately report suspected nutrition problems and oral lesions.

---

loose dentures and sore gums may not want to eat or talk. A vicious circle begins: not eating causes major weight loss, which in turn causes dentures to shift and fit less well. This condition causes even more discomfort and further lessens the desire for eating and communication. Nutrition problems also are caused by persistent swallowing problems (dysphagia), illness, and a poor diet. Whatever the cause, when nutrition is compromised, speech, energy, and health are severely at risk.

Pain from cavities, food lodged in the gums, cold sores, or ill-fitting dentures should never be underestimated. Anyone who has had even the tiniest canker sore on the tip of the tongue knows how painful and how distracting it can be. Residents with poorly tended gums and teeth are at greater risk of bacterial infections, which change blood coagulation variables. These changes can trigger a stroke.[7] Finally, social communication opportunities are lost because of the chronic bad breath caused by inadequate mouth care. Other people are not as likely to come close to or linger with residents who have halitosis (Recommendation Box 2-11).

4. *Clinical depression.* The primary symptoms of depression are withdrawal and impaired communication. Depressed elders have an increased number of physical complaints, changes in sleep patterns and appetite, loss of interest in activities, slowing of speech and motor movement, and pervasive sadness, helplessness, and hopelessness.

Research indicates that those who have least control over their own lives (e.g., nursing home residents) experience the most stress and depression. Most residents experience depression at some time during their nursing home stay,[8] and nearly all

> ### RECOMMENDATION BOX 2-12
>
> **Recommendations for Reducing the Effects of Depression on Communication**
>
> - Advocate for mental health consultations for residents who appear chronically or severely depressed.
> - Do not assume that someone can be "jollied" out of depression.
> - Encourage residents to participate in activities and discourage isolation.
> - Urge friends and family to visit the resident regularly. Let them know their company is important to the resident. Persons with confidantes have a lower incidence of depression than do persons without someone to confide in (see In-Service 117).

> ### RECOMMENDATION BOX 2-13
>
> **Recommendations for Reducing the Effects of Balance and Movement Problems on Communication**
>
> - Include canes, wheelchairs, and willing escorts in your list of communication aids and encourage their use.
> - Begin transport to social events early to allow on-time arrival and comfortable seating (Box 2-1).

persons with early to middle stage Alzheimer's disease experience depression. Yet elderly persons in nursing homes have little contact with mental health specialists. Although a resident is old and has Alzheimer's disease, direct treatment or counseling for depression and stress should be available. Mild antidepressants (e.g., sertraline hydrochloride [Zoloft]) have been found effective for some patients, as have behavioral treatments such as validation therapy,[9] in reducing depression and anxiety. Direct treatment can relieve the symptoms of the communication disorders that result from depression. Sometimes having a good friend or confidante available can reduce the symptoms (Recommendation Box 2-12).

5. *Balance and movement problems.* Staying balanced and moving about safely are enormous challenges for many nursing home residents. Arthritis, osteoporosis, paralysis, pain, weakness, and fear of falling contribute, directly or indirectly, to communication problems. For example, limitations in movement and balance decrease the ability of residents to groom themselves. Washing, styling hair, shaving, or putting on makeup require an agility that persons with Alzheimer's disease no longer have. Balance and movement problems also play a major role in restricting residents' communication opportunities in other ways. Patients who have limited ability to move may have difficulty turning to see a speaker's face and therefore miss the message. A person with poor balance must pay more attention to avoiding a fall than to listening to someone speak. An individual with Alzheimer's disease who cannot get around because of balance and movement problems is at higher risk of isolation, withdrawal, depression, and more rapid deterioration (Recommendation Box 2-13 and Box 2-1).

BOX 2-1 Allowing Time for Transportation

A nursing home in the Bronx receives a grant to determine the effectiveness of a new group communication therapy called the Breakfast Club. The treatment requires that residents with Alzheimer's disease be transported to a homelike kitchen setting each morning at 8:30 to join the group. Residents from the fifth floor are routinely 10 to 20 minutes late because the elevator operator in their wing refuses to change his routine to accommodate the special project. "This is my elevator," he asserts, "and they'll get there when I get them there!"

▶ **QUICK TIP SUMMARY**

Communication Breakdowns Resulting From Sensory Impairments, Speech and Language Disabilities, or Medical Problems Not Related to Alzheimer's Disease

Elderly nursing home residents have a variety of problems that negatively affect their desire and ability to communicate. If residents have Alzheimer's disease as well, their problems are more than doubled.

Sensory Impairments
- Hearing loss: Conductive hearing loss, sensorineural hearing loss, tinnitus (ringing in the ears), recruitment (sensitivity to loud noises)
- Vision disorders: Cataracts, glaucoma, macular degeneration, loss of acuity

Speech and Language Disabilities
- Aphasia
- Dysarthria
- Dysphagia
- Voice disorders
- Tracheostomy

Medical Problems
- Chronic illness: Diabetes, arthritis, heart disease, atherosclerosis, emphysema
- Drug and medication problems: Symptoms such as slurring, dry, painful mouth, and confusion
- Problems with oral hygiene and nutrition: Painful mouth, halitosis, or low energy
- Clinical depression
- Balance and movement problems

COPING WITH SUDDEN CHANGES IN COMMUNICATION PATTERNS

Sudden changes in a resident's communication pattern can be an important signal to staff members that something is wrong. The ability to interpret a sudden change could avert a medical or emotional crisis.

Sudden Changes in Speech If a patient's speech is suddenly more difficult to hear or understand, if words are mumbled or missing, or if speech is stuttered or lacking altogether, the patient may be entering a later stage of Alzheimer's disease. However, these symptoms also can signal one of the problems listed in Table 2-3.

TABLE 2-3 How to Respond to Sudden Changes in Speech	
COMMUNICATION CHANGE	INDICATIONS/ACTIONS
Speech becomes slurred; words are indistinct, "mumbly." *Or* The patient is suddenly unable to speak and may show facial droop or drooling.	Could be sign of impending stroke or a reaction to medication. **Report to charge nurse or physician immediately**.

TABLE 2-4 How to Respond to Sudden Changes in Language	
COMMUNICATION CHANGE	INDICATIONS/ACTIONS
Conversational rudeness increases dramatically; and attempts to communicate in previously functional ways decrease. *Or* Communication and behavior patterns change from reasonably compliant to agitated, repetitive, even combative.	May signal pain or impending illness. Monitor carefully. May need more social conversational opportunities to stimulate and maintain current communication ability. May need different level of activity. Provide more activities or less demanding activities.
Reverts to first language.	Not unusual for elderly patients. Ask family to teach staff a few words in the patient's first language. Write important words on index cards (e.g., "bathroom," "hungry"). Bring in taped music sung in the native tongue to calm and entertain the patient. Locate a staff member or volunteer who speaks the same language.
Becomes restless or distraught during group activities that were formerly enjoyed.	Language level of group may now be too complex. Simplify language; decrease rate of speech. Decrease longer conversations; increase the number of short (e.g., 30-second) exchanges.
Becomes mute or near mute with no other signs of deterioration due to disease. Appears more withdrawn; eats less.	May be depressed. Try more one-on-one communication and acceptance of complaints or distress. Seek counseling for patient. *Or* May have sores in mouth caused by ill-fitting dentures or excessively dry mouth. Resident is at risk of bacterial infection. **Report the changes to the charge nurse or physician immediately**.
Increases cursing, swearing, or use of abusive language.	May be a sign of mental decline or emotional upset. Do not take abuse personally. Look for physical, emotional, and environmental causes. Listen for the real emotional message behind the tirade.
Language suddenly becomes "wild" or hallucinatory.	Change may be caused by drug reactions or interactions. **Report to charge nurse or physician immediately.** Seek to eliminate auditory and visual overload.

Sudden Changes in Language If a resident is suddenly "rude" when he or she had previously joined in social communication, if a resident rapidly changes from talking occasionally to seldom speaking, or if language that was once functional is suddenly full of hallucinations, the cause of the change should be investigated (Table 2-4).

Sudden Changes in Voice

If a patient exhibits unexpected changes in voice quality, a process independent of Alzheimer's disease is in operation. The change should be taken seriously and addressed (Table 2-5).

TABLE 2-5 How to Respond to Sudden Changes in Voice	
COMMUNICATION CHANGE	INDICATIONS/ACTIONS
Voice becomes very weak or "wobbly" and more difficult to hear.	May be a sign of physical deterioration, illness, or impending illness. Monitor carefully.
Voice remains hoarse or "raspy" for 3 weeks or longer.	A chronically hoarse voice may signal a serious condition such as polyps or cancer of the vocal cords. **Report immediately**.
Voice is wet-sounding or "gurgly," especially after eating or drinking.	May signal swallowing problems. Must be monitored closely to guard against aspiration. **Report immediately**.

GOOD PRACTICE 2-1

Responding to Other Communication Problems or Sudden Changes in Communication Abilities

Directions: Using information from In-Service 2, complete the following scenarios. Discuss your responses as a group.

1. One morning Alf's speech is very slurred and "mumbly." He also is drooling slightly from the right side of his mouth. You should _____ because _____.

2. Rhoda is a Holocaust survivor who came to the United States after World War II. Today most of her words are in Polish or Yiddish. To make her happier and your job easier, you could _____ _____.

3. Vera is bedridden, has no speech, and must have her pureed diet spoon-fed to her each meal. During feeding sessions, she often moans and makes primitive noises that have a wet, "gurgly" sound. She sounds congested and coughs frequently. You should _____ because _____.

4. Asher's conversations with you have become increasingly "wild" and hallucinatory. Some of the things he says are scary. You should _____ _____.

5. Angelina has a very hoarse, "raspy" voice. She has been in your charge for 15 months and has always sounded this way. You should _____ _____.

6. Since her fall last month, Mrs. Stewart has been afraid to go to activities she used to enjoy. She remains in her room and is becoming increasingly isolated. "I'm just not up to it," she says. You should _____ _____.

7. Mr. Leong used to enjoy quietly watching the Today show every morning, but lately he complains he can't see the screen. "There's something wrong with the damned thing!" he bellows. His inability to see the TV has put an additional burden on everyone's morning routine. You should _____ _____.

Continued

GOOD PRACTICE 2-1

Responding to Other Communication Problems or Sudden Changes in Communication Abilities – cont'd

8. Last month Fred's daughter, who used to visit him every week, moved to Arizona. Around the same time, his roommate and best friend, Jack, was moved to another floor of the nursing home because he had COPD. Fred is becoming increasingly sad and seldom leaves his room any more. You should _____ _____ .

9. Mr. Povich is constantly telling staff to "Stop mumbling!" He is becoming more suspicious and paranoid. He talks so loud that his voice can be heard all the way to the lobby. You should _____ _____ .

10. Dorothy is frail, ill, and agitated. Generally she is among the first to be put to bed. As soon as she receives her medications at night, she falls into a deep sleep. Her son comes to visit two or three nights a week after work, depending on his shift, and sits silently by her side while she sleeps. She seems unaware of his presence. You should _____ _____ .

GOOD PRACTICE 2-2

Case Study of a Communication-Impaired Resident

Directions: Work individually or in teams of two or three. Identify a resident in your facility with whom you have difficulty communicating. Fill in the background information to the best of your knowledge. Provide a brief description of each of the communication problems listed in the guidelines below. Consult In-Services 1 and 2 and the Introduction to this book to describe this resident's communication profile to the other participants in the in-service.

Initials of Resident: _____ Age: _____ Sex: _____
First Language: _____ Level of Education: _____
Previous Occupation: _____
General Background Information (approximate number of months in facility, family history, etc.): _____
_____
_____

  I. Communication Problems Caused by Sensory Impairments
     Hearing impairment or tinnitus _____
     Vision disorders _____
  II. Communication Problems Caused by Speech and Language Disabilities
     Aphasia _____
     Dysarthria _____
     Dysphagia _____
     Voice disorders _____
     Tracheostomy _____
 III. Communication Breakdowns Caused by Medical Problems
     Chronic illnesses _____
     Drugs and medication problems _____

Continued

GOOD PRACTICE 2-2

Case Study of a Communication-Impaired Resident – cont'd

      Problems with oral hygiene and nutrition _____

      Clinical depression _____

      Balance and movement problems _____

IV. Communication Problems Caused by Aging

      Loss of independence _____

      Loss of livelihood and social role _____

      Loss of physical attractiveness _____

      Loss of energy _____

      Loss of family and friends _____

      Loss of familiar environments _____

      Loss of first-language partners _____

 V. Communication Breakdowns Caused by Alzheimer's Disease

      Problems with memory _____

      Problems with understanding _____

      Problems with expressive language _____

      Problems with social skills _____

      Empty speech, stereotypical or repetitive speech _____

      Mutism, continual crying out _____

VI. Reducing Communication Problems for the Resident

      How could you reduce the resident's communication problems caused by the following:

Sensory impairments? _____

_____

Speech and language disabilities? _____

_____

Medical problems? _____

_____

Aging? _____

_____

Alzheimer's disease? _____

_____

REFERENCES

1. Fein DJ: The prevalence of speech and language impairments. *ASHA* 25:37, 1983.
2. Weinstein B, Amsel L: Hearing loss and senile dementia in the institutionalized elderly, *Clin Gerontol* 4:3, 1986.
3. Gilhome-Herbst KG, Humphrey C: Hearing impairment and mental state in the elderly living at home, *Br Med J* 281:903, 1980.
4. Tonkovich JD: Communication disorders in the elderly. In Shadden B, editor: *Communication Behavior and Aging: A Source Book for Clinicians*, Baltimore, 1988, Williams & Wilkins.
5. Colton RH, Casper JK: *Understanding Voice Problems: A Physiological Perspective for Diagnosis and Treatment*, Baltimore, 1996, Williams & Wilkins.
6. Vogel D, Carter JE: *Effects of Drugs on Communication Disorders*, San Diego, 1994, Singular.
7. Valtonen VV: Infection as a risk factor for infarction and atherosclerosis, *Ann Med* 23:539, 1991.
8. Folstein M, Mchugh P: Dementia syndrome of depression. In Katzman R, Terry R, Bick K, editors: *Alzheimer's Disease: Senile Dementia and Related Disorders*, New York, 1978, Raven.
9. Feil N: Validation therapy, *Geriatr Nurs* 13:129-133, 1992.

PART **II**

How Environments Impair Communication

Making Changes in the Physical Environment That Support Communicaton

PREMISE
The overall design of the living space, the choice of objects, and the arrangement of furnishings within that physical space can magnify the communication problems of persons who have Alzheimer's disease. Carefully selected adjustments to the physical environment have a positive effect on a resident's willingness and ability to communicate. An environment that maximizes residents' retained abilities also conserves time and energy for professional caregivers.

LEARNING OBJECTIVES
- Describe a communication-impaired environment and contrast it to a communication-supportive environment.
- Describe five environmental factors that interfere with good vision and discuss how these factors reduce effective communication.
- Describe three barriers to good hearing and discuss how these barriers affect a resident's ability to communicate effectively.
- Describe two factors relating to aroma and taste that are potential barriers to a resident's enjoyment of dining and recreation; identify positive taste and smell experiences that stimulate efforts to communicate.
- Identify environmental factors that operate as barriers to good communication within

the participant's current work setting, and discuss possible low-cost solutions.
- Describe at least one innovation in environmental design for persons with Alzheimer's disease.

DEFINITIONS   **Communication-impaired environment**   "A communication-impaired environment is one where there are few opportunities for successful, meaningful communication."[1]
Physical environment   The physical environment is made up of the nursing facility's buildings and grounds and all the objects within that space. Physical environment also refers to the way space is used and decorated and to the sights, sounds, smells, tastes, and tactile sensations that each place uniquely communicates.

- *"The less competent the individual, the greater the impact of environmental factors on that individual."* [2]
- *"The environment affects individuals and individuals affect their surroundings. The environment is not simply a passive backdrop in which older people live, but an active contributor to what older persons will do and how well they function."* [1]

CREATING A NURSING HOME ENVIRONMENT CONDUCIVE TO COMMUNICATION

As the foregoing quotations suggest, environmental factors can either magnify or reduce the communication problems of persons who have Alzheimer's disease. In-Service 3 highlights environmental conditions that discourage effective communication in nursing homes and other institutions. We have included many recommendations to offset these problems, but not every suggestion will work in every setting, or for all residents. As you learn to observe your facility's physical setup with a more discerning eye, we encourage you to use the recommendations as a starting point for your own ideas. Practical solutions work best if you and your colleagues tailor them to the residents who are under your personal care.

It is not enough to convert a poor communication environment into a good one and consider the job well done. If you want to prevent gradual and almost unnoticed return to a physical environment that hinders communication, include plans for monitoring those policies and procedures that alter residents' environments.

Factors Interfering with Good Vision

1. *Poorly arranged or inadequate lighting.* Poor lighting increases stress, fatigue, and agitation in the elderly. Persons who must concentrate on safety because of poor lighting are less likely to pay attention to communication. When lighting is inadequate or poorly arranged (e.g., glaring, unfiltered light or light reflecting from shiny surfaces), elderly residents must make more effort to read facial cues, recognize words on signs, or gaze at pictures. They find it more difficult to gauge distances and depth, so they experience greater difficulty making their way from place to place (Recommendation Box 3-1).

2. *Lack of visual accessibility.* When persons with Alzheimer's disease cannot see the nurses' station or people passing by, they may feel isolated, frightened, or paranoid. If they cannot see the door that clearly designates "BATHROOM," they are less likely to remember to use it. The incidence of incontinence increases when visual access is denied (Recommendation Box 3-2).

3. *Inadequate signs, labels, and information displays.* Examples of printed materials that are insensitive to residents' way-finding needs are signs placed too high for residents to see, name tags with small print, or directories and bulletins filled with

---

RECOMMENDATION BOX 3-1

Recommendations for Improved Lighting

- Place table lamps at a lower level to improve accessibility, and increase the number of and locations of lights. (**NOTE:** The recommended lighting level for elderly persons is 50-100 foot-candles.)[3]
- Encourage family members to furnish cool-heat light therapy lamps for residents who enjoy reading or looking at picture albums.
- Allow residents to operate lights in their personal spaces whenever possible. Choose lights or lighting controls that respond to light touch or are sound sensitive (e.g., responsive to a clap of the hands).
- Avoid high-gloss finishes, even in visitors' areas. Minimize table glare with table coverings. Define table edges with contrast-colored tape or with a tiny raised lip.
- Use floor and wall colors that absorb rather than reflect light (e.g., beige walls and royal blue floors add contrast and brighten the environment).
- Define changes in floor levels (e.g., stairs, gaps between elevator and unit floor, ledges, and thresholds) with contrasting colored tape.
- Remind family members, staff, and volunteers to use good lighting when speaking to residents. Keep the light source on the speaker's face and seat residents with their backs to the light.

RECOMMENDATION BOX 3-2

Recommendations for Improving Visual Accessibility

- Position the head of the resident's bed so that the hallway and the door to the bathroom can be seen. If the patient tends to wander, consider installing a dutch door and leave the top open.
- Place a large "BATHROOM" sign on all bathroom doors.
- Paint each bathroom door a single distinctive color and remind the resident often, "Yes, here's the bathroom, it has the bright red door."
- Make special trips with the resident to the windows and describe the outdoor scene, especially bird and animal activity and weather changes.
- Turn off the resident's television if he or she is clearly not watching. Avoid using television as "companionship" or passive caregiving.

---

a confusing array of activities and notices. Written communication for the resident not only has to be visually accessible but also should make the resident's comprehension level a priority. Residents with no reading skills need alternative signals to assist them with way finding. Residents who retain rudimentary reading and comprehension skills should not be insulted with printed material that is, for them, unreadable. Such disregard promotes rather than reduces wandering and limits patient function, independence, and access to information. Signs and information that ignore residents' needs send negative signals to visitors and to potential consumers (Recommendation Box 3-3).

4. *Too little visual stimulation.* When there is too little visual stimulation, patients have fewer things to talk about, and their responsiveness to visual stimuli decreases. Nutrition also can be affected by a lack of visual stimulation. Food that is presented in a boring way decreases appetite (Recommendation Box 3-4).

5. *Too much visual stimulation or clutter.* Visual overstimulation, such as constant television, high traffic patterns of rapidly moving staff and visitors, wildly

RECOMMENDATION BOX 3-3

Recommendations for Improving Way-Finding Signs and Information Displays

- Wear giant name tags with large, bold print. Point to your name, or repeat your name and the resident's name frequently.
- Place room labels and all printed information meant to assist with way-finding at two eye levels: one for residents who walk and one for those in wheelchairs.
- Include a large personal photograph of each resident at the entrance to that person's room.
- Code important areas or persons by using distinctive and consistent visual cues such as same-colored bright scarves, quirky hats, a special shawl, or ribbon to mark each bed.
- Design announcement boards appropriate for the residents, ones that can be easily adjusted to eye level, have clean spaces and large print, and use only a few words (e.g., CHURCH SERVICE 10:30). Include simple line drawings that suggest the activity (praying hands), and limit color coding to key messages or activity locations (blue border for chapel, green for outdoors, orange for activity room). Refer the resident to these announcements frequently.
- Keep residents' eyeglasses clean.

RECOMMENDATION BOX 3-4

Recommendations for Increasing Visual Stimulation

- Allow plenty of visual and physical access to the out-of-doors.
- Build a video library of restful scenery, cooking shows, humor (*I Love Lucy* never grows old!), and musical groups singing hymns and old favorites. Advertise for donations in your nursing home newsletter.
- Use hallways and common gathering places as areas for attractive displays of pictures, murals, plants, or aquariums. Vary these displays often enough to heighten residents' interest.
- Put up poster-sized pictures of children and grandchildren in residents' rooms and print the subjects' names under the posters.

RECOMMENDATION BOX 3-5

Recommendations for Decreasing Visual Overstimulation or Clutter

- Clear table surfaces and storage spaces so that items can be organized and clearly labeled for easy access. Encourage residents' reliance on labels and familiar storage spaces to find personal items. "Your glasses are in the second drawer, Fred. [Pointing to label on the drawer.] That's right, the *second* drawer. Open it and see."
- Keep residents' possessions labeled or coded clearly enough to be recognizable by residents and staff alike.

patterned pictures on the walls, and clutter everywhere, leads to agitation, stress, distraction, and confusion for residents and staff members alike (Recommendation Box 3-5).

Factors Interfering with Good Hearing

1. *Too much noise.* Without exception, environments cluttered with noise hinder successful communication. Conditions that create noise pollution include:

- The nature of building materials (e.g., hard surfaces and lack of sound-absorbing materials)
- The arrangement of the physical plant (e.g., location of elevators, ice machines, and heating or air conditioning vents)
- The location of the facility in the neighborhood (e.g., nearby highways, construction, and playgrounds)
- Operational factors (e.g., 18-hour television noise, recorded background music [Muzak], and noisy paging systems)
- Staff practices (e.g., loud voices and group conversations, calling to colleagues down the hall)
- Patient disruptions (e.g., crying out, constant moaning, and sundowning behaviors)
- Resident limitations (e.g., hearing loss and memory deficits, both of which require louder and more frequent repetition from speaking partners)

All of these factors interfere with the ability of residents (and staff and visitors) to attend, listen, concentrate, and understand.

Noise interferes with hearing aid performance and causes ringing in the ears (tinnitus). It interrupts sleep and increases residents' anxiety, agitation, and irritability. Furthermore, noise begets noise: The noisier the environment, the louder people must speak to be heard. Residents' inappropriate cries and moans are sometimes caused or increased by a physical environment that is either overly stimulating or (when the resident has sensory deprivation due to impaired hearing and vision) lacking enough stimulation[4] (Recommendation Box 3-6).

2. *Lack of sufficient amplification where it is necessary to hear sound and voice.* When they cannot hear important sounds and voices, residents become less attentive and may not respond. Listening and processing auditory information take more physical and psychological effort than those of us who hear well can appreciate. These residents may find it easier not to try to listen. Inability to hear because of too much noise or too little sound amplification causes a person to feel embarrassed, isolated, depressed, and paranoid (Recommendation Box 3-7).

RECOMMENDATION BOX 3-6

Recommendations for Decreasing Noise Distractions in the Nursing Home

- Use a low-pitched, modulated speaking voice.
- Establish a policy among staff of approaching one another when speaking rather than calling across the hall or from room to room.
- Monitor the volume of televisions, radios, and paging systems. Eliminate paging systems wherever possible.
- Teach and encourage residents to use earphones with their televisions, radios, or audio tape players.
- Experiment with sound-absorbent materials such as carpet samples or curtains in areas of high traffic and noisy distractions: hallway telephones, ice machines, bathing rooms, elevators.
- See In-Service 12 for ideas for managing the noise levels of late-stage dementia residents who cry out.
- Brainstorm with colleagues to reduce or eliminate auditory distractions on your particular shift or in your specific setting.

3. *Lack of pleasurable or soothing auditory stimulation, lack of familiar sounds and voices.* Human beings find the sounds of music, nature, and familiar voices soothing. When ordinary sounds are missing from their living environment for too long, residents are deprived of opportunities that might calm them and stimulate distant memories (Recommendation Box 3-8).

RECOMMENDATION BOX 3-7

Recommendations for Ensuring Adequate Amplification of Sound or Voice

- Reduce or eliminate competing noises from the environment (see Recommendation Boxes 3-6 and 4-8).
- Move the resident to a quieter and less distracting place when explaining something important.
- Remind all caregivers, including volunteers and family members, to speak to residents face to face at eye level and in a low-pitched voice.
- Check hearing aids frequently to see that they are clean and in good working order. To lengthen the life of batteries, store them in the refrigerator.
- Suggest that families of hearing-impaired residents purchase earphones for better television, radio, or compact disc player reception or that they activate the printed captions option on personal televisions.
- Install amplification devices on telephone receivers.

RECOMMENDATION BOX 3-8

Recommendations for Increasing Pleasurable and Soothing Auditory Stimulation

- Ask family members to bring audiocassettes of familiar voices: friends, relatives, pets, favorite hymns, and short excerpts from church, temple, or mosque service. Simulated presence therapy (Simpres) is a personalized audio tape recording by a beloved relative in the format of a one-sided "telephone conversation" with pauses to simulate waiting for the resident's response. Simpres tapes, played repeatedly over a headset, have been found to decrease agitation and withdrawal and to improve the mood of a person with dementia.[5]
- Collect a library of audiocassettes that have soothing sounds of nature, quiet music or chant, the Psalms, or familiar poetry. Sometimes tape-recorded "white noise," such as a hissing sound of steam escaping under pressure, is soothing to residents who engage in chronic disruptive vocalizations.[4] These may be purchased through a catalogue of audiology supplies or where electronic "sleep machines" are sold.
- Invite volunteers to be personal readers for Alzheimer's disease patients. Although a resident with dementia may not comprehend the words, he or she may still be calmed by the voice and personal attention.
- Purchase an audio tape (teacher's store or speech-language pathology catalogue) or open the window and call attention to familiar environmental sounds, such as birdsongs, children's laughter, church bells, rain, and distant train whistles.

Factors Interfering with Enjoyment of Aromas and Tastes

1. *Lack of pleasant aromas.* Few things make us stop and say "Ahhh" like the aroma of chocolate chip cookies, fresh coffee, roses, or newly mown grass. A living environment that seldom offers homey and familiar aromas robs residents of stimulation for pleasant sensory experiences. Even worse, unpleasant odors (e.g., pungent cleaning chemicals, urine and feces, "cover-up" air fresheners, and stale air) discourage visitors from lingering and deprive the residents of (odor-free) conversation among themselves. The presence of noxious odors also makes eating less pleasant for everyone (Recommendation Box 3-9).

2. *Lack of positive taste experiences, staff inattention to residents' taste and food preferences, unpleasant dining experiences.* In homes throughout time and across cultures, mealtime has traditionally been an occasion for family and friends to express hospitality, to gather and to share stories. For persons who have Alzheimer's disease, mealtimes should still be a prime opportunity to experience the pleasure of eating together and socializing.[6] Hovering staff who need to hurry the process along, ugly plastic food trays, tepid and unimaginative food, and poorly thought out resident groupings serve to dampen enthusiasm for conversation and for eating.

As people grow older, their sense of taste deteriorates. People will not eat what they do not like to eat no matter how eager they seem to be for the lunch bell to ring. If, in addition, everything that surrounds the daily experience of eating is tiresome, residents are even less likely to eat well. Staff should concentrate their efforts on improving conditions rather than writing off mealtimes as just another routine because "the residents don't know what they're eating anyway." You might not be able to directly improve the quality of food in your facility, but you can try to present food to patients in as appealing a manner as possible and in a way that suggests dining ambiance rather than institutional drudge (Recommendation Box 3-10).

RECOMMENDATION BOX 3-9

Recommendations for Increasing Positive Aroma Experiences and Decreasing Institutional Odors

- Encourage visitors to bring pleasant room sprays, fabric deodorizers, colognes, shampoos, and lotions that the resident enjoys and can tolerate.
- Find ways to release and call attention to enjoyable aromas (e.g., popcorn, coffee, fresh-baked bread and cookies), especially just before mealtime.
- Open the window or go outdoors and call attention to the smell of newly cut grass, fresh air just after a rain, outdoor barbecues, or lilacs.
- Avoid using strong-smelling cleaning agents in the residents' dining area just before meals.
- Refer to Recommendation Box 3-2 to remind patients to use the toilet and thereby avoid the lingering odor of urine.

RECOMMENDATION BOX 3-10

Recommendations for Increasing Positive Taste Experiences and Decreasing Unpleasant Eating Experiences

- Use words that describe pleasant aromas and tastes just before and during meals. Invite residents to notice different textures and visual aspects of their food. Name the ingredients in a cookie or a stew. Talk about how certain dishes are prepared.
- Insist that feeding assistants know and use considerate, safe feeding techniques.[7]
- Be alert to indicators that the patient's diet needs medical review and revision (e.g., choking, regurgitation through mouth or nose, "watery" sound in throat).
- Avoid large portions of food served too rapidly.
- Make sure food temperature is moderate.
- Alternate flavors, textures, and temperatures with each spoonful.
- Name the food before each bite, or invite the resident to guess what the previous bite was.
- Serve meals "family style" to residents who are independent eaters to give them some control over their food choices and to encourage them in the use of procedural memories (see In-Service 1).
- Keep a food warmer or microwave oven in the dining area to rewarm food that has grown unappetizingly cold and congealed.
- Make certain all residents practice or receive thorough oral hygiene after every meal, especially if they will lie down within the next hour.
- Ask family members to bring in favorite dishes or treats that are within the resident's dietary restrictions.
- Develop a pleasant dining atmosphere. Collaborate with dietary staff and occupational therapists to vary visual surroundings and presentation of food.[8]
- Brighten lighting (without increasing glare) to improve food consumption and reduce agitation during meals.[9]

► **QUICK TIP SUMMARY**

Physical Environmental Factors That Affect Communication

Factors Interfering with Good Vision
- Poorly arranged or inadequate lighting, glaring unfiltered light, shiny surfaces
- Lack of visual accessibility
- Missing or inadequate signs and information displays, small illegible print or too much print
- Too little visual stimulation
- Too much visual stimulation or clutter

Factors Interfering with Good Hearing
- Too much noise
- Lack of proper amplification where it is necessary to hear sound and voice
- Lack of pleasurable or soothing auditory stimulation, lack of familiar sounds and voices

Factors Interfering with the Enjoyment of Aromas and Tastes
- Lack of pleasant aromas, poor control of noxious odors
- Lack of positive taste experiences, staff inattention to residents' tastes and food preferences, unpleasant dining experiences

INNOVATIVE FACILITY DESIGN AND ENVIRONMENTAL STIMULATION

Research and clinical experience characterize Alzheimer's disease as an illness that requires proportionately less medical intervention and considerably more financial, caregiving, and environmental support. Increased attention to facility design[3] and new concepts of environmental stimulation have inspired several successful models for quality long-term care of residents with dementia.

1. *Holistic facility design.* The Heritage Woods program in British Columbia, Canada,[10] is based on the concept that caregiving for residents with Alzheimer's disease should rise above the traditional large-group institutional design. The facility is six cottages in a natural-appearing neighborhood setting, each cottage housing 12 to 13 residents. The designers' philosophy is that the total environment of the facility should act as a therapeutic tool. For example, each cottage kitchen is set up as a major activity center easily seen from residents' bedroom doorways. Smaller groupings of residents appreciably reduce the level of noise, traffic, and distraction. Plumbing, furnishings, decor, and dining implements are "domestic and home-like."

Resident grouping, choice of staff, and program selection are governed by a unifying philosophy. Special attention to hiring and retention of staff pays off because direct-care professionals stay longer at Heritage Woods and get to know the residents well. At the same time, fewer behavior problems with residents result in lower staff turnover and less need for high staff-to-resident ratios. Grouping of residents according to abilities and needs has improved program efficiency.

2. *The Eden Alternative.* In recent years, Dr. Bill and Judy Thomas of upstate Sherburne, New York, have conceived and promoted a vision of long-term care in which the living environment is "both organic and humanistic with gardens and vines, animals and children, all generations in contact with each other."[11] They have dedicated themselves to changing the basic culture of nursing home environments on the basis of 10 foundational principles they describe as the heart and soul of the Eden Alternative. Three of the principles are as follows: (1) "Three plagues account for the bulk of human suffering in a human community: loneliness, helplessness, and boredom"; (2) "Loving companionship is an antidote to loneliness, and easy access must be provided"; and (3) "To give care lovingly makes us stronger; to receive care gracefully is a pleasure and an art. A healthy community promotes both." The Thomases instruct nursing home personnel in how to implement these holistic principles in gradual yet practical steps through intensive workshops, conferences, and retreats at their Summer Hill Farm Retreat Center.

3. *Gardening therapy.* Besides the obvious benefits of sunshine and fresh air, attention to the therapeutic use of outside environments can support resident treatment goals and provide spontaneous fun, interesting activities, and opportunities for varied companionship. Gardening encourages a variety of sensory stimuli, improves sleeping and eating patterns, and fosters a sense of well-being.[12] Attractive and functional outdoor design can affect almost every aspect of residential living for a person with dementia.

Beauty and function are not enough, however. The layout and construction materials must accommodate persons who wander and become lost easily and ensure the safety of aging residents with sensory, mobility, and balance problems. Furthermore, the loveliest, safest, and healthiest garden is useless if residents cannot get to it easily from their living quarters. Careful planning for the compatibility of indoor-outdoor passages will prevent staff from complaining that outdoor activities are "Too much trouble!"

Accessibility also means that residents should be able to dig in and garden if they desire. A variety of small, self-contained "garden plots on wheels" are on the market. These are adjustable for standing or sitting, so that residents do not have to bend over as they plant, weed, harvest, and chat.[12] Well-designed, attractive outdoor spaces offer many opportunities for caregivers and care receivers to share a wide range of potentially life-enriching activities.

4. *The Snoezelen multisensory room.* Snoezelen therapy is a multisensory approach to calming and soothing persons with dementia (as well as persons with other types of cognitive, neurologic, and sensory disorders).[13,14] The term *Snoezelen* is a combination of two Dutch words that mean "to snooze" and "to sniff." Lead researcher Dr. Jason Staal, a psychologist at Beth Israel Medical Center in New York City, has found that Snoezelen behavior therapy reduces socially disturbed behavior, produces relaxation responses, improves mood, facilitates verbal expression, and enhances attention and concentration in persons with dementia.

Placing geriatric patients in a room filled with quieting stimuli, from pleasant aromas and warm temperatures to pastel lighting, soft blankets, and peaceful music, provides them with experiences that are at their level of understanding. The therapeutic value is based on previous research findings that sensory preferences such as favorite flavors, colors, aromas, or music tend to remain intact longer than specific memories or language skills.[13]

GOOD PRACTICE 3-1

First-Impression Visualization

Directions: Speak slowly to allow participants enough time to develop their images. Give the group the following instructions:

We are going to take a guided visualization, or mental trip. I will ask you to close your eyes and picture the scene I describe. Afterward, when I ask you to open your eyes, please do not speak until you have written down some important first impressions. *[Pause.]*

Now, close your eyes. Pretend for the moment that you have never been to the nursing facility in which you now work. Instead, you are a first-time visitor, coming to see a friend who is a resident here. Imagine yourself driving into the parking lot. As you step out of your car and approach the visitors entrance, look around for the first time at the buildings and grounds. Take your time. What do you see? *[Pause.]*

Enter the building. Notice some details about the receiving area, then locate the receptionist. Ask how to find your friend. Walk down the halls or go up the elevator or stairs to the correct unit and room. Take your time. What are directional signs, bulletin boards, notices, and personal identification badges like? *[Pause.]*

Pay attention to the sounds and smells along the way. *[Pause.]*

Notice the tempo of movement among caregivers and residents. *[Pause.]*

Notice any sensations you have whenever you touch anything. What catches your attention about decor, room arrangements, nursing stations, and residents' rooms that you pass? *[Pause.]*

Observe the personnel and the patients whom you meet—their eye contact, facial expressions, comments to you and to each other. What is the traffic like? Enter your friend's room. What is it like? Would you like to spend a number of months or years in this room?

Continued

GOOD PRACTICE 3-1

First-Impression Visualization — cont'd

Now open your eyes. Please do not speak yet. Write down the first three impressions that you, as a guest, have just had about the facility in which you work.

1. _____
   _____

2. _____
   _____

3. _____
   _____

When you have finished writing, let's compare impressions.

GOOD PRACTICE 3-2

Brainstorming: One Way to Identify Resources for Improving the Communication Environment

Directions: Rules for Brainstorming

1. Break into groups of three or four persons. Each group should select a recorder.
2. Express ideas in a rapid-fire manner.
3. Express as many ideas as possible within a very short time (e.g., 90 seconds per category).
4. Do not judge or criticize anyone's idea.
5. Encourage "wild and crazy" ideas and laughter.

TOPIC: List several ways in which your unit could use the following "windfall" resources:
A donation of 50 indoor plants (25 of these are in hanging baskets) _____
_____
_____

A donation 100 carpet sample squares _____
_____
_____

Three volunteer hours apiece from each of the following:
A carpenter _____
_____
A plumber _____
_____
An interior decorator _____
_____
A mason _____
_____
A heating/air conditioning specialist _____
_____
A sign maker _____
_____
A photographer _____
_____
An audiologist _____
_____

Continued

GOOD PRACTICE 3-2

Brainstorming: One Way to Identify Resources for Improving the Communication Environment — cont'd

When the small groups have brainstormed several possibilities for each category, come together again as one group and compare answers. Choose two or three ideas that generated the most interest (or laughter) and experiment with a plan for implementation.

GOOD PRACTICE 3-3

Role Playing Mealtime Feeding Assistance

Directions: Two class participants are needed, one to be Madeline, the "resident," and one to be Dan, the "feeding assistant." Madeline can self-feed but is very slow, forgets she is taking a bite midway to her mouth, and turns her attention to other activities in the room. The menu today is milk and coffee, beef stew, chunky applesauce, pumpernickel bread with tiny seeds, and Neapolitan ice cream with a chocolate chip cookie. Dan is supposed to encourage Madeline to self-feed and to assist her physically only if necessary. However, he also has to see that Madeline eats well and in a timely manner. Begin the role play as the resident and the feeding assistant enter the dining area together. Take at least 5 minutes to enact the role play. Discuss the behaviors and the interaction between Madeline and Dan, take suggestions from the audience, and then repeat the role play with another pair of participants. Which recommendations from the text of In-Service 3 were most useful?

_____
_____
_____
_____

How will you change your dining room interactions with the residents as a result of this role play? _____
_____
_____

GOOD PRACTICE 3-4

The Experience of Being Fed

Directions: Materials needed: several small containers of applesauce, ice cream, or pudding, and if possible one warm-to-hot item such as boiled vegetables or mashed potatoes; spoons; and napkins. Warm, damp washcloths also may be a good idea. Divide into teams of two. One partner, the caregiver, feeds the person playing the resident *at least five spoonfuls* of food. The resident is unable to self-feed and has very little if any verbal communication skills. Both partners should have the experience of feeding and being fed. Then in large group, discuss these questions:

- How did you feel when you were the one being fed (e.g., out of control, pampered, helpless, invaded, disregarded)?

Continued

GOOD PRACTICE 3-4

The Experience of Being Fed — cont'd

- How would you describe the physical aspects of the feeder's skills (e.g., rate of food presentation, placement of spoon on your tongue, amount of food on the spoon, position of the feeder's body in relation to yours)?
- What words, amount of eye contact, gestures, or facial expressions did your feeder use to make the experience pleasant?
- Did the experience of being fed affect your desire to eat in any way (i.e., did it seem to affect the taste of the food or your enjoyment of eating)?
- As a result of this experience, would you change your approach to feeding residents? In what ways?
- How would you now advise or supervise others in feeding protocol?

GOOD PRACTICE 3-5

Working with Cognitively And Hearing-Impaired Residents

Directions: Discuss in the large group:

- How many residents in your charge would you estimate have a hearing loss?

_____

- This number is what percentage of the total number of residents for whom you care (25%? 50%? Almost all?)? _____
- Think of one of the hearing impaired residents for whom you care. Then select two recommendations from Recommendation Boxes 3-6, 3-7, and 3-8 or from the section of In-Service 3 titled "Factors Interfering with Good Hearing" that you could use to enhance your communication with this person. Copy them in the spaces below and place a star beside the recommendation you can begin implementing today. Share with the class.

_____

_____

_____

REFERENCES

1. Lubinski R: Environmental considerations for elderly patients. In Lubinski R, editor: *Dementia and communication*, Philadelphia, 1991, BC Decker.
2. Lawton MP: *Environment and aging*, Monterey, Calif., Brooks/Cole, 1980.
3. Hiatt L: *Nursing home renovation designed for reform*, Oxford, England, 1991, Butterworth Heinemann.
4. Sloan P: Managing the patient with disruptive vocalization, II. Presented at the 5th Annual Alzheimer's Disease Education Conference: Shaping Alzheimer's Care: the Power of Change, Chicago, 1996.
5. Camberg L, Woods P, Ooi W: Evaluation of simulated presence: a personalized approach to enhance well-being in persons with Alzheimer's disease, *J Am Geriatr Soc* 47:784, 1999.
6. Robinson A, Campbell J, Williams S: Improving nutrition and enhancing the mealtime experience in a variety of care settings. Presented at the World Alzheimer's Conference, Washington, DC, 2000. Educational session F-7.
7. Womach P: *Scoop it. Mold it. Pipe it! Dysphagia textures with thickeners to include HACCP guidelines*, Bellvue, Wash., 1996, Challenge Books.
8. Hellen CR: *Alzheimer's disease: activity-focused care*, 2nd ed, Boston, 1998, Butterworth-Heinemann.

9. Koss E, Gilmore G: Environmental and functional ability of AD patients. In Vellas B, Fitten, LJ, editors: *Research and practice in Alzheimer's disease*, New York, 1998, Springer Publishing.

10. Convey M, Sudbury F: Daring to change for better residential care. Presented at the World Alzheimer's Conference, Washington, DC, 2000. Educational session G-11.

11. *The Eden Alternative: human values in aging*, Sherburne, N.Y., 2001, The Eden Alternative.

12. Brawley E, Carman J: Creative therapeutic gardens for individuals with Alzheimer's disease. Presented at the World Alzheimer's Conference, Washington, DC, 2000. Educational session F-18.

13. Mulvihill K: Psychedelic room helps dementia patients. Available at: http://www.brain.com/Merchant2/merchant.mv?Screen=PROD&Store_Code=W&Product_Code=body_17610. Accessed January 12, 2002.

14. What is the Snoezelen Worldwide Foundation? *Global News*. Available at http://www.swwf.com. Accessed January 12, 2002.

Making Changes That Support Communication in the Psychosocial Environment

PREMISE

"Although it is unrealistic to assume that lifelong social rules can be completely retained, it is possible to cultivate a social environment that encourages self-sufficiency, independence, contribution, and self-expression to the degree possible for the individual."[1]

The formal and informal social "rules" of a nursing home can create a psychosocial environment in which residents have little desire or opportunity for communication. In-Service 4 examines the psychosocial factors that prevent residents' cognitive, social, and spiritual needs from being met and that limit social interaction. Each section includes recommendations for improving the psychosocial environment.

LEARNING OBJECTIVES

- Define the terms *communication-impaired environment* and *psychosocial barriers*.
- Describe at least seven of the 10 potential psychosocial barriers to good communication presented in In-Service 4.
- Identify psychosocial barriers in your work setting (shift, unit, and facility). Consider in detail one situation that warrants immediate attention or one that might be quickly or easily improved with recommendations in In-Service 4.
- Discuss the difference and the overlap between *spirituality* and *religious orientation*. Consider the formal and informal roles of spiritual support in long-term care settings and what they mean to caregivers.

DEFINITIONS   **Communication-impaired environment**   "A communication-impaired environment is one where there are few opportunities for successful, meaningful communication."[1]

Psychosocial barriers   Psychosocial barriers to communication exist when (a) the environment and the staff members working within that environment do little to support the preserved cognitive and memory abilities of the patient, (b) residents are not socially accepted or treated with respect by staff members or other residents, (c) basic needs for privacy and personal space assume low priority in the daily operation of the facility.[1]

OVERCOMING PSYCHOSOCIAL BARRIERS IN THE NURSING HOME ENVIRONMENT

One point to be made about psychosocial environments that support good communication for Alzheimer's residents is that the caregiver and the care receiver are inextricably bound together. What enhances the resident's interpersonal skills or motivation to communicate reflects the quality of caregiving and hence the self-esteem of the professional caregiver.

Factors Interfering with Preservation of Cognitive Function

1. *Too few activities appropriate for persons with Alzheimer's disease, inaccessibility of activities for residents, inadequate transportation to and from activities.* When the remaining cognitive skills of a person with Alzheimer's disease are not maximized and carefully challenged, the resident has less reason to talk and less to talk about. In facilities where activities are infrequent, lack variety, or are insensitive to the residents' cognitive levels, dementia patients languish from boredom and inactivity. A direct care staff passively contributes to the "not-enough-activities" syndrome if it has no interest in, provides no input to, or relies totally on therapy consultants for the planning and follow-through of appropriate activities. Unless residents are reminded and assisted in getting to and from activities, even the most exciting events will be poorly attended. Efficient transport planning is a key component in the goal of keeping residents involved and interested (Recommendation Box 4-1).

RECOMMENDATION BOX 4-1

Recommendations for Providing Accessible Activities at Appropriate Levels for Persons with Alzheimer's Disease

- Request an in-service training session on adapting activities to the residents with Alzheimer's disease in your care.
- Advertise your need for persons in the community to help transport residents to and from activities. Invite groups who meet regularly and have common interests but are not characterized by outreach volunteer activity (e.g., the local historical society, the quilting club, the county speech and hearing association, a hiking club, a young people's theater group).
- Ask family members to list activities that their relatives might enjoy or that could be adapted from previous interests.
- Encourage residents to observe activities even though they may not wish to participate.
- Look for opportunities during the residents' daily routine to engage them in paying attention to and caring for others (e.g., to care for plants, pets, and other residents, to call others to an activity, to distribute music sheets, or to help tuck someone into bed). Believe that everything a resident with Alzheimer's disease does all day long has the potential to be a meaningful activity.[2]

2. *Lack of awareness of residents' personal histories.* Being chronically unaware of a resident's personal history severely limits the staff's choice of topics and opportunities to encourage healthy social conversation with a dementia patient. The resident's cultural preferences and practices may be forgotten, less because of memory deficits than because they were deemed unimportant. Habitual disregard for the resident's unique history lessens the humane character of the professional caregiver's work and places the resident at risk of lowered self-esteem, depression, isolation, and loneliness (Recommendation Box 4-2).

3. *High rate of absenteeism and turnover among nursing home personnel.* For persons with dementia, bonding to caregivers in the nursing home is difficult enough. So many "nurses" to keep track of, different people on different shifts, the embarrassment of forgetting what to say, and a resistance to building new communication partners after so many losses. In many areas of the country, the rate of staff turnover is 90% and higher.[4] Personnel most likely to develop the deep relationships with residents suffering from Alzheimer's disease are "here today, gone tomorrow," leaving their patients vulnerable to feelings of confusion, abandonment, isolation, and loneliness (Recommendation Box 4-3).

RECOMMENDATION BOX 4-2

Recommendations for Appreciating Residents' Personal and Cultural Histories

- Complete a Resident Social Communication Profile (Good Practice 4-1) on each resident in your immediate care. If you are a shift or unit supervisor, make this a requirement for every new employee on the floor.
- Ask family members or someone from the same cultural background to educate you and your coworkers on the cultural practices, traditional foods, and holiday decorations or ceremonies that might have been part of the resident's past. Use this personal history in conversation with residents.
- Use the memory books or wallets (see In-Service 11) that family or staff members have made with the residents.[3] Refer to them daily.

RECOMMENDATION BOX 4-3

Recommendations for Helping Residents Deal with Absenteeism and Staff Turnover

- Assemble a photo album of direct care staff members who work on the unit. Take head shots for clarity of facial features. Wear a distinctive item (smock, hat, scarf, pin) for the picture. Place pictures in a protective plastic sleeve. Print first name below each picture in large block letters. Secure the book to a surface near the nurses' station for the residents' easy access. Look through the book frequently with residents and talk about what the persons in the picture are wearing, when they come on shift, and personality characteristics that the residents might recognize.
- Add new photographs as new personnel arrive; keep photos of departed staff for a while to remind residents that "Sarah left to have a baby"; "Jane found a new job"; "Harry moved away. We miss him." This helps reduce feelings of abandonment and confusion.
- Provide closure to residents when you are leaving for longer periods (vacation) or not returning at all. Try to impress on the residents who you are, say goodbye, and that you will miss them.
- Leave a small memento, perhaps a tiny pillow or handkerchief that has a whiff of your favorite cologne.

Factors Interfering with Social Interaction

1. *Poor arrangement of rooms and furniture.* Although the arrangement of rooms and furniture is a characteristic of the physical environment, the effects are felt primarily in the psychosocial realm. Unimaginative placement of chairs and objects within a physical space makes social interaction with others difficult to impossible (e.g., wheelchairs lined along the wall back to front, chairs placed distantly on the periphery of a room, or side-by-side seating in the dining area or across a wide table).

If the ambiance is coldly institutional and boring, persons with Alzheimer's disease, so easily influenced by the mood of either persons or spaces, are less inclined to take initiative and interact socially with each other. They are more likely to vie for time and attention from their busy caregivers. Drab decor discourages visitors from lingering or returning (Recommendation Box 4-4).

2. *Unnecessarily restrictive institutional rules or unspoken policies.* Some facilities have rules or unspoken (informal) policies that conveniently serve the staff but are stuffy, outmoded, or generally not in keeping with the culture of the residents. These restrictions may reflect outdated nursing home philosophies. They may have built up gradually and unnoticed. They may reflect the self-protective needs of an overworked staff. Some examples: discouraging close male-female friendships, interfering with legitimate expressions of intimacy, or dissuasion from discussing "taboo" topics, such as death, loss of a roommate, deepening medical problems, sex, or depression. When residents have no legitimate outlet for their questions or needs, they may respond with high levels of anxiety, frustration, and anger. Their pent-up feelings are liable to erupt into catastrophic reactions (see In-Service 10). The psychosocial environment is even less healthful for persons with Alzheimer's disease if a belief prevails that professional counseling is unnecessary or useless for them.

Of course, operational policies and procedures are necessary in any group living situation. A disturbed resident may simply not comprehend restrictions that he or she is unused to. Frequent reassessment of psychosocial allowances and restrictions is needed so that the delicate balance is maintained between the medical-custodial goals of the staff and the human social and communication needs of residents (Recommendation Box 4-5).

3. *Overuse of impersonal, task-related communication and "ordering."* Communication problems are more likely to occur if the staff seldom takes time for social conversation or quiet companionship with individual residents. When adult patients are constantly "ordered" or told what to do, they rebel. Residents' refusals to comply can cause staff members to try to "help" the task along (e.g., putting the resident's socks on for him after fruitlessly demanding he dress himself). Learned

---

RECOMMENDATION BOX 4-4

Recommendations for Arranging Rooms and Furniture to Promote Social Interaction

- Place chairs so that they face each other or are arranged in a "conversational circle," especially in common areas or when residents are in groups or waiting for services (e.g., hair dresser, podiatrist, physical therapist). Leave enough space in the circle for wheelchairs.
- Set up a "conversational focus" in the center: a coffee table with flowers or coffee service, staff picture book, a basket of small Beanie Baby animals, handkerchiefs, or scented pillows.
- Strive to make the atmosphere in visiting areas welcome and homey. Develop an "adopt-a-space" program and give prizes to the unit staff or shift who creates the most inviting area for families and friends to converse.

helplessness frequently grows out of too many staff orders. Sometimes, a resident's agitation and anger escalate, and she begins heaping verbal abuse on the hapless caregiver. Catastrophic reactions increase. Cycles such as this once begun are difficult to reverse (Recommendation Box 4-6).

4. *Lack of attention to residents' personal hygiene and appearance.* When residents' personal hygiene and appearance are left unattended (e.g., uncombed hair, dirty fingernails, or unpleasant breath and body odors), potential communication partners are less likely to approach or stay to socialize. Residents themselves are less likely to seek social interaction when they feel unkempt. In addition to sensory discomfort, patients who are deprived of this normal avenue of care and touch feel isolated, lonely, and neglected. A resident's poor personal appearance also tends to make family members unhappy with the staff's quality of caring, no matter how busy they are (Recommendation Box 4-7).

RECOMMENDATION BOX 4-5

Recommendations for Overcoming Restrictive Institutional Practices

- Recognize that at least some unnecessarily restrictive practices and taboos exist in every institution. Challenge yourself and coworkers to regard them as barriers to healthy staff-resident communication and to courageously ferret them out.
- Encourage residents to provide emotional support to one another.
- Advocate for programs and counselors that will help residents and staff cope with sensitive issues (e.g., spirituality, death and dying, personality clashes, and sexual disinhibitions).

RECOMMENDATION BOX 4-6

Recommendations for Reducing Impersonal Task-Related Talk and "Ordering"

- Communicate with residents even if you are too busy to sit down. Chat quietly while you change sheets, arrange a tray, or comb hair.
- Increase your use of touch to soften routine task talk and to keep the resident from feeling that you are "just doing a job."
- Invite a friend to volunteer as a Communication Partner to a resident with Alzheimer's disease (see In-Service 11). Lend the volunteer this book as a guide.
- Develop alternative ways of persuading residents to comply (see In-Services 10 and 11 for techniques for reducing resistance and refusal).

RECOMMENDATION BOX 4-7

Recommendations for Improving Residents' Personal Appearance and Encouraging Social Interaction

- Organize a "looking good" group where family members, volunteers, or residents who function at higher levels can assist with the grooming needs of residents functioning at lower levels.
- Require residents to practice or receive thorough oral hygiene after each meal. Check regularly that this has been done. *This recommendation is a priority for the resident's health and safety as well as for social-hygienic reasons (see In-Service 2).*

Factors Interfering with Residents' Rights and Need for Privacy and Personal Space

1. *Lack of private places.* When they have no access to private areas in which to be with friends or family, residents lose opportunities for close companionship and intimacy. The personal affairs of the residents and their families are unprotected from public scrutiny. This leads to frustration, bottled-up emotions, and embarrassment on the part of the relatives if not the resident. The resident's sense that everything he or she does or says must be done "in public" is demeaning even when the person only poorly understands what is going on (Recommendation Box 4-8).

2. *Failure to respect patients' rights to privacy and personal space.* One indication that attitudes and behaviors of staff or visitors have become institutionalized is that staff members fail to respect residents' rights to privacy and personal space (e.g., failing to knock before entering residents' rooms, talking in front of residents as if they were not there, or not explaining procedures that are being, or about to be, performed, and referring to a person as a bed, a room, a disease, or a case). These and similar ways of treating residents insult the humanity of the caregiver as well as that of the care receiver, because it reduces persons to objects and nursing homes to warehouses (Recommendation Box 4-9).

3. *Inadequate procedures for protecting personal property and treasures.* Staff grow understandably weary of residents with Alzheimer's disease who make constant claims of loss or theft or who cry that their personal items are not treated with respect. Yet nursing homes need to be especially vigilant in their protection of a demented person's personal treasures against theft, breakage, or mysterious

---

RECOMMENDATION BOX 4-8

Recommendations for Creating Private Places

- Set aside quiet corners or rooms where families and residents can find privacy.
- Locate telephones for resident use where they are accessible yet screened from view and surrounded by sound-absorbent materials.
- Install telephone jacks in residents' rooms so that a telephone can be brought to the resident, or have cordless telephones available for patient use. Even residents who no longer speak may enjoy hearing a familiar voice.

RECOMMENDATION BOX 4-9

Recommendations for Respecting Residents' Rights to Privacy and Personal Space

- Refrain from talking about residents in their presence as if they were not there. Avoid remarks about who or what a person with Alzheimer's disease "used to be" in her presence.
- Knock and wait 1 second before entering private areas.
- Use conversational courtesies when interrupting an activity or conversation (e.g., excuse me, please, thank you).
- Use the person's name when speaking both with and about her.
- Explain or ask permission before searching through the resident's personal belongings, even when you are "sure" the resident does not understand.
- Talk about what you are doing while you work with the resident, or explain procedures about to be performed, even when you are "sure" the resident does not understand.

> ### RECOMMENDATION BOX 4-10
> **Recommendations for Protecting the Property of Residents with Alzheimer's Disease**
>
> - Familiarize yourself with your facility's policy on personal property protection for residents and discuss with the rest of the unit staff how effective the policies seem to be for your setting.
> - Conduct frequent and stringent audits on complaints of mysterious disappearances.
> - Caution family members to limit to a precious few the number of personal possessions that they bring. Too many mementos create clutter and are hard to keep track of.
> - Discourage family members from bringing expensive personal possessions for the resident.
> - Refer to the sections on wandering, pilfering, and paranoia in In-Service 10 for communication that reassures and redirects the resident's concern.

disappearance. If the staff develops an attitude of ignoring such claims because "the person has Alzheimer's disease," catastrophic reactions and incidents of paranoia escalate rather than decline. Family members who notice a careless attitude about their relative's possessions are liable to develop a distrust that could lead to damaging public complaints. Residents and families need to feel that their possessions are protected (Recommendation Box 4-10).

▶ **QUICK TIP SUMMARY**

Psychosocial Factors that Interfere with Communication

Factors Interfering with Preservation of Cognitive Function
- Facility provides too few activities at the Alzheimer's disease resident's level, insufficient transport to and from activities.
- Staff members ignore resident's personal history or disregard cultural or religious preferences and practices.
- High staff turnover and absenteeism preclude bonding between caregiver and resident.

Factors Interfering with Social Interaction
- Poor room and furniture arrangements discourage social interaction; decor is drab and boring.
- Institutional "rules" restrain or discourage friendships and intimacy.
- Staff uses primarily task-related communication, orders the residents, seldom takes time for social conversation or quiet companionship.
- Residents' personal hygiene and appearance are frequently unattended.

Factors Interfering with Residents' Rights and Needs for Privacy and Personal Space
- Institution lacks sufficient space for private conversation or solitude.
- Staff's attitude regarding resident's right to respect and privacy is invasive.
- Nursing home has inadequate procedures for protecting residents' personal possessions; claims of loss or theft are not taken seriously.

Meeting the Resident's Spiritual Needs

1. *Spiritual yearning versus religious practice.* The awareness that we are more than only flesh and blood, the search for meaning under the burden of great disaster, the sense that events and people are guided by a wisdom greater than our own, the idea that we are connected with all others and with nature: these are expressions or aspects of our spiritual nature. Spiritual yearning undergirds much of our behavior

even if we do not perceive it. Human beings have many dimensions, and we must look at our humanity in a holistic way, acknowledging every aspect, including the spiritual.[5]

Across time and cultures, one way that humans have attempted to realize their spiritual goals is through organized religion and religious practices. A religion is based on a specific set of doctrines—beliefs—about God or the supernatural and is expressed through a system of personal and communal rules of behavior, rituals, and prayers. Some persons who contract Alzheimer's disease are devout members of a certain religion, (e.g., Catholic, Jewish) or have had spiritual experiences that brought a new and fulfilling dimension to their lives. Others have no apparent interest in either spiritual or religious connections. Within an institution, staff members also hold religious or spiritual beliefs and practices that range from "deep" to "none." How can we best acknowledge and support the former without offending or intruding on the latter?

Given the diversity among caregivers and care receivers, many nursing homes that have no specific religious orientation rely solely on families and clergy to meet the spiritual needs of individual residents. This cautious policy springs from politically correct and well-meaning intentions but sometimes winds up short-changing everyone.

Openness to residents' spiritual needs can change the psychosocial atmosphere of an entire unit. A staff that is actively alert to matters of the spirit will find more residents who, with encouragement, respond to or even welcome spiritual support. A caregiver's attention to spiritual comfort may turn out to be the best avenue for maintaining communication through the course of the illness. The freedom to provide spontaneous and unembarrassed support of a resident's spiritual yearnings can refresh a caregiver's professional commitment as much as it soothes and reassures the care receiver. As families evaluate quality of care practices, a caregiver's sensitivity to their relative's spiritual needs take on special importance.

2. *Communicating spiritual support.* If neither the family nor the resident has indicated a religious preference, or if you have received unmistakable signals from relatives that "God talk" and religious symbols are unwelcome, this attitude must be respected. Aside from such clear messages, it is unfair to assume that persons without specific religious orientation have no desire for spiritual solace. Professional caregivers can help move the resident into a place of greater peace and calm by intentionally communicating attitudes of loving kindness and consolation without making reference to religious doctrine. The following are examples of hope-filled phrases:

CASE ILLUSTRATION

INTERVIEW

Dr. Wu, how would you design a program to accomplish this goal [of caregiver and Alzheimer's patient sharing spiritual needs and resources]?

First I would train professional caregivers to research and understand the religious history of each patient and family. Second, I would help them know how to communicate effectively on spiritual topics. . . . Caregivers must not be uncomfortable in discussing the topic of spirituality. *They are to be facilitators, not priests or clergy.* Third . . . we [need] professional clergy and members of the faith community who are trained to work with this population.

Excerpt from an interview with David Wu, PhD, Director or Dementia Services, Fuller Theological Seminary, Pasadena, Calif. As reprinted in "SNALF Expert Opinion," World Alzheimer's Congress 2000, Washington, DC, July 3, 2000.

- I'll keep you in my prayers.
- Sleep with the angels.
- Do not be afraid. Take heart.
- Thank you for all the good things you have done in your life.
- How courageous you are.
- You are loved.

Take a moment from your rounds to simply be present with the person and "hold her in the light." Place your hand lightly, quietly on the resident's shoulder or hand. Communicate with wordless intent that you wish her to feel great peace and calm, warmth, and well-being. In the midst of a stressful day, such moments remind us that connecting spiritually with our residents is a rare privilege and one we would not wish to miss.

If either family or resident has indicated a religious preference, the professional caregiver's role may be more specific. Religious objects should be kept within eye-level view of the patient and referred to frequently by name ("the cross by your bed," "the prayer shawl you wore in temple"). Sometimes these objects have a faint lingering aroma that conjures up the sacred space to which they belong. Place the object on the resident's pillow for a moment, near his nose, and encourage him to breathe in the spirit. Refer to religious experiences that the person may have had as a child, especially if the two of you are members of the same religion (Recommendation Box 4-11).

RECOMMENDATION BOX 4-11

Recommendations for Respecting and Responding to Spiritual Yearnings

- Speak to the family about attaching a familiar prayer card to the head of the bed so that any companion can read it either silently or aloud with the resident.
- Remind the family—for admission may have been some time ago—that they are welcome to bring in familiar or beloved religious objects, including compact disks of hymns and excerpts of prayers or sermons. Such objects encourage staff and other visitors to offer spontaneous spiritual comfort.
- Decorate and officially bless a chapel area, or designate a private room as a sacred place for prayer. Typical religious objects—rosary, Bible, Koran, yarmulke, icon, crucifix, small religious statue, veil, (unlit) candle, holy water, prayer book or card—should be stored here and available to the accompanied resident.
- Schedule regular Saturday and Sunday religious services. Rotate denominational (specific faith), nondenominational (no reference to a specific faith), and ecumenical (combining prayers from several faiths) types of services. Encourage volunteers to bring in midweek Bible study and hymnfest activities. Religious services and spiritual activities should be physically and cognitively accessible to residents; levels of cognition and transport plans should be in place just as they are for other nursing home activities.[6]
- Provide religious and spiritual support for residents with dementia so that they can participate in group activities with music (familiar hymns, chants, preacher's voice), touch (sign of the cross, holy water, hands folded in prayer), aromas (flowers and, with caution, incense), and auditory (psalms, prayers, even just the word *amen*) stimuli.[6]
- Hold short memorial services for residents who have died. Fellow residents will sense the ritual even if they do not comprehend the particulars: that the nursing home marks the end of life with dignity, honors courage in the face of great struggle, and blesses the final journey.

GOOD PRACTICE 4-1

Resident Social Communication Profile

Directions: Use this questionnaire as a way of familiarizing staff members to new nursing home residents and as a resource for engaging residents in social conversation. The information can be obtained from the resident, the resident's record, or from family members. All three may have to be consulted.

The decade in which the resident was born; the resident's mother's name _____
_____

The cultural or ethnic background in which the resident was raised _____
_____

The city, state, and country in which the resident was raised _____
_____

A childhood memory _____
Veteran status; during which war; where stationed _____
_____

If married, spouse's name; where married _____
Where the resident lived and worked most of his or her adult life _____
_____

Resident's occupation; retirement date _____
Children's and grandchildren's names _____
_____
_____

Religious preference; nominal, occasional, or regular participation in church activities before admission _____
Favorite television shows _____
_____

Hobbies, special interests, musical preferences _____
_____

One or two things the resident cares deeply about _____
_____

One or two things the resident intensely dislikes _____
_____

Other important information _____
_____
_____

GOOD PRACTICE 4-2

Resident Trivia

Directions: This activity takes a little preparation by both students and instructor before the in-service but is well worth the effort. The game itself, Resident Trivia, should take approximately 15 minutes: 2 or 3 minutes to assemble teams, 7 minutes to process the patient information, and approximately 5 minutes of play. The instructors are the moderators.

Before the In-Service

1. *Participants:* As a "ticket" to In-Service 4, each participant must fill out a resident social communication profile (Good Practice 4-1) on three residents. A resident may not be profiled by more than one participant. Collect the resident profiles at the beginning of the in-service.

2. *Instructor:* Before class, write each of the 14 questions from the resident social communication profile on a separate 3-by-5 index card (e.g., Card 1: Decade resident was born? Mother's name? Card 10: Religious preference? Card 14: Hobbies, special interests, musical preference?). If you have more than eight participants, make two sets of questions.

Assemble Teams, Learn Resident Profile Information

3. Divide the class into two teams of two to four players each. If possible, group the teams by floor or unit (e.g., all members of Team A work on Unit 4, all members of Team B work on Unit 8.) (**NOTE**: The game still works if you cannot do this.) With more than eight participants, assemble four teams (C and D), and enlist a second moderator.

4. Distribute two resident profiles to each team. Be sure each resident is known by at least one member of a team. Make note of which teams receive which resident profiles. Devise a score sheet.

5. Allow 5 to 7 minutes for team members to learn the information on the profiles. Then collect all profile sheets from the teams and begin the competition.

Playing The Game

6. As moderator, pose a question from the index cards, first to one team and then to the other: "Team A, what was Tom's occupation before he retired?" "Team B, what is Ethel's religious preference?" "Team A, what branch of the army was Harvey in?" "Team B, what is Merv's favorite thing to eat?"

7. Keep the game moving rapidly. Limit playing time to 5 minutes. Limit participants' thinking time to 8 seconds per question. Cycle through the questions at least two times. Award 5 points for each correct answer.

8. Give a humorous prize to the winning team: a lottery ticket for all to share, a package of peanuts, small ribbons to pin on their uniforms, or play money.

9. Play the game at other communication in-services to strengthen quick recall of the residents' personal history. Increase the challenge by distributing three resident profiles to each team.

10. Secure the Resident Social Communication Profiles after each play. Caution participants about confidentiality.

REFERENCES

1. Lubinski R: Environmental considerations for elderly patients. In Lubinski R, editor: *Dementia and communication*, Philadelphia, 1991, BC Decker.
2. Hellen C: *Alzheimer's disease activity-focused care*, Boston, 1998, Butterworth-Heinemann.
3. Bourgeois MS: Evaluating memory wallets in conversations with persons with dementia, *J Speech Hear Res* 35:1344, 1992.
4. Harrington C et al: Experts recommend nurse staffing standards for nursing facilities in the United States, *The Gerontologist* 40:1, 5-16, 2000.
5. Wu D: A spiritual paradigm for understanding Alzheimer's disease. Presented at the Spring Conference of the California Association of Homes and Services for the Aging, Burlingame, Calif., May 9-10, 2000.
6. Carlson D, Hellen C: Undo the box—celebrate the gift: spirituality and activity, *Alzheimers Care* Q 1:56-66, 2000.

PART III

Face to Face: The Communication Challenges Encountered by Professional Caregivers

Communcation Strengths and Problems of Professionals Who Care for Persons with Alzheimer's Disease

---

IN-SERVICE OUTLINE

Premise

Learning Objectives

Definitions

Communicating Strengths of Professionals Who Care for Persons with Alzheimer's Disease

Communication Problems of Professionals Who Care for Persons with Alzheimer's Disease

▶ QUICK TIP SUMMARY: Communication Problems of Professional Caregivers

A Final Note on the Communication Problems of Professional Caregivers

GOOD PRACTICE 5-1: Communicating with Others: What's My Personal Communication Style?

GOOD PRACTICE 5-2: What Is My Communication Style as a Professional Caregiver?

GOOD PRACTICE 5-3: Adapting Your Communication Style to the Patient's Needs

---

PREMISE

Professional caregiving demands enormous amounts of physical, mental, and emotional energy. When your nursing home residents have Alzheimer's disease, they offer little cooperation in completing tasks and give few thanks for your efforts. Interactions seem to be discouragingly one-sided. Working with Alzheimer's disease patients has been likened to "being exposed to a severe long-term, chronic stressor."[1] Many professional caregivers find it difficult to leave that stress behind when they go home.

One of the primary causes of the stress is the breakdown in communication between caregivers and the patients for whom they care. Alzheimer's disease patients have multiple deficits that contribute to this breakdown, but the resident accounts for only half of every interaction. The caregiver is the other half. The fact is, the persons in your care may not be the only ones with communication problems. Healthcare workers are at least as likely as members of the general population to have problems that interfere with communication.

In-Service 5 examines the positive and the negative aspects of caregiver communication that are most likely to influence the behavior of patients with Alzheimer's disease. You will assess your personal communication strengths in working with patients who have Alzheimer's disease and learn about ways to overcome or compensate for your communication weaknesses.

LEARNING OBJECTIVES
- Describe in detail your personal communication style.
- Identify at least two communication strengths in your personal communication style that contribute to quality care of residents with Alzheimer's disease.
- Identify one change in your personal communication style that might improve caregiving skills.
- Identify one professional communication skill that if practiced by all class participants would improve communication and caregiving in your current settings.

DEFINITION
Communication style   The set of verbal and nonverbal behaviors that a person typically uses to send or receive messages. Personal communication style varies depending on the people involved, the circumstances, and the person's communication goals for the moment. For example, a 16-year-old girl may coax the car keys from her father in a childlike way, skillfully shift her style to "mature woman" with her 17-year-old boyfriend, and change again to "silly teenager" with her girlfriends. Seasoned and sensitive caregivers can adapt their communication styles to compensate for the communication deficits of persons with Alzheimer's disease.

COMMUNICATION STRENGTHS OF PROFESSIONALS WHO CARE FOR PERSONS WITH ALZHEIMER'S DISEASE

Professional caregivers have numerous communication strengths on which to draw that can be used to help Alzheimer's disease patients in their struggle to communicate. For example, when nursing assistants speak and move in a relaxed manner, the behaviors of residents are more flexible, calm, and cooperative. Residents also respond better when assistants use a personal rather than an authoritarian way of speaking. Box 5-1 is an example of how one caregiver changed her communication style to meet the particular needs of her patient.

Your work with Alzheimer's disease patients will go more smoothly and be less stressful when you do the following:

1. Acknowledge your own communication strengths and weaknesses
2. Are willing to eliminate or change a personal communication style that hinders your work with persons with Alzheimer's disease or with others who also care for the patients
3. Understand the communication losses and retained abilities of patients with Alzheimer's disease
4. Believe that if you use good communication skills, the patient's cooperation will increase and troublesome behaviors will decrease

---

BOX 5-1   Adapting Communication to a Patient's Needs

Every day Jack Phillips would put on his coat and tie, ready to go to work as he had done for forty years. We called on nursing assistant Mimi Girard, who knew best how to reason with him. "No, Jack, no work today, breakfast first," she coaxed, "then a shower, okay?" He paused, trying to figure this out, then asked, "Is the car in the garage?" "Yes, Jack," she assured him, "the car is safe and sound."

Somewhat settled, he walked to the day room. Getting him there was more than "assist residents to day room" as listed in the job manual, and coaxing him to take off his coat and tie was more than "give shower." To carry it off took knowing each other and an exchange based on familiarity within partnerships of caretaking.

From Diamond T: *Making gray gold*, Chicago, 1992, University of Chicago Press.

5. Are willing to take responsibility for communicating with the person with Alzheimer's disease
6. View the resident as an individual with likes and dislikes and a personal history that can be used to help you care for the resident with greater confidence
7. Can recognize and respond quickly to the patient's efforts to communicate
8. Can adapt your personal communication style to meet each patient's communication needs
9. Are sensitive to subtle changes in the patient's communication or other behaviors as a crisis-prevention skill
10. Can maintain a calm communication style during crisis, especially when the resident is being abusive
11. Are willing to ask for help in tough communication situations
12. Are willing to use stress management techniques when your personal tension level becomes too high

COMMUNCATION PROBLEMS OF PROFESSIONALS WHO CARE FOR PERSONS WITH ALZHEIMER'S DISEASE

Most of us think that our personal communications styles are more than adequate to get us through everyday situations. We might not be great public speakers, but usually our acquaintances know what we are trying to say. However, a communication style that works well under ordinary circumstances might not be the best one to use when working with a person with Alzheimer's disease. Why not? A caregiver's way of speaking can enhance a resident's ability to respond appropriately, but it can also destroy relationships and jeopardize the resident's sense of cooperation and security.

The following seven factors in a caregiver's communication style can significantly affect the communication success of a patient with Alzheimer's disease.

1. *Speech, language, voice, and hearing characteristics.* Every adult exhibits a unique combination of speech, language, and vocal traits that together form a sort of "acoustic fingerprint"—the voice we recognize on the telephone. Even among normal speakers, some persons mumble or speak in a soft voice; others talk rapidly, have elaborate vocabularies, or use long, complex sentences. Although their friends can follow what they say, these persons would have difficulty communicating effectively with Alzheimer's disease patients. A caregiver who uses little or no body language, eye contact, or touch is also at a disadvantage with persons with Alzheimer's disease. Persons with Alzheimer's disease rely on the emotional messages of nonverbal communication to function socially, even when they no longer understand speech.

Listening skills are crucial to successful communication with persons with Alzheimer's disease. As a patient's cognitive condition deteriorates, his or her language becomes more difficult to understand and interpret. Greater effort must be made by the listener to pay attention and listen mindfully; otherwise important information is missed or misread. Poor listening habits and careless attention to patients' utterances invite even more rapid decline in their communication skills. Poor listening habits also create barriers between the caregiver and residents' families and between the caregiver and coworkers.

Some caregivers have diagnosable communication disorders that go beyond poor communication style. An estimated 10% of all adults have some type of clinical communication disorder—dysarthria (slurred or unclear speech), a stutter, or perhaps a chronically hoarse voice. Hearing loss is the most prevalent of these communication disorders. As a person ages, he or she is more prone to loss of hearing. Persons with uncorrected hearing loss may speak in voices that are too soft or too loud for the hearing comfort of others. Their speech becomes less

---

RECOMMENDATION BOX 5-1

Recommendations for Overcoming Your Own Speech, Language, or Hearing Problems

- Consult a speech-language pathologist if others often ask you to repeat what you say or accuse you of mumbling. A professional can find the cause and help you improve the clarity of your speech.
- Consult a certified audiologist to rule out hearing loss if you frequently have to ask others to repeat. Follow the advice of that professional, no matter how insignificant the loss may seem to you.
- Take a course to improve your listening skills if you are often criticized because you have not listened to or remembered important messages. Many good programs are available on audiotape (see In-Service 8 for a definition and explanation of empathic listening skills).
- Join a community theater group, a poetry reading club, a Toastmasters speaking group, or a Dale Carnegie course if you sense that others miss your meaning because you rarely use nonverbal communication to support your message. Such recreational and self-help activities teach participants to deliver a message with greater emphasis and confidence. They also serve as excellent antidotes to job stress.

---

precise and more difficult to understand. The reluctance of persons with hearing loss to ask others to repeat may cause listeners to unfairly judge them as "vague," inattentive, or forgetful. Many of the symptoms of hearing loss are the same as those of early-stage Alzheimer's disease.

Healthcare employees with any of these *uncorrected* communication impairments will have trouble communicating with coworkers, friends, or family but most especially with persons who have Alzheimer's disease. If you suspect that you might have even a mild hearing loss, it is better to do something about the problem than to jeopardize your job and your personal relationships (Recommendation Box 5-1).

2. *Gender, status, and age factors.* Perceived differences in gender, status, age, and social customs govern the way people speak to each other. We speak more casually with friends and more formally with elders, authorities, or persons to whom we wish to show respect.

American culture is inclined toward negative attitudes about aging and the elderly and places a high value on youth and beauty. A caregiver who views older, female, or dependent persons as having less worth may be tempted to address them in a patronizing manner, especially if those persons have dementia. Any display of bias relating to gender or age inevitably creates serious communication problems on the job. If you persist in speaking to persons of a certain age, sex, or status with less respect, including telling jokes about people with dementia, you will quickly undermine your effectiveness in the nursing home with residents and staff. Everyone responds negatively to an environment in which a toxic speaking style prevails, particularly if he or she is the target of such bias (see In-Service 7 for the definition of *toxic talk*) (Recommendation Box 5-2).

3. *Cultural and linguistic differences.* A caregiver's cultural background is one of the strongest influences on communication style. First, there are the obvious differences in pronunciation between persons who speak "standard American English" and those who speak a dialect or English as a second language. Accent differences, limited vocabulary, and grammatical errors can cause communication breakdowns among staff members with different linguistic backgrounds, between foreign-born employees and nursing home residents, and among foreign-born residents of different cultures.

> **RECOMMENDATION BOX 5-2**
>
> **Recommendations for Overcoming a Communication Style That Reflects Gender, Status, or Age Bias**
>
> - Know your biases relating to gender and age differences. Leave bias jokes and ethnic slurs outside the door of your workplace, or leave the workplace.
> - Avoid using the same trendy language with your elderly residents that you use with your peers.
> - Reject an attitude that suggests "parent-child" or "I'm OK, but you don't know what you're doing" when speaking with a resident with Alzheimer's disease.

> **RECOMMENDATION BOX 5-3**
>
> **Recommendations for Overcoming Cultural and Linguistic Differences**
>
> - Understand your own cultural frame of reference, and explore the ways it is similar to but different from that of residents and coworkers.
> - Advocate for diversity training programs in your workplace; attend and learn from them. Cover for coworkers so that they can attend and learn too.
> - Seek accent improvement if you have trouble being understood. Tutoring can be found in the communication or English as a Second Language Department of a local college. Some speech-language pathologists specialize in accent reduction. Consult the Yellow Pages.
> - Attend adult education courses in English as a Second Language or effective communication. High schools and community colleges offer these classes free or at low cost. ProLiteracy Worldwide (formerly Literacy Volunteers of America) offers English instruction free of charge.

Communication styles that are richly rewarded by one culture may raise serious objections in another. In some cultures, people are encouraged to tell stories, show emotion, and assert themselves. In others, the use of broad gestures, direct eye contact, and long speeches would be considered rude. We are all products of our unique upbringing; most of our differences cannot and should not be erased. Nevertheless, they can and should be studied, appreciated, and accepted by one another within the nursing home community. If cultural differences become the subject of prejudice in your nursing home, effective communication among residents and staff will be at risk (Recommendation Box 5-3).

4. *Personality factors.* Introversion and extroversion are two personality traits that have definite effects on the communication styles of caregivers. Persons who are introverted may be unwilling to reach out and support communication with a person with Alzheimer's disease. Extroverted persons may not have the patience to listen with empathy, or they may have a communication style that excites or agitates patients.[2]

Other personality traits, such as tendencies toward denial or depression, feelings of embarrassment or low tolerance of a patient's deviant behavior, sensitivity to criticism, or inability to deal with conflict, will negatively influence interactions with patients. A person who seeks to be in control of every situation is unlikely to be flexible enough to communicate successfully with Alzheimer's disease patients. A person who is quick to anger will find the need for constant restraint exhausting (Recommendation Box 5-4).

RECOMMENDATION BOX 5-4

Recommendations for Managing Troublesome Personality Factors

- Evaluate your personality traits through one of several available means: self-help or Meyers-Briggs workshops, human resources seminars or counseling sessions, or self-help books and questionnaires.
- Seek "how-to" books, audiotaped courses, or classes or groups that concentrate on improving interpersonal communication. Many weekend or evening workshops specialize in building these skills in a friendly and nonthreatening manner.
- Keep a journal of your observations and feelings. Keeping a journal is viewed by many experts as one of the most effective ways to work through personal issues, and it is free. Check out books from the library or your church, synagogue, or spiritual community center on how to get the most from writing about your personal journey.
- Seek professional counseling for persistent or serious depression, anxiety, or rage.

5. *Education and experience.* Certified nursing assistants (CNAs) frequently comment that they do not receive enough training in the management of human relationships when working with an Alzheimer's population.[2,3] Continuing education is vital for both job performance and job satisfaction. It introduces new vocabulary, techniques, and ideas. It provides a fresh outlook and new motivation to perform better on the job. Unless you enrich your daily experience with continuing education, your enthusiasm will falter and your caregiving style will become less effective.

Many nursing assistants discover that experience is not always the best teacher. Bad experiences have a way of building barriers to communication. If you care for a resident who has been combative, the fear and hostility that you feel as you approach that person again may show in your body and verbal language. The resident senses your reaction and responds, not unexpectedly, in like manner. A vicious circle of miscommunication has begun. Professional caregivers have to be resilient and view such experiences as "lessons learned" rather than "getting burned." Trying times will occur, but they should not be more burdensome because of inadequate training and negative experiences. Continuing education should bolster your ability to cope with tough situations and turn them into positive experiences (Recommendation Box 5-5).

6. *Situational influences.* Many situational factors govern how well a caregiver communicates with persons with Alzheimer's disease. You will notice great differences in your communication style and in the responses of your patients depending on whether the setting is public or private, noisy or quiet, task-oriented or social, routine or emotionally charged. For example, many times the pace of nursing home operations conflicts with the pace of the residents who live in the home. The needs and routines of caregivers and patients seem to exist on different time tracks. Compare the nursing assistant's urgent pleas: "Come on, I haven't got all day" and "Please, Mrs. Cohen, finish your tray. The girls downstairs are going to pick up soon" with the resident's slow replies: "What did you say, dearie?" and "You're walking too fast. I can't keep up." Your awareness of these differences and your ability to adapt your speaking style often is crucial for good patient care (Recommendation Box 5-6).

7. *Responses to the burdens of professional caregiving.* Nursing home employment has many aspects that feel burdensome: absenteeism, understaffing, the limitations of new trainees, double shifts, low pay, heavy physical labor, the demands of record-

---

RECOMMENDATION BOX 5-5

Recommendations for Maximizing Education and Experience

- Apply and advocate for as much in-service training as possible. Stretch your own educational goals beyond state or federal requirements.
- Stimulate your ideas through professional reading. Professional journals and periodicals are full of information and tips for making your job easier and more satisfying.
- Develop an open mind for bad and good experiences. Good experiences give you confidence; unpleasant ones teach valuable lessons. Adopt the attitude "What did I learn from this that will help me do better or be more effective the next time?"

RECOMMENDATION BOX 5-6

Recommendations for Overcoming Situational Factors

- Understand how your particular work environment affects communication. Study the environmental factors that affect communication as discussed in In-Services 3 and 4. Make adjustments so that you and your residents can have the best conditions possible for communicating.
- Guard against letting your choice of words, tone of voice, and body language reflect the exasperation you feel when you are in a hurry and the resident has all the time in the world.

---

keeping, and scheduling. The list seems endless. The responses to communication efforts of a person with Alzheimer's disease also can become part of the burden. The patients' topics of conversation are not intellectually challenging. Repetitive questions, constant moaning and crying, and confusing, pointless answers may only inspire your irritation or boredom.

It is not unusual for professional caregivers to have multiple stresses within their own lives. Nursing assistants make up 85% of all nursing home personnel and provide up to 90% of direct care to residents with Alzheimer's disease, and they have the highest rate of turnover among nursing home employees, averaging 97% to 100% each year.[4,5] The reasons for the high turnover rate are multiple. Pay for CNAs averages little more than minimum wage, below the poverty level in most of the United States,[5] and many CNAs moonlight or work two jobs. Many are single heads of household or grandparents raising grandchildren. Many are immigrants and speak English as a second language. Many have minimal education and are working in their first job with little or no experience with the structure and accountability required in the managed care environment. The Bureau of Labor Statistics has reported that close to 90% of assaults and violent acts by patients against staff in nursing homes involve CNAs.[6] In short, as a group, nursing assistants in the United States are undertrained, underappreciated, underpaid, and overworked.

Hidden (and not so hidden) feelings of exhaustion, frustration, and resentment begin to show in caregivers' behavior. Some caregivers stop trying to communicate with patients except when they need to get a job done. And most residents, sensing a caregiver's emotional hardening, respond poorly to this treatment. Research has revealed that tolerance in caring for persons with Alzheimer's disease is related less to the severity of the patients' problems than to the caregivers' own perception of the burden.[7] In short, how well you respond to your Alzheimer's disease patients depends on how overwhelmed you feel about having to deal with them at all (Recommendation Box 5-7).

RECOMMENDATION BOX 5-7

Recommendations for Overcoming the Burdens of Professional Caregiving

- Examine your support systems. Join or start a once-a-week discussion group for caregivers in your facility. Perhaps you can start by meeting colleagues for coffee after work on a regular basis.
- Cultivate or return to some leisure activities to lessen your stress. Your heart, soul, and body may be crying out for better balance. Make some time for *you*.
- Update your continuing education. Training in new ideas and techniques could give you the coping tools and regeneration you need.
- Seek career counseling if you have a persistent feeling of "What's the use?" about your job. You may need a total change of careers. Or you may do better working with a different type of patient or in a different environment. Decide which path to take and begin to act on your decision right away, so that you can feel in control of your life once again.
- Seek professional counseling if the rest of your life seems out of control. Take care of yourself as well as you would your residents.

▶ **QUICK TIP SUMMARY**

Communication Problems of Professional Caregivers

Healthcare workers are at least as likely as the general population to have problems and impairments that compromise their communication with Alzheimer's disease patients. These problems may relate to the following:
- Speech and language characteristics
- Gender, status, and age biases
- Cultural and linguistic differences
- Personality factors
- Education and experience
- Situational influences
- Response to the burdens of professional caregiving

FINAL NOTE ON THE COMMUNICATION PROBLEMS OF PROFESSIONAL CAREGIVERS

The important point to remember is that communication success or failure does not rest entirely with the skill level of the Alzheimer's disease patient alone. Success or failure rests heavily on *your* communication skills as well.

GOOD PRACTICE 5-1

Communicating with Others: What's My Personal Communication Style?

Directions: Look at how, when, and under what conditions you communicate most comfortably. Below is a set of 15 questions that probe your typical style of interacting with others. Circle the answer that most closely describes your communication style. Use the scale at the end of the questionnaire to interpret your score. **Important: Do not place a value judgment on your personal style of communication. Rather, be aware of your characteristics so that you can adapt them toward more effective interpersonal skills.**

Continued

GOOD PRACTICE 5-1
Communicating with Others: What's My Personal Communication Style? — cont'd

1. I like my work environment to be
   a. Quiet all the time
   b. Quiet, interrupted by occasional conversation
   c. Generally quiet, but sometimes filled with conversation and music
   d. Generally alive with people and noise interspersed with regular quiet periods
   e. Full of people, activity, and as much music as possible

2. The number of "social" or "personal" conversations as opposed to business conversations that I have on an average day at work is
   a. None
   b. One
   c. Two
   d. Three
   e. Four or more

3. I consider myself
   a. A recluse
   b. Shy
   c. An average communicator
   d. A better-than-average communicator
   e. A "real talker"

4. People tell me that my rate of speech is
   a. Very slow
   b. Deliberate
   c. Average, or no comments
   d. Rapid
   e. Too fast

5. People tell me
   a. I talk too softly.
   b. I sometimes cannot be heard.
   c. Very little about how loud I am; I must sound normal.
   d. I sometimes talk too loudly.
   e. I speak pretty loudly most of the time.

6. People tell me
   a. They cannot understand my speech.
   b. I often mumble, or my accent is "thick."
   c. Very little about my pronunciation. It must be normal.
   d. I am a very good speaker.
   e. I should go on the stage!

7. I would rate my vocabulary as
   a. Limited
   b. Adequate for daily needs, but new words often stump me
   c. Average. I do alright.
   d. Sophisticated, college graduate level
   e. Good enough to do the *New York Times* crossword puzzle in ink without a dictionary

Continued

GOOD PRACTICE 5-1

Communicating with Others: What's My Personal Communication Style? — cont'd

8. My use of body language is
   a. Minimal. I talk with my mouth only.
   b. Infrequent. I sometimes gesture with my hands.
   c. Frequent but limited. I gesture mainly with my hands.
   d. Ample. I use gesture and touch to make a point.
   e. Flourishing. I use all I have to get my message across.

9. The acuteness of my hearing
   a. Is something I've never thought about
   b. Sometimes seems like a problem, but I've never had it checked
   c. Has been checked. I could use a hearing aid but do not wear one.
   d. Has been checked, is currently adequate (with or without an aid)
   e. Is excellent. I never miss a thing.

10. My use of humor is
    a. Rare. People tell me I take life too seriously.
    b. Passive. I enjoy humor but can't tell a joke.
    c. Occasional. I rely on it once in awhile.
    d. Well developed. I have a good sense of humor.
    e. Constant. I have a great sense of humor, although I perhaps overdo it once in a while.

11. I maintain eye contact during conversation
    a. Rarely. I seldom look people in the eye.
    b. With difficulty; especially with authority figures
    c. Most of the time with friends and peers but not with certain people who make me uncomfortable
    d. Fairly easily and fairly often with most people
    e. All of the time. I enjoy "staring people down."

12. I rely on touch when I communicate at work
    a. Seldom. It makes me uncomfortable.
    b. Occasionally with close colleagues
    c. Sometimes, when I know the people well
    d. Often, when it seems appropriate to get a message across
    e. Frequently. I consider touch a primary means of communication.

13. I feel responsible for starting the conversation or introducing a new topic
    a. Seldom, if ever
    b. Occasionally
    c. About half the time
    d. More often than not
    e. Always, it seems to me

14. As a listener, I
    a. Am primarily a "good ear" and not a talker
    b. Prefer to listen but talk if I have to
    c. Enjoy listening and responding to what I hear
    d. Prefer to talk but listen if I have to
    e. Am primarily a talker. I get impatient if I have to listen too long.

Continued

GOOD PRACTICE 5-1

Communicating with Others: What's My Personal Communication Style? — cont'd

15. Relative to my personal communication style,
    a. I feel uncomfortable most of the time about the way I speak or sound.
    b. I occasionally make errors or have trouble being understood.
    c. I wish I could improve.
    d. It may not be the best, but I'm not going to change it now.
    e. It is adequate, but I'm always looking for ways to improve.
    f. It is quite good. I am generally pleased with how I speak and sound.

SCORING

Score 1 point for every *a*, 2 for *b*, 3 for *c*, 4 for *d*, 5 for *e*, 6 for *f*, and total the results.
- 60-75: Very extroverted communication style, may need to develop listening skills
- 40-59: Outgoing talker, expectation of leadership role
- 20-39: Good listener, may want to develop more speaking initiative
- Less than 20: Very introverted communication style, may have difficulty taking responsibility in communication situations

---

Modified from Ostuni E, Santo Pietro MJ: *Getting through communicating when someone you care for has Alzheimer's disease*, Vero Beach, FL, 1991, Speech Bin.

GOOD PRACTICE 5-2

What Is My Communication Style as a Professional Caregiver?

Directions: Circle the answer that best describes the communication style you use with most of your residents. Take the time to read each of the choices carefully.

1. When I am with residents, I usually
   a. Don't say much
   b. Use primarily task talk*
   c. Mix task talk with social conversation to make the task more pleasant for both of us

2. When talking with residents, I
   a. Keep moving
   b. Once in awhile stand briefly by the resident's bed (chair) as I work
   c. Sit down at least once a week and direct my attention solely to that resident for a few moments

3. I routinely refer to the residents
   a. On a first-name basis ("Ida," "Joe") or as "honey," "sweetie," "good girl," or "naughty boy"
   b. Formally as "Mrs. Jones," "Mr. Smith"
   c. By the name that the resident and family prefer and with adult praise such as "charming," "endearing," or "nice work"

4. When I need to get an Alzheimer's disease patient to do something, I
   a. Do as much of the task as I can to save the aggravation of trying to explain it
   b. Tell the patient in no uncertain terms what he or she has to do and that I won't put up with any nonsense

---

*Task-talk: A command style of language used to get residents to do something: "Roll over," "Swallow," "Sit up," "Move your arm," and so on (see In-Service 9).

Continued

GOOD PRACTICE 5-2

What Is My Communication Style as a Professional Caregiver? — cont'd

    c. Get the patient's attention first then present one instruction at a time and praise the resident for successful completion of each step

5. If residents have low-verbal skills, I
    a. Rarely try to communicate
    b. Say something once in a while just to hear my own voice
    c. Talk or sing to them frequently and stay alert to any response they make to my communication

6. When family and friends visit, I
    a. Stay out of the resident's room when visitors are present, avoid family members as much as possible
    b. Treat family members politely but do not get involved in long conversations
    c. Get to know family members and observe them with the resident

7. When I am with patients and coworkers at the same time, I
    a Don't say much to either
    b. Talk mainly to my coworker
    c. Try to include both coworker and resident in a conversation

8. When a coworker needs to talk to me about a confidential matter and I am with a resident, I
    a. Talk to my coworker as if the resident weren't there
    b. Leave the resident abruptly to finish the conversation
    c. Signal to the resident that I must leave but will return soon

9. When talking about a resident with Alzheimer's disease to others, I
    a. Don't think it matters what terms I use to describe the resident's behaviors, strengths or weaknesses, or where I am when I say it
    b. Use only professional terms to describe the resident. That way it doesn't matter to whom I talk or where
    c. Use positive and professional terms to describe resident behaviors and carefully select to whom and where I speak

10. The responsibility for helping to maintain the communication skills of Alzheimer's disease patients and making them feel as secure and content *through communication* belongs to
    a. Family members, friends, and chaplains who know the patient best
    b. Speech-language pathologists and other therapists who provide specialized communication treatment and programs
    c. Every single staff person who comes in contact with the resident but especially me

GOOD PRACTICE 5-3

Adapting Your Communication Style to the Patient's Needs

Directions: In this role play for two, one participant plays the part of the patient with Alzheimer's disease described below. The other plays himself or herself as a caregiver communicating in his or her own style as determined in Good Practice 5-2. Observers rate the *appropriateness* of the caregiver's communication style with this particular patient. This is not a value judgment of the style itself but of the appropriateness of the style the caregiver uses with this particular patient.

Continued

> **GOOD PRACTICE 5-3**
>
> **Adapting Your Communication Style to the Patient's Needs — cont'd**
>
> *Scene:* Breakfast in the nursing home dining area
>
> *Patient:* Maude is an 82-year-old former homemaker who appears very fragile and weepy this morning. She knows exactly what she wants for breakfast and how she wants it cooked and served but she can only express herself in "empty speech" (see In-Service 1). She is becoming increasingly agitated as she attempts to tell you what it is she needs but is not getting in the dining room. Maude has a moderate hearing loss in both ears.
>
> *Caregiver:* Your job is to get Maude to eat her breakfast and not upset the other residents in the dining room.
>
> *Observers:* Rate the appropriateness of each aspect of the caregiver's communication style with this particular patient on a scale from 1 to 10 (for a review of elements of communication style, see Good Practice 5-1). Add the 10 scores for an overall percentage of 100. Be prepared to support your number ratings.
>
> Rate of speech _____
> Loudness of speech _____
> Clarity of speech _____
> Level of vocabulary _____
> Amount and style of body language _____
> Use of sense of humor _____
> Amount of eye contact _____
> Use of touch _____
> Quality of listening _____
> Quality of feedback _____
>
> *Caregiver:* How did the ratings of the observers compare with your own assessment of your personal communication style? (see Good Practice 5-1).

REFERENCES

1. Schulz R, Visintainer P, Williamson GM: Psychiatric and physical morbidity effects of caregiving, *J Gerontol* 45:181-191, 1990.
2. Diamond T: *Making gray gold*, Chicago, 1992, University of Chicago Press.
3. Peppard N: *Special needs dementia units: design, development and operation*, New York, 1991, Springer.
4. Richter J, Bottenberg D, Roberto K: Communication between formal caregivers and individuals with Alzheimer's disease, *Am J Alzheimers Care Relat Dis Res* 8:20-26, 1993.
5. *The nursing facility sourcebook*, Washington, DC, 1997, American Health Care Association Facts and Trends.
6. Cohen-Mansfield J: Turnover among nursing home staff: a review, *Nurs Manage* 28:59-64, 1997.
7. Brunk K: Random acts of violence: how CNAs cope with abuse from residents, *Contemp Long term Care* 28:59-64, 1997.
8. Zarit S, Orr N, Zarit J: The hidden victims of *Alzheimer's disease: families under stress*, New York, 1985, New York University Press.

6

Multicultural Issues in Nursing Homes

IN-SERVICE OUTLINE

Premise

Learning Objectives

Definitions

Company Culture in Nursing Facilities

▶ QUICK TIP SUMMARY: What Constitutes a Company Culture?

Impact of Cultural and Ethnic Issues on Communication in a Nursing Home

▶ QUICK TIP SUMMARY: Cultural Diversity in Nursing Homes

Fostering Good Communication in Multicultural Settings

GOOD PRACTICE 6-1: Paired Interviews

GOOD PRACTICE 6-2: Discussion Questions about Cultural Diversity

GOOD PRACTICE 6-3: Discovering Your Company Culture

PREMISE

A person's cultural background has a profound impact on all aspects of his or her communication. It shapes not only the way a person speaks and sounds but also how he or she uses gestures and touch, what topics are considered taboo, and how the person relates to authority. Such communication practices bind people together within a single culture but can become a source of serious conflict between persons from different cultures. In nursing homes both the uniting and the dividing forces of culture can operate. The uniting company culture created by a single purpose (care of the resident) intersects and sometimes collides with the myriad multiple cultures represented by caring versus cared for, work status, age, gender, and ethnic, regional, and religious experiences of employees and residents. The dynamics of such a complex cultural mix profoundly affects the mood or psychosocial environment of all those who work and live within the narrow spaces of long-term care facilities.

To meet the growing demands of providing care for the nation's elderly, nursing homes hire an increasing number of persons from ethnic minority groups every year. Today these facilities face the challenges that have been fostered by cultural diversity. Whether the differences are between staff members, between staff members and residents, or between residents, diversity issues are best addressed through sensible policies of openness, education, and enrichment (Box 6-1).

BOX 6-1   Challenges of Cultural Diversity

Mrs. Fast beckoned to me to come closer so that I could hear her voice, still weak from a recent stroke. "Honey," she rasped, "I think I'm losing my hearing." "What makes you think so?" I asked. Whatever Mrs. Fast's impairments, poor hearing did not seem to be one of them. "I can't understand a word those two people are saying." I glanced at the two aides, a man and a woman chatting cheerfully as they changed Mrs. Fast's bed. They were conversing in Polish.

LEARNING OBJECTIVES

- Define the term *company culture*. Identify two or three company culture practices in your current work setting.
- Identify several major cultural differences between staff members and residents in your work setting. Explain how these create both breakdowns and alliances in communication.
- Discuss some differences in communication style among coworkers that arise from having grown up in particular cultures and languages.
- Recommend at least three ways to support a favorable communication climate among culturally diverse persons in your facility.

DEFINITIONS

Culture   The "customary beliefs, social forms, and material traits of a racial, religious, or social group."[1] When we were children, the habits and associations of our culture were taught to us by a small circle of people: our family, our teachers and classmates, and a few neighbors. Later we may have joined another religion, moved to a different geographic region, and socialized with persons from a variety of backgrounds. Yet even as we stretch to adapt to new surroundings, we retain the stamp of our early cultural beginnings.

Ethnicity   Ethnicity pertains to "a large group of people classified according to a common racial, national, tribal, religious, linguistic, or cultural origin or background."[1] *Ethnic* is a descriptive term that signifies a particular group and their cultural practices (e.g., the ethnic food of Guatemala or the ethnic dances of a Native American Indian tribe). *Ethnicity* (or *ethnic*) is a narrower, more precise term than is *culture*. We use *ethnic* when referring to genetic markers and blood relationships and when speaking about traditional behaviors and beliefs. *Culture* has a broader interpretation and is less strict in suggesting race or parentage. For example, we speak of the Asian culture, but under this umbrella term are widely diverse ethnic groups from India, Japan, Korea, or any of the countries that form the Pacific Rim. Other particular places or groups, such as the Wild West, Silicon Valley, Wall Street, or the homeless, have clear cultural definitions but lack ethnicity such as blood relationship or genetic markers.

Company culture   Every organization has a subtle but unique personality, one that vigorously promotes its own acceptable ways of behaving, speaking, and sometimes dressing. To begin, company cultures are rooted firmly in their product or service (fast food restaurants versus legal firms), their mission statements, and goals ("to provide friendly service to our neighbors" versus "to provide legal services to the indigent"), and in their hiring requirements and practices ("minimum age 16 years, speaks fluent Spanish" versus "extensive courtroom experience and Colorado board certification required"). However, company culture goes beyond products and services, missions and goals, and employee credentials. Organizations vary widely in their personalities even when on the surface they appear be similar, as for example, two nursing facilities. The friendliness of "old" employees to new recruits, the strictness with which rules are enforced, the way certain practices are frowned on and others are encouraged, the pride or resentment that arises when staff members describe their jobs to outsiders—such characteristics are not formally written in the procedures manual, but they operate powerfully to give each workplace a personality that is like no other.

COMPANY CULTURE IN NURSING FACILITIES

One of the strongest influences that shapes company culture is language. The first level of culture is defined by the technical vocabulary that all employees have to know to work together efficiently. Healthcare professionals must learn a large number of medical terms that are essential for everyday communication in a nursing facility. Persons new to the profession or those who speak English as a second language have to work hard to become fluent in "medicalese."

Apart from the medical vocabulary, employees in every facility develop a second type of "lingo" or familiar way of speaking. These words and phrases (sometimes accompanied by meaningful facial expressions) are understood best by people who have worked closely together and have experienced similar joys and hazards. In-jokes often grow out of these experiences. In-jokes can be a healthy way for employees to deal with tough situations, or they can hurtfully exclude those who were not "there," who don't "get it," or who are not with the in-crowd. Language helps create a culture in which people are expected to understand and to talk as everybody else does in the workplace (e.g., on this unit, this floor, this department). New employees raised in ethnically different countries or neighborhoods experience a heavy burden when trying to conform to American cultural standards, to a cumbersome healthcare vocabulary, and to a particular company culture.

Employees are not the only ones who must adjust to the company culture in a nursing facility. The persons experiencing the greatest culture shock on entering institutional life are new residents. If those residents, uprooted from their previous lifestyle and culture, also are disoriented because of Alzheimer's disease, adjustment can be overwhelmingly difficult in the first days and weeks (Box 6-2).

BOX 6-2   A Culture of Concern Keeps Staff

The program enabled us to achieve a staff turnover rate of 30.65% for fiscal year 1997, compared to a state average of 149%. . . . How did we do it? We began about three years ago to focus on development of a mission that truly "grabbed the heart." It stresses five attributes: community, competence, human dignity, service, and vision. We then created an orientation and training program that fulfilled this mission.

From Chapman J: A culture of concern keeps staff, Nursing Homes Cleveland 48:51-52, February 1999.

▶ **QUICK TIP SUMMARY**

What Constitutes a Company Culture?

A company culture is
- The products and service, mission and goals, and hiring requirements and practices of the organization
- The formal or professional language of the workers
- The informal, inside ways of expression and jokes based on common experiences of coworkers
- Explicit and subtle codes of conduct that govern topics and styles of communication, dress, and staff relationships

IMPACT OF CULTURAL AND ETHNIC ISSUES ON COMMUNICATION IN A NURSING HOME

The effects of cultural and ethnic diversity on the lives and relationships of persons who live and work within a nursing home are countless. Staff members need to be aware of how these differences influence communication and how effective communication techniques can help them avoid misunderstandings.

1. *Cultural differences between staff members and residents.* In many nursing homes, particularly in urban areas, a large percentage of direct care and support staff employees are African or Caribbean American, Hispanic, or Asian. One New York City home recently reported that its employees represented 84 nationalities. In recent years, the U.S. nursing home industry has aggressively recruited healthcare professionals from other countries, such as the Philippines, to offset the increasing number of unfilled entry-level positions. Thus many immigrants who work as nursing assistants and who provide the bulk of direct care to residents are still learning the language and becoming acclimated to the culture, whereas the community of current American residents is on average 90% white and mainly of European or North American heritage.

Age differences create another culture gap. If a generation is 20 years, residents who are in their 80s are easily two, three, even four generations apart from their caregivers. The two groups have grown up in different worlds. Besides being a lot older, the one demographic characteristic that caregivers and care receivers share is that they are both predominantly female. Otherwise in terms of nationality, ethnicity, language, life experience, and age, they are on opposite ends of the spectrum.[2,3]

When a resident has Alzheimer's disease, the communication barriers are formidable in any setting. Cultural differences between staff members and residents in the nursing home intensify the potential for communication breakdown. Yet the caregiver, spurred by economic and career needs, and the resident, impelled by medical, physical, and emotional needs, must learn to communicate with one another (Box 6-3).

2. *Cultural differences among staff members.* Diversity training has been slow to enter nursing homes despite the increasing prevalence of culturally diverse staffing patterns. The Hebrew Home for the Aged in Riverdale, New York, developed a diversity program and gained national attention in an article by I. Fisher titled "With Care, Nursing Home Bridges Racial Gulf" published in the *New York Times* on January 12, 1993: "To the Home's administrators, the program was long overdue, not because racial tension was so bad there, but because they felt that fewer misunderstandings would improve patient care."[4]

Misunderstandings between staff members with diverse cultural histories can disrupt the quiet routine required by Alzheimer's disease patients. Most caregivers,

---

BOX 6-3   Cultural Differences between Staff and Residents

The nurses from the Philippines were well-trained and highly qualified, but they were from another country and language and this generated some communication gaps. Sometimes they did not understand American colloquial slang and customs.

Art Loudes, who was 79, sang in his room "You are My Sunshine" and "Clementine" with full voice but almost no teeth. To someone not familiar with the song, his singing was only a jumble. Charge Nurse Alvarez, in the United States less than two years, took him for demented, made a comment to the effect, and infuriated him to a frenzy. When she realized her mistake, she apologized.

From Diamond T: Making gray gold, Chicago, 1992, University of Chicago Press.

no matter what culture they come from, are conscientious in their effort to do a good job and would be surprised to hear that their communication style is a possible cause of problems. Yet this can be the case. Each culture thoroughly trains its children in the style of verbal and nonverbal communication that is unique to that society. As adults, these same people may not understand how choice of words or tone of voice could negatively affect persons from other cultures. Consider the many ways that cultural "rules" for communication determine the following:

Eye contact	Opening, closing a conversation
Personal space	Gender, age, and status roles
Appropriate topics for discussion	Interrupting
Turn-taking in conversation	Use of touch
Laughter, humor	Celebrations, accepting gifts
Acceptable silence	Politeness
Customs for dating, courting	Forms of personal address
Family versus company loyalties	Beliefs about illness and death
Forms of personal address	Rituals of greetings and farewells

To illustrate, an American-born, English-speaking nursing supervisor might consider the averted gaze of a nursing assistant from a Spanish or Asian culture to be a sign of insolence or inattention. Giggling is an acceptable response in some cultures, yet may be seen as totally inappropriate in the United States. People from different cultures have a strong sense of personal space—Americans prefer approximately 3 feet between themselves and their speaking partners. If conversational partners press closer, we feel invaded ("Get outta my face!"). If a conversational partner moves outside the 3-foot space, we believe they are being distant or trying to end the conversation.

A few other examples: (1) Coworkers in an American nursing home could misinterpret as ungracious the practice in many cultures of never opening a gift in front of the giver. (2) Americans sometimes are uncomfortable with European openness in discussing personal information such as age and salary; conversely, Europeans may view the common American question "Where do you work?" as "None of your business!" (3) When a firm handshake, which is prized by Westerners as a sign of personal strength, is met with the looser handshake of a person of Asian descent, "limp" translates to "wimp." (4) Professional caregivers from the United States may underestimate the educational backgrounds or skill of persons trained in other countries because of the new arrival's difficulty passing English-language examinations.

At the same time that the majority group is busy judging others by Western standards, cultural opinions surface among minority groups. American assertiveness may be viewed by foreign-born persons as overbearing, informal manners of speaking and behaving as rude, and the day care and "television" method of raising children as shocking. Many non-U.S. cultures do not believe in putting their sick and elderly relatives in institutions. They feel that the family should be the cradle of care. Raised with different values, some employees are caught between the need for a job and disgust for the American custom that places elderly persons in nursing homes.

3. *Cultural differences among residents.* The residents themselves are not immune to old prejudices and ways of behaving, which often are aggravated by the closeness and regimentation of institutional living. Having Alzheimer's disease exacerbates difficulties in expressing oneself tactfully about delicate issues. One of the more obvious deficits is the Alzheimer's disease patient's loss of ability to use polite forms and "bridges" that we normally use to soften blunt statements. When residents quarrel over cultural biases, staff members need tact and understanding to help mend residents' feelings and prevent future incidents (Box 6-4).

BOX 6-4   Cultural Differences Among Residents

Alice, a three-year resident of Marymount Nursing Home, has been an enthusiastic member of the home's communication partners program. Her job is to escort her communication partners to activities. "Good morning, Mr. Levin," she begins cheerfully, "I'm here to walk with you to church." "Get outta here," Levin bellows, "It's synagogue. Don't you know that by now? I go to synagogue." Both residents withdraw angrily from the Communication Partners program.

▶ **QUICK TIP SUMMARY**

Cultural Diversity in Nursing Homes

- Effective communication is at risk when persons from different cultures work and live together in a closed community.
- In many nursing facilities, at least 30% to 40% of direct care staff members are from different countries, races, and cultural backgrounds. In some homes, the percentage is far greater.
- Certified nursing assistants, who compose the highest percentage of culturally diverse employees, currently provide 80% to 90% of the care for residents with dementia.
- Today's residents are 90% white, American- or European-born, and English-speaking.
- Finding compatible methods of communication that span cultural differences is critical if the staff wants to provide a smoothly functioning environment for residents with Alzheimer's disease.

FOSTERING GOOD COMMUNICATION IN MULTICULTURAL SETTINGS

Most people find that as they gain greater understanding of their colleagues' backgrounds and their residents' histories, they are able to temper their own negative reactions with more empathy and restraint. It all becomes part of maturing into the job and the work setting. Keep this thought in mind: "We cannot change people's race or nationality. Most people would not want to change their religion. The one thing that we all have influence over is our own attitude. . . . What you can do is to try to appreciate this [culturally different] individual and focus on providing quality care in spite of your differences."[5] Tables 6-1, 6-2, and 6-3 address various communication styles.

No matter who you are or what your cultural upbringing, be on constant lookout for good ideas for refining your personal communication style. Improving personal and professional communication skills should be a continuing education goal for everyone (Recommendation Boxes 6-1 and 6-2).

TABLE 6-1 Communication Styles of African Americans	
CHARACTERISTIC COMMUNICATION STYLE	HOW TO RESPOND IN CONVERSATION
NONVERBAL	
Generally judge the feelings of others by reading their nonverbal communication	Do not rely on lengthy verbal accounts.
When listening, tend to look away from person speaking; when speaking tend to look at the listener	Do not assume the person is not listening to you if he or she loses eye contact.
Tend to stand close to people when talking	Allow the speaker to determine personal distance, or say "I need a little more room to think about this."

Continued

TABLE 6-1 Communication Styles of African Americans – cont'd	
CHARACTERISTIC COMMUNICATION STYLE	HOW TO RESPOND IN CONVERSATION

VERBAL

Animated, confrontational, and heated interpersonal style	Expect active style of communication. Be alert to good resident-caregiver fit.
Frequently interrupt during friendly conversation	Accept interruptions as style and not rudeness, or offer "One second, let me finish."
Disagreement often indicated by silence	Avoid interpreting silence as agreement.
Personal questions perceived as invasion of privacy	Avoid intrusive or direct questioning style.
A cool attitude often covers true feelings.	Do not accept cool demeanor as reflection of true feelings.
Family and personal problems and relationships not readily discussed with outsiders	Respect speaker's right to privacy.

Modified from Randall-David E: *Strategies for Working with Culturally Diverse Communities and Clients*, Bethesda, Md, 1989, Association for Care of Children's Health.

TABLE 6-2 Communication Styles of Traditional Hispanics and Latinos	
CHARACTERISTIC COMMUNICATION STYLE	HOW TO RESPOND IN CONVERSATION

NONVERBAL

Tend to stand close to people when talking	Allow speaker to determine personal distance. Or say "I need a little more room to think about this."
Usually make physical contact in greeting by shaking hands, embracing, or back patting	Shake hands when greeting Hispanic or Latino person.
Often touch people when speaking	Avoid pulling away and rejecting friendly gesture.
Eye contact generally avoided when speaking to authority figure; prolonged eye contact seen as disrespectful	Avoid direct or prolonged eye contact. Do not interpret lack of eye contact as inability to relate socially.
Manner of interaction tends to be indirect.	Remember that low key indicates respect and not a lack of feeling.
Latinos expect elders to be treated with utmost respect.	Address elderly Hispanic persons more formally than younger adults.

VERBAL

Commonly show delays in responding to questions	Allow time for reply; do not hurry the speaker.
Do not usually interject, interrupt, or affirm in conversation	Do not assume that conversation is not being followed when feedback is limited.
Hesitant to share personal or family information with strangers	Avoid intrusive or direct personal questions, especially in front of others.
Are generally nonconfrontational	Make a point of establishing trust, support, warmth, and caring.
Women may be more emotionally expressive than men.	Be aware of possible gender differences and gauge communication accordingly.

Modified from Randall-David E: *Strategies for Working with Culturally Diverse Communities and Clients*, Bethesda, MD, 1989, Association for Care of Children's Health.

TABLE 6-3 Communication Styles of Traditional Asians	
CHARACTERISTIC COMMUNICATION STYLES	HOW TO RESPOND IN CONVERSATION
NONVERBAL	
Women do not shake hands in traditional cultures.	Do not be the first to extend your hand when meeting an Asian woman for the first time.
Asians consider it inappropriate to be touched by strangers.	Communicate sincerely in a nonphysical manner.
Traditional religions do not allow touching the head.	Do not touch the head of any Asian person, especially an elder.
Direct eye contact is disrespectful.	Establish only fleeting eye contact.
Pointing at people or objects, especially with toes or foot, is considered rude.	Do not cross your legs or stand with one foot on a chair when in conversation with an Asian.
Waving with palms facing upward can be interpreted as sign of contempt.	Avoid waving.
Smiling, laughing, or giggling is an acceptable way of covering embarrassment or avoiding conflict.	Do not assume that smiling indicates agreement or pleasure. The opposite might be true.
Emotional restraint is highly valued.	Avoid being too lively or casual. This might be interpreted as rudeness.
VERBAL	
Tend to speak in a quiet voice	Match conversational style with a quiet tone. Watch the speaker's face carefully to read lips and eyes. Find a quiet spot to exchange important information.
Generally speak in a nonconfrontational and self-deprecating style	Do not interpret low-key style as low self-esteem. To avoid offending, do not raise issues that evoke strong feelings or conflicts.
Do not share personal feelings openly	Respect the need for privacy.
Generally defer to others in interactions	Invite equal participation in conversations.
Often nod and utter words of assent ("I see") to indicate they are listening	Do not necessarily take words of assent as agreement.

Modified from Randall-David E: *Strategies for Working with Culturally Diverse Communities and Clients*, Bethesda, MD, 1989, Association for Care of Children's Health.

The guidelines in Tables 6-1, 6-2, and 6-3 were developed for persons in American social service agencies either traveling to other countries or working with immigrant families in the United States. Many of the statements are truer of persons who live in local communities in which these cultures and languages still predominate or who are first-generation immigrants. They may not be as characteristic of second-generation persons who have grown up in neighborhoods or gone to schools in which the culture is primarily American and the first language is English.

RECOMMENDATION BOX 6-1

Fostering Good Communication in Multicultural Settings: For Employees Who Are United States-Born Speakers of English as a First Language

- Learn to correctly pronounce the names of coworkers from foreign countries. Use the person's given name unless he or she offers a nickname. Do not assume it is acceptable to "Americanize" a name just because it would be easier for you to pronounce.
- Observe your foreign colleagues' care of residents with Alzheimer's disease. Their style of communication, though different, may be very effective. If so, learn by trying to vary your style rather than correcting theirs.

Continued

RECOMMENDATION BOX 6-1

Fostering Good Communication in Multicultural Settings: For Employees Who Are United States-Born Speakers of English as a First Language — cont'd

- Tolerate differences in communication styles if they do not interfere with patient care or hurt another's feelings. If an individual's way of speaking or behaving puzzles you, tactfully show an interest in learning why they express themselves as they do.
- Trust that foreign-born employees or speakers of English as a second language mean to say the right thing even if they do not achieve the best results. Remember that few staff members would jeopardize their jobs by being intentionally rude.
- Consider carefully who should counsel a coworker whose culturally based communication style, in your opinion, interferes with quality patient care. If you are friendly with each other, the coworker may appreciate and be able to act on your quiet advice without feeling hurt. However, if you feel the employee is seriously compromising patient care, go directly to your supervisor.
- Express respect and praise for your coworker's sincere efforts to develop more effective ways of communicating. An honest compliment from you as a peer goes a long way toward establishing a positive communication environment.
- Develop and openly support a communication ethic of multicultural acceptance. Be vigilant in discouraging toxic talk that involves racial slurs, jokes, and embarrassing questions (see In-Service 7). In an atmosphere that tolerates racist toxic talk, only a few may be guilty, but all staff members are responsible.
- Support your facility's programs in diversity training and participate in these programs with an open mind. Advocate for in-service training that is well adapted to and concentrates on the diversity issues that characterize your workplace.
- Develop mentoring programs between American-born staff members and persons who speak English as a second language or between experienced members of culturally different staff members and new immigrant recruits.

RECOMMENDATION BOX 6-2

Fostering Good Communication in Multicultural Settings: For Employees Raised in Culturally Different Environments or Who Speak English as a Second Language

- Do not assume that a communication breakdown between persons of diverse cultural backgrounds is always the fault of the nonnative speaker of English. Check again. There is a good a chance that the faulty interaction does not have its roots in cultural differences. While keeping an open mind about the need to improve your communication style, do not be too quick to blame yourself or to let others blame you for every misunderstanding.
- Keep a cool attitude when dealing with ethnically inspired insults from residents who have dementia. Persons with Alzheimer's disease lose the ability to inhibit or soften "rude" statements. Although their efforts to communicate are colored by racial slurs and outdated notions about ethnic differences, they may be unaware that they no longer live where others would agree.

Continued

RECOMMENDATION BOX 6-2

Fostering Good Communication in Multicultural Settings: For Employees Raised in Culturally Different Environments or Who Speak English as a Second Language — cont'd

- Never argue with a resident who has spoken offensively. It will not change his or her mind, can easily make things worse, and leaves you open to accusations of verbal or psychological abuse (see In-service 7). When a resident's bitter remarks repeatedly hurt and frustrate you:
  - Speak with your supervisor (should someone else take care of the resident?).
  - Look closely and systematically at the antecedents (could events or persons other than you be triggering the outbursts?).
  - Evaluate your own style of communication and behavior toward the resident. Invite a mentor or friend to help you do this objectively.

GOOD PRACTICE 6-1

Paired Interviews

NOTE: People can work together for months or years before feeling comfortable or interested enough to learn about their coworkers' cultural, religious, or ethnic backgrounds. This short exercise works best in groups of four to ten persons and can reveal pleasant surprises, even to those who think they know each other well.

Directions: Divide the group into pairs (1-2, 1-2, or apples-oranges, apples-oranges, etc.) Every "1" finds a "2" (but not the person sitting in the next chair) or every "apple" finds an "orange." Using the following list of questions, have the two persons in each team interview one another. Emphasize oral exchange of information. Participants then use the information about each other to introduce their partners to the rest of the group. Keep the atmosphere informal, friendly, and accepting. Allow ample time for questions and spontaneous conversation at the end. Encourage people to probe for differences in regional and family cultures, not just national and ethnic differences.

Name _____ [Interviewers, make sure you learn how to pronounce your partner's name correctly!]

Where were you born? _____

Where did you spend most of your childhood? _____

Tell me about something special you used to do or play as a child, with your family or with neighborhood friends. _____
_____

Think of one special holiday that your community celebrated. Was special food served on that holiday? _____
_____

What views did your childhood community have toward the elderly? How were they treated? How were they cared for if they were sick or frail? _____
_____

If you could have one wish in the world, regardless of cost, what would it be? _____
_____

GOOD PRACTICE 6-2

Discussion Questions about Cultural Diversity

Directions: The following questions, intended for small group discussion, relate to the cultural practices in communication that might arise in the nursing home and health care setting. You may want to create additional questions that relate to the diverse cultural communication issues in your particular setting.

- Give examples of gestures that are widely recognized and used in your culture. Are gestures used lavishly, moderately, or seldom to get ideas across?
- How are touch and personal space used in your culture? How is the use of touch related to the status of persons (e.g., parent/child, teach/student, man/man, woman/woman, and public display versus private)? How does distance between speakers depict role, status, and emotion?
- How is eye contact used in your culture?
- How important is tone of voice in your language? What are the social rules regarding use of a loud or a soft voice?
- Describe communication styles that people are expected to use with authority figures.
- What is the family structure like in your society regarding care for the elderly? What are your culture's expectations regarding home care versus hospital or institutional care? How does your society feel about people who grow "senile"?
- What are your culture's beliefs and practices about death and dying?

GOOD PRACTICE 6-3

Discovering Your Company Culture

Directions: Use the following questions for small group discussion.

- Does your staff have "in-house" words or names for the following:
  - Certain safety, medical, or hygiene procedures?
  - Particular patients or groups of residents?
  - Specific physicians or administrators?
  - Employees who exhibit certain behaviors, or the behaviors themselves?
- Relate at least one joke often told by you and your coworkers as a reference point for humor, trouble, overwork, etc.—a joke that no one outside your workplace would appreciate.
- Compare the cultures of previous settings in which you have worked with your coworkers' descriptions of places where they have been employed:
  - How easy was it to get to know and be comfortable with your colleagues?
  - Was staff encouraged to work with or against each other?
  - Was it as good on the "inside" as it appeared to be from the "outside"?
  - What was the cultural mix and how did it affect the interactions of staff members and residents?

REFERENCES

1. *Webster's Tenth Collegiate Dictionary*, Springfield, MA, 1994, Merriam-Webster.

2. Harrington C, Carrillo H, Thollaug S, Summers P: *Nursing Facilities, Staffing, Residents, and Facility Deficiencies, 1991-1997*, report prepared for the Health Care Financing Administration, San Francisco, 1999, University of California.

3. Strahan G: An overview of nursing homes and their current residents. *1995 National Nursing Home Survey: Advance Data from Vital and Health Statistics*, #280, Hyattsville MD, 1997, National Center for Health Statistics.

4. Fisher I: With care nursing home bridges racial gulf. *New York Times*, January 12, 1993.

5. Pillemer K, Hudson B: *Ensuring an Abuse-Free Environment : A Learning Program for Nursing Home Staff*, Philadelphia, 1991, Coalition of Advocates for the Rights of the Infirm Elderly.

The Toxic Effects of Verbal Abuse and Communication Neglect

IN-SERVICE OUTLINE

Premise
Learning Objectives
Definitions
Causes of Verbal Abuse and Communication Neglect
The Responsibility and Risks of Reporting Abuse and Neglect
GOOD PRACTICE 7-1: Self-Assessment: Hidden Feelings That Influence Attitudes, Actions, and Communication: A Group Discussion Activity
GOOD PRACTICE 7-2: Clarifying Information for Reporting an Incident of Abuse or Neglect
GOOD PRACTICE 7-3: Scenarios for Discussion

PREMISE

The most extreme examples of inappropriate or ineffective communication that caregivers can exhibit are verbal abuse and communication neglect. Acts of aggressive speech and the withholding of social speech, both classified as forms of psychological mistreatment, occur in nursing homes at least four times more often than do acts of physical abuse.[1]

Every nursing home employee is responsible for prevention of any type of abuse or neglect. This unprofessional and illegal behavior is discussed in this in-service in the hope that the more you know about verbal abuse and communication neglect, the more you will work to prevent it. This in-service also introduces the term *toxic talk*, a way of speaking that, although not illegal, has major implications in the development or prevention of verbal abuse and neglect.

LEARNING OBJECTIVES

- Identify the differences between verbal abuse and communication neglect.
- Describe toxic talk and explain why it creates a ready environment for verbal abuse and neglect.
- List at least three ways in which verbal abuse, communication neglect, and toxic talk can be prevented.
- List all possible reasons that these three violations of good communication must be stopped immediately if detected by anyone (employee, volunteer, visitor) in a nursing home.
- Discuss the reasons for and against reporting known or suspected cases of abuse or neglect.

DEFINITIONS   **Verbal abuse**   One of several types of psychological mistreatment in which one person speaks to another with the intention of causing emotional pain. A verbal abuser also attempts to control the other's behavior through violent words. Examples include the following:

- Yelling or cursing angrily to scare a resident into action
- Threatening to throw something at or to hit a resident
- Threatening to punish a resident if he or she does not follow directions (e.g., "I'll lock you in your room," "No food for a week," or "I'll put rats in your bed")
- Making fun of or playing humiliating practical jokes on a resident (Box 7-1)

Communication neglect   Neglect that occurs when caregivers avoid looking at, talking to, or touching a resident in ways that suggest deliberate withholding of warmth and nurturing. Communication neglect can be an intentional act, as when the staff member wants to "punish" a patient for some "bad behavior," or it can be an unconscious attitude, as when a patient is "just one more job to get done." In some settings, for example:

- Residents are treated as objects or called by the name of their disorder or prosthesis (e.g., "Go get that new diabetic in room 103 for a bath" and "Take those wheelchairs down to lunch," referring to patients as "wheelchairs").
- Staff concern for efficiency and numbers overshadows the patients' need for comfort and companionship.
- Tasks are performed in a cold, detached, and dehumanizing way.
- Residents are subjected to frequent, long-term, and unrelieved periods of "time out" for inappropriate behavior.
- Signals or cries for help are ignored.
- Environment (e.g., no private places for visiting), schedules, and staff attitudes (that the presence of guests "interrupts important tasks") discourage visitors from coming to see the residents.

When the foregoing attitudes and practices are the rule rather than the exception, administrative or accrediting agencies find good cause for investigating a facility for incidents of psychological abuse (Box 7-2).

Toxic talk   An unhealthy form of communication that conveys an attitude of disrespect for a person's humanity, right to privacy, and self-determination. It is a way of speaking to and about residents that severely undermines the morale and the communication ethic of the entire environment. The intention is not to emotionally harm or coerce, as with verbal abuse, or to ignore or punish, as with communication neglect, but to insinuate that the resident is not worth considerate humane treatment (Box 7-3). Toxic talk is characterized by tone of voice, style of speaking, or careless disclosure of confidential information. Toxic talk may take place to or in front of a resident, among staff members, or with outsiders. Examples of toxic talk include the following:

- Using a sarcastic or surly tone of voice or a habitually curt form of speech: "Whatsa matter, ya deaf?" "What? You're wet again? Yuk!"
- Discussing the resident's "bad" behavior or illness within that person's hearing (even though you are "sure" he or she can no longer understand): "She makes my life miserable with her constant whining. I don't know what she wants, and frankly I don't care anymore either." "His doctor says the cancer is everywhere. This guy's a dead duck."
- Talking about a patient in an insulting or otherwise unprofessional manner to other staff members: "He's nothing but a worthless bag of s—." "She doesn't have a brain left in her head." "Uh oh, here comes ol' motor-mouth Mabel."
- Talking about patients by name or other identifying details to persons outside the facility, especially if the remarks are demeaning or reveal confidential information.
- Reprimanding or insulting a coworker or speaking ill of another employee in the presence of residents, visitors, or volunteers.

Toxic talk may not be against the law, but it is certainly injurious. It creates a feeling of disrespect for the residents among the employees of the facility. It reflects poorly on the professionalism of the individuals who indulge in it. It pollutes the environment and undercuts the moral fiber of any work team. It can easily destroy community trust, involvement, and investment. Worst of all, toxic talk reduces caregiver sensitivity and sets the stage for acts of verbal abuse or communication neglect. Employees at every level of the workforce should guard against the destructive effects of toxic talk.

BOX 7-1   Verbal Abuse

Margaret, a 76-year-old widow with Alzheimer's disease, can never remember whether she has eaten a meal. She prowls the unit foraging food from the tray cart, searching for an occasional stray snack, and begging for additional helpings. The staff worries about her consumption of unauthorized food. They waste precious time hustling her away from the rooms of other angry residents, and she is gaining too much weight. In exasperation, one nursing assistant tells Margaret that she will put poison in the woman's food if she doesn't stop eating so much. "Maybe she'll stop if we all tell her the same thing," suggests the nursing assistant hopefully. "Sounds like a treatment plan to me," agrees her colleague.

BOX 7-2   Communication Neglect

We sat tidying up some charts. As I glanced over Mary Karney's vital signs, I remembered the incident when she was crying on the bed, and I was told to keep moving. Here were the records of her life signs; they made it clear that formally, the nursing assistant's job had nothing to do with talking with Mary. It had, in fact, been more efficient and productive not to do so, the faster to collect the measurements. To stay and give Mary Karney an emotional outlet for her trouble was supplanted by the act of taking vitals and moving on. . . . Tasks produced numbers that, rather than folded in as part of human relations . . . dictated the form of interaction between staff and residents.

From Diamond T: *Making gray gold*, Chicago, 1992, University of Chicago Press.

BOX 7-3   Toxic Talk

Three staff members from The Manor just off the night shift collapse wearily in the diner booth and watch the waitress pour their coffee. "Anna drove me nuts last night, screaming and yelling," says Maggie, shaking her head. "She's a real pain in the butt, all right, but she is nothing compared to that daughter of hers," adds Sarah. "Moaning and bitching all the time. She doesn't like her mom's diet, there aren't enough activities, her TV is tilted so she can't see it. I just tune out," Rita yawns, "How come she's in this dump anyway? Isn't she Mike Penfield's mom, that lawyer guy who's building the big mansion up on Spring Street?"

June, the waitress, finishes pouring the coffee. She has a date that night with Anna Penfield's nephew. At a nearby table, two reporters from a local newspaper lean forward slightly. Their newspaper has built its readership by exposing scandal and abuse in the county's institutions. A member of The Manor's board of directors and her husband sit quietly in the booth behind the three tired employees, scraping up the last of their eggs. Their eyes meet.

CAUSES OF VERBAL ABUSE AND COMMUNICATION NEGLECT

Research on abuse in nursing homes has shown that acts of verbal abuse and communication neglect occur more readily in work settings where

- State laws and agencies do not provide adequate oversight and protection of the rights of residents with dementia or of their caregivers.
- Managers and administrators fail to create and enforce policies that support caregivers and residents or that enhance the working conditions and climate of the workplace.
- Personnel are less experienced, especially in crisis prevention and intervention.
- The staff does not receive specific training in how to prevent verbal abuse and communication neglect.
- Staff members are under work-related stress and are approaching "burn-out."
- Employees have a history of resorting to violence to solve problems.
- Staff members are repeatedly provoked by combative or verbally aggressive residents[1-4] (Box 7-4).

Abusive incidents of all types occur more often when the residents are abusive to the staff. A high rate of resident aggression can be a sign that staff members abusively handle or speak insensitively to patients on a regular basis. This interrelatedness between care receiver and caregiver abuse sets up a dangerous cycle of violence.

Recognizing that physical and psychological abuse are chronic problems in long-term care facilities, the Coalition of Advocates for the Rights of the Infirm Elderly (CARIE) developed an abuse prevention curriculum designed specifically for nursing assistants.[5,6] The program has three major objectives: (1) to increase staff awareness of actual abuse and potentially abusive situations, (2) to equip nursing assistants with appropriate conflict intervention strategies, and (3) to reduce staff-resident conflict and abusive behaviors by staff members.

An eight-module training manual provides text and role-playing opportunities for participants to test various methods of coping with difficult resident care situations. Throughout training, nursing assistants are encouraged to share their own examples of troublesome or provocative patient behavior. The curriculum was tested in 10 nursing homes in the Philadelphia area. Results from the pretest-posttest assessment of 114 nursing assistants were positive. Attitudes toward elderly charges improved, and there was significant reduction both in patient aggression toward staff members and in nursing assistants' aggression toward their patients.

Programs such as the one developed by CARIE are meaningful in the prevention of abuse, but they do not constitute the only solution to this complex issue. In long-term care facilities where abuse, neglect, and attitudes that support toxic talk

---

BOX 7-4 Staff Predisposition to Abuse and Neglect
These patients often are the defenseless targets of long-term care staff who, guided by the belief that a loss of cognitive ability diminishes a person's humanity, dismiss residents with dementia as beyond help and unworthy of care. Other times, patients are victims of staff with criminal records and unchecked violent behavior. . . . [However] nearly every expert on the front lines of long-term care agrees that ignorance and exhaustion, more often than malice, are usually to blame in cases where dementia patients suffer.

From Foote J: Dementia: abuse and neglect compound the suffering of many elderly, *Star Ledger*, 7 May 1995, Middlesex edition.

are the norm, the problem is a systemic one that requires the attention and action of the administration (Box 7-5).

No matter how poor the living and working conditions, poor conditions can never justify abusive acts, verbal or otherwise. As a professional caregiver, you must take personal responsibility for your attitudes and the behavior that flows from those attitudes.

THE RESPONSIBILITY AND RISKS OF REPORTING ABUSE AND NEGLECT

Up to this point we have spoken only of *verbal* abuse and *communication* neglect because (1) this is an in-service training manual about communication skills; (2) *verbal* abuse and communication neglect occur more frequently than do *physical* abuse and neglect, and (3) acts of physical abuse and neglect usually are preceded by a history of psychological, that is, verbal, abuse and neglect. Both psychological and physical categories define illegal acts that carry penalties if the accused parties are found guilty.

If you suspect abuse or neglect, whether verbal or physical, the thing *not* to do is to confer with everyone on your shift and then run immediately to the facility chief executive officer or the police! Do speak immediately to your supervisor. If this is not possible, report your suspicions immediately to someone in administration with whom you feel comfortable and who knows and trusts your judgment. The matter will probably be taken out of your hands and be dealt with through the proper channels.

Should you still feel dissatisfied, there are other means of recourse. Two organizations have been established that are authorized by state or federal legislation to receive and process claims and to help the victim and ameliorate the abuse: Adult Protective Services (APS) and the Long Term Care Ombudsman Program (LTCOP). These agencies have literature that explains how to lodge a complaint and how the investigative process works. In some states, APS has a separate law that specifically addresses institutional abuse.[7,8]

Many state laws *require* citizens to report abuse and neglect. Still, an employee accepts a great responsibility by reporting an incident that is potentially embarrassing, scandalous, or harmful to the public image and financial health of the institution. Reporting suspected abuse or neglect is a communication act that touches all aspects of professional caregiving: your personal system of ethics and values, the safety and care of the residents, your daily interaction with coworkers and supervisors, and the position of the nursing facility within the community. Company culture can harbor a strong self-protective countercurrent that dis-

---

BOX 7-5 Systemic Predisposition to Abuse and Neglect

Training is obviously important, but the presumption that the lack of it is responsible for the abuse is a naive conclusion. Caregivers do not learn to be abusive in lieu of proper training necessarily. Their behavior may be the result of chronic stress, pathological influences, inadequate supervision, uninspiring management, environmental conditions, or faulty recruitment and selection procedures.

Abuse is a human and a systemic problem. . . . To achieve freedom from abuse, the total context of caregiving must be examined and redesigned.

From MacNamara RD: *Freedom from abuse in organized care settings for the elderly and handicapped: lessons from human service administration*, Springfield, IL, 1988, Thomas.

BOX 7-6 Reasons to Report Incidents of Abuse and Neglect

Nursing assistants in the CARIE training sessions are asked to consider the following possibilities in not reporting cases of observed or suspected abuse and neglect:

- The resident could be seriously injured.
- The resident could become ill or die.
- The situation between the resident and the employee could become worse.
- The employee could abuse other residents.
- You could be contributing to the escalation by not saying anything.
- The situation could be discovered by the newspapers.
- You (the coworker) could be legally involved (be accused of being accessory to the crime, because you knew and did not report), if the situation is uncovered later.
- You could have it on your conscience.[5, 6]

Perhaps you can think of other possibilities.

---

courages people from "blowing the whistle." Whistle blowers, people who notify authorities of suspected wrongdoing by fellow workers, have much soul-searching to do before stepping forward (Box 7-6).

Even though you are sure you are acting in the best interests of the residents and of your profession, you must not expect your report to be popular in the eyes of coworkers, supervisors, or administrators. You could be the victim of backlash (e.g., you are correct under the law but lose your job, are shunned, and receive threatening notes). Objectively assess the possible legal, emotional, and financial costs to you and your family. Develop plans for shouldering these responsibilities. Seek support from friends and relatives. Federal regulations and state laws protect persons who blow the whistle with legitimate or plausible complaints. These laws do not protect persons who turn out to simply be disgruntled employees. You must have good evidence to back up your claim. In the long run, you are not the one who has to decide whether a law has been broken. *Professional investigators will determine whether abuse has actually occurred.*

Results of studies from the fields of business and engineering indicate that illegal practices decline where workers know that reporting such incidents is accepted and encouraged as a fair procedure to deal with the problem. Reporting suspected or known acts of verbal abuse or communication neglect is one way that you might be called on to keep your work environment and your caregiving profession abuse free (Recommendation Box 7-1).

RECOMMENDATION BOX 7-1

Recommendations for Preventing Verbal Abuse, Communication Neglect, and Toxic Talk

- Personally guard against toxic talk inside and outside the workplace. This unpleasant style of communicating is more contagious than the common cold; others around you are quick to respond in like manner. No one expects you to be bubbly and sparkling all day every day, but you can develop a habit of pleasant communication with residents and coworkers. Watch your tone of voice carefully; choose your words with the same caution that you would choose a car.
- Understand the disease process. Aggressive behaviors are expressions of a severely compromised brain and are not an outburst of personal hostility toward you, even if you are the one being called names. This knowledge should be one deterrent of impulsive or defensive reactions.
- Know your limitations. Disgust, contempt, fear, superiority, anger, frustration, and disappointment are but a few of the emotions you will experience in this job. Yet you and you alone are responsible for your actions. You can and must be in command of your own behavior, especially when you are trying to cope with a resident's anxiety or anger.
- Trust your experience. In tough communication situations, seasoned caregivers learn to stay calm and decide whether to handle the problem directly, to wait a while, or to ask someone else for help.
- Establish an informal "buddy system" with someone on your shift who will come to your assistance when you need it, someone whose "hot buttons" are not pushed by certain residents the way yours are. Offer to help your buddy in the same way. The buddy system builds teamwork and decreases the likelihood of an abusive incident.
- Observe coworkers who are skilled in coping with unexpected crises and difficult communication situations. Watch how they use verbal and nonverbal body language to defuse the situation or accomplish a difficult task.
- Read and know well the resident's bill of rights, which according to a federal mandate, must be posted in every long-term care facility.[8]
- Educate yourself on your state's legal definitions of abuse and neglect and the state laws that protect the elderly in institutions.
- Know your state's legal requirements for reporting suspected abuse or neglect and the consequences of *not* reporting such incidents. Inquire about the reporting procedure in your facility. Is there a procedure or form for reporting? Is there a taboo against even asking for the form?
- Speak to a trusted supervisor or someone in your administrative hierarchy first and in strict confidence. Do *not* air your complaints and questions to anyone and everyone who will listen. It is irresponsible and terrible to have slandered the reputation of someone who turns out not to be guilty.

GOOD PRACTICE 7-1

Self-Assessment: Hidden Feelings That Influence Attitudes, Actions, and Communication: A Group Discussion Activity

Directions: **Part I:** Fill in (a) the resident's initials, (b) the resident's behavior that irritates you (e.g., repetitive moaning, resistance, incontinence), (c) your feelings when this behavior occurs (e.g., rage, disappointment, inadequacy), and (d) how you are tempted to react (e.g., throw a plate, quit, curse, cry).

When (a) _____ does or behaves like (b) _____ I feel (c) _____ , and I'd like to (d) _____ .

Directions: **Part II:** Write in possible causes for your feelings and professionally acceptable solutions for dealing with both the feelings and the residents who trigger them. Discuss and compare your answers with those of others in your group.

One reason the resident's behavior might be occurring: _____
_____

One part of my behavior that I could change, one new thing in my approach that I might try: _____
_____

One change in the environment that might help: _____
_____

One other person who might be helpful and in what way: _____
_____

GOOD PRACTICE 7-2

Clarifying Information for Reporting an Incident of Abuse or Neglect

Directions: In the following decision tree, report the incident only if all answers to the questions are "yes."

Today's Date: _____ Date of Incident:_____

1. Describe the incident as clearly as you can: _____
_____
_____
_____

2. Did you actually see or clearly overhear the incident? Yes/No
3. Can you identify the resident involved? Yes/No
4. Can you identify the staff member involved? Yes/No
5. Are you able to clearly describe the incident? Yes/No
6. Do you believe that it was the worker's intent to hurt the resident emotionally or physically? Yes/No
7. Do you believe it was the worker's intent to inappropriately neglect, ignore, or socially isolate the resident? Yes/No
8. Do you believe you are doing the right thing by reporting the incident? Yes/No

GOOD PRACTICE 7-3
Scenarios for Discussion

Directions: Break the group into teams of three or four persons. Assign a scenario to each of the teams. Ask each team to answer the following five questions. Then reassemble the group for general discussion.

DISCUSSION QUESTIONS

- Does this scene depict verbal abuse, communication neglect, toxic talk, or appropriate communication behavior? Why or why not?
- If your group is in doubt about how to judge a scenario, work out the solution by completing the following statements:
  - It depends on whether _____.
  - If *this* is so, then it probably is _____.
- If the situation seems to be a case of verbal abuse or neglect, how would you suggest solving the problem?
- If the scene does not seem to be abuse or neglect, can the situation be improved to benefit the resident or the caregiver?
- Has anyone in your group ever witnessed or experienced a similar situation? What was the outcome? Do you think this outcome was fair? Is it better than the one you are now considering?

Scenario 1: Max has a habit of accosting visitors to his unit and asking for cigarettes. He is very aggressive, peering myopically at the surprised guests and holding on to their sleeves. When Agnes is on duty, she steers Max firmly into his room and sits him down in a chair. "It's very rude to ask strangers for anything. Don't leave this room until I say you can." Then she closes the door firmly. Max has arthritis in his hands and cannot open the door easily by himself. He is terrified of being in a closed room by himself.

Scenario 2: George, a certified nursing assistant, is having a hard time getting Julius washed up. Julius flails and thrashes about, and sometimes George's jaw or shin gets in the way. In frustration George yells, "Stand still, dammit." George's loud voice and stern face startle Julius, and for a moment he stands meekly while George scrubs away. Then Julius begins to thrash and protest again. This time, George's voice booms, "Sonovabitch! You stand still or you're gonna have soap in your eyes, in your mouth, up your ass. I'll make sure of it."

Scenario 3: Angelica helps 82-year-old Mathilde into her room. Wordlessly, Angelica undresses Mathilde, slides a nightgown around the thin body, and guides Mathilde into bed. Angelica takes Mathilde's vital signs, charts the results, and switches off the light. Before leaving the room, she turns with her face in the shadows and asks the still figure on the bed, "Do you want a glass of water or anything before I leave?" Mathilde, who has poor vision and hearing, returns the gaze but says nothing. Angelica shrugs and leaves the room.

Scenario 4: It is 2 AM, and Evan's voice echoes endlessly down the hallway: "Mother, mother! I hafta go to the bathroom." The words are slurred, but Stewart and Marie have heard them often and have no trouble figuring out what the old man is yelling. Marie complains, "That guy's voice is driving me crazy, like fingers on a blackboard. Can't anything shut him up?" Stewart looks up from the chart he is writing in. "Aw, what's the use? He's on his way out anyway. Besides, when he's gone, we'll just get another screamer. They dump all the worst ones onto this unit."

Continued

GOOD PRACTICE 7-3

Scenarios for Discussion — cont'd

Scenario 5: Joe lies helplessly in his bed, his body and mind almost spent from the ravages of Alzheimer's disease. A few staff members stand at the nurses' station charting the last bits of patient information before going home for the night. "I heard he was a real hell-raiser in his day. Mama told me about all the women in town he screwed," muses Suzanne. "It wasn't just girls from what I heard," adds Eric with a cynical tone of voice. "When he was more alert, I made sure I knew where his hands were." Rose, just 2 days into the job and only 1 week away from graduation, listens wide-eyed and wide-eared. Today, when she was changing Joe's sheets, his hand had sort of "wandered" even though his eyes were closed. She sure doesn't want that dirty old man feeling her up.

Scenario 6: "Time for lunch." Helen's voice and touch on Madge's back cause Madge to startle and look up. "I always make Madge jump that way if I really want her to do something. If I get face to face with her, she just ignores me."

Scenario 7: Beside the bed: "Get your pants on. Not that way. Here, this way. God, you're stupid. Finally got 'em on? Let's go." Walking down the hall: "Family's waiting. Got ants in their pants. Hurry up. They haven't got all day, neither do I." In the elevator: "Wait'll I tell 'em how bad you've been this week. They'll never wanna see you again. D'ya think they really care anyway?" Entering the reception area: "Here he is at last. Sorry he looks so goofy. Had a hard time getting him dressed again." To herself on the way back to the unit: "Man that guy is slow. How'd I get stuck with such a loser?"

Scenario 8: Guests are shocked to hear the way Vera speaks to Nat, who sits slumped over in his wheelchair. Vera squats low on the floor so that she can see Nat's face and calls in a loud, low-pitched voice, "Nat, wake up. It's me, Vera. Time for lunch." Nat stirs as Vera taps his arm. "I'm putting a pillow under your elbow. Sit straight. Good." Her voice carries down the hall. "Heads up, we're on our way." As they approach Nat's dining room table, Vera moves around to the front of the wheelchair again and blares to a more erect and alert Nat: "Looking good, Nat. Have a nice lunch." He nods in acknowledgment. "I'm glad I don't live here," shudders the visitor to her husband. They have come to the nursing home to see the husband's convalescent brother. "I sure would hate to have someone yell at me all the time like that."

REFERENCES

1. Pillemer K, Bachman-Prehn R: Helping and hurting: predictors of maltreatment of patients in nursing homes, *Res Aging* 13:74, 1991.
2. MacNamara RD: *Freedom from abuse in organized care settings for the elderly and handicapped: lessons from human service administration*, Springfield, IL, 1988, Thomas.
3. Tellis-Nayak V: *Nursing exemplars of quality: the paths to excellence in quality nursing homes*, Springfield, IL, 1988, Thomas.
4. Office of Evaluation and Inspections: *Resident abuse in nursing homes*, Washington, DC: Office of Inspector General, Department of Health and Human Services, 1990.
5. Pillemer K, Hudson B: Model abuse prevention program for nursing assistants, *Gerontologist* 33:128, 1993.
6. Talerco K, and others: *Elder mistreatment in nursing homes: detection and intervention strategies training manual for trainers*, Philadelphia: 1996, The Coalition of Advocates for the Rights of the Infirm Elderly (CARIE).
7. American Bar Association Commission on Legal Problems of the Elderly: Information about laws related to elder abuse. Available at: www.elderabusecenter.org/laws/index.html. Accessed: 9 February 2002.
8. *Nursing Home Reform Act of 1987*, Public Law 100-203.

Communicating with Families: Same Goals, Different Goals

PREMISE   Many professional caregivers report that their interactions with the families of patients are among the most difficult of their daily duties. In a study of nursing assistants, Richter et al.[1] found many nursing assistants thought that "communicating with the family was the greatest barrier in care of the person with Alzheimer's disease." Nursing assistants commented that families frequently disrupted patient care and were very demanding. Nursing assistants made statements such as, "It's hard to be nice to the families," "Family members complain and yell," "Relatives want attention," and "Families discuss their feelings of guilt, and I don't know what to say to them." Rather than viewing the family as a resource, nursing assistants in Richter's study perceived them to be a major source of stress. At the same time, many family members view nursing homes and nursing home staff with feelings ranging from ambivalence to suspicion, anger, or even contempt. Founded or unfounded, these feelings between professional caregivers and family members must be dealt with if residents with Alzheimer's disease are to be provided the best treatment and if you want to reduce your stress in caregiving.

This in-service addresses the question "Why is it so difficult to communicate with residents' families?" by exploring the problems that families bring to the nursing home along with their relatives who have Alzheimer's disease. We will also examine the barriers that staff members bring to encounters with families.

LEARNING OBJECTIVES

- Recognize comminication difficulties that family members may experience when talking to nursing home staff.
- Describe at least three communication problems of direct care staff that may upset family members.
- Role play at least four specific responses that represent empathetic listening skills with a troubled family member.
- Explain why empathetic listening skills can improve any communication situation.

DEFINITIONS

Family caregiver   For the purposes of this in-service, the person in the resident's family who takes primary responsibility for the resident's affairs. Most often this is a female relative, usually the "dutiful daughter." Frequently this is the person who was providing direct care before the resident entered the nursing home. One third of primary family caregivers are elderly themselves.

Caregiver burden   The result of the physical, psychological, and financial stresses that Alzheimer's disease places on family caregivers. The degree of the burden experienced depends on many interacting factors, but all family caregivers carry a burden.

Empathic listening   A nonjudgmental response that captures the essential theme or feelings expressed by the speaker.[2] Empathic listening offers the potential for building rapport and mutual understanding between speaker and listener. It does not necessarily indicate agreement or sympathy with the speaker. An example of listening to a family member with empathy might be "It sounds as if you feel the staff is taking advantage of your willingness to help."

PROBLEMS THAT FAMILY MEMBERS BRING TO ENCOUNTERS WITH NURSING HOME STAFF

1. *Negative perception of nursing homes.* According to one study, at least three fourths of family caregivers of frail, elderly persons believe that "people go to a nursing home only when there is no other place to live."[3] Family members seem to be unaware of any benefits that a nursing home might provide. Eighty percent of caregivers 70 years or older see a nursing home as the place of last resort. Less-educated persons, those in poorer health, and those with lower incomes are the most resistant to nursing home placement.

2. *Personal communication problems.* The average age of family caregivers of Alzheimer's disease patients is 57 years. One third are older than 65 years. More than two thirds are women.[4] Elderly family caregivers themselves are at risk of all of the personal communication problems that accompany aging (see In-Services 2 and 5). Many of them are coping with their own hearing loss, depression, aphasia, Parkinson's disease, and other disorders.

3. *Long-standing interpersonal communication problems with the patient.* By the time a patient enters a nursing home, family members have already experienced profound communication breakdowns and distress. These changes in communication are not as likely to bother the nursing home staff in the same way that they upset family caregivers.

a. Loss of reciprocity in the relationship, loss of mutual give and take. One daughter reported, "I am stunned by the realization that I'm still playing the role of the criticized child, but she's not playing 'mommy' any more."[5]

b. Asynchronies. When a resident's cycles of sleeping and eating become disturbed, any of the family caregiver's social relationships that centered on mealtimes and bedtimes grind to a halt. For most people, these are the times that in the past had nourished the relationship.

c. Deterioration of social life. As the patient's condition worsens, family caregivers begin to function within a more narrowly constricted social environment. For most family caregivers, this restricted social life does not expand when the patient enters the nursing home.

d. Emotional scars from previous violence. By the time the patient enters the nursing home, communication between family caregiver and patient may have deteriorated so severely that domestic violence has occurred. Research studies have documented patient-to-caregiver physical abuse in 16% to 33% of cases and caregiver-to-patient violence in 5% to 23% of cases. The emotional scars of physical abuse are not erased by institutionalization.[6]

4. *Confusion over new role.* Once the patient has been admitted to the nursing home, the role of the family in the patient's care changes radically. In the transition, the family member's status changes from primary caregiver to visitor, from insider to outsider, and from high control to low control over the patient's care. At the same time, most family members continue to have frequent contact with their loved ones after admission and perceive that their burden of care continues after institutionalization. In truth, "the family is often working through feelings of loss, guilt, and helplessness and may have a strong need to continue the caregiving role after a loved one has been admitted to the nursing home."[7]

Family members generally view themselves as protectors of or advocates for their loved ones in the nursing home and want to provide as much of the hands-on care as possible. However, families usually are not oriented to the procedures of a long-term care facility and learn only by trial and error what duties they may and may not assume. Some family members believe that too many patient care duties are still left to them even though they are paying a large amount of money to the nursing home. Other family caregivers may feel insulted because they are allowed to do so little. According to Maas et al.,[7] family members react to ambiguous situations with hostility toward staff, disagreements over the use of services, criticism of the care provided, and less-frequent visits. They also react with increased guilt, health problems, and more use of drugs and medications.

5. *Emotional and spiritual neediness.* Families of Alzheimer's disease patients must make emotional and spiritual adjustments during the course of the disease. The most common are as follows:

a. The need to deal with their own feelings of guilt and sadness at having institutionalized the patient. Many Alzheimer's disease patients remain at home far beyond the point at which admission to the nursing home might have been optimal and far beyond the breaking point for family caregivers. Usually there is dissension in the family over the placement, and often the person who makes the final decision is berated by the patient and by the rest of the family. The feelings of guilt, anger, and mourning that this process engenders do not suddenly evaporate after the admission. They reappear in the family caregiver's search for reassurance, denial of earlier problems, and defensiveness in interacting with professional caregiving staff.

b. The search for remaining connectedness to the resident. Because it is so difficult to deal with the loss of communication with a mate, a parent, or a sibling, most family members continue to work hard to stay connected with the resident. They state with conviction, "I'm sure he knew it was me sitting with him even though he couldn't say my name." Connectedness is extremely important to them.

c. The search for meaning in the disease. By the time an Alzheimer's disease patient enters the nursing home, family members have spent a great deal of effort trying to find some meaning in their loved one's illness. After they have turned over their caregiving role to the institution, this search for meaning may become all-consuming.

d. The need to grieve over the slow loss of a loved one and to deal with the eventual death. Under any circumstances, death is the most difficult event that humans face. Psychologists tell us that most people find it more difficult to deal with the deaths of their loved ones than with their own deaths. Family caregivers of persons with Alzheimer's disease have already begun to deal with this reality. Their loved ones are slipping away day by day, yet many nursing homes barely acknowledge the pain of death and the need to grieve. Some do not even offer a memorial service when a resident dies. This silence discredits the importance of the family's loved one and the enormity of the family's feelings of grief.

e. The need to grieve over personal losses of health, quality of life, financial resources, and affection that occur over the course of long-term caregiving. Perhaps the most poignant adjustment of all for caregivers is to the reality that, even though responsibility for the loved one has been delegated to a nursing home, the personal toll for years of caregiving has been life changing and, in some ways, permanent. The primary caregiver has had to constantly redefine his or her life in the knowledge that the partner can no longer accept or confer affection and moral support. The illness endlessly soaks up vital savings and investments and arbitrarily turns simple pleasures and social routines into nightmare performances. Inevitably, the primary caregiver's quality of life and health status suffer. Once the patient is relocated or gone forever, the family member has to confront those personal losses and grieve for them.

▶ **QUICK TIP SUMMARY**

Communication Problems That Family Caregivers Bring to the Nursing Home

1. Negative perceptions of nursing homes. At least three fourths of Americans see nursing homes as a last resort.
2. Personal communication problems of the family caregiver: Caregivers also suffer from hearing loss, depression, Parkinson's disease, and other problems associated with aging.
3. Additional long-standing communication problems with the Alzheimer's disease patient, such as
   a. Loss of reciprocity
   b. Asynchronies—loss of mealtime and bedtime relationships
   c. Deterioration of social life
   d. Emotional scars from previous domestic violence
4. Confusion over the transition in role from primary caregiver to visitor
5. Spiritual and emotional neediness, which includes
   a. Need to deal with feelings of guilt and sadness at having institutionalized the patient
   b. Need to remain connected to the patient
   c. Need to find meaning in the disease
   d. Need to grieve over the slow loss of a loved one
   e. Need to grieve over personal losses of health, quality of life, financial resources, and affection

PROBLEMS THAT NURSING HOME STAFF MEMBERS BRING TO ENCOUNTERS WITH FAMILY MEMBERS

What is it that members of the nursing home staff do, or do not do, that causes communication with family members to break down? Family members who participated in the study by Maas et al.[7] reported that what caused them the most dissatisfaction with the nursing home was the failure of staff members to solicit their help with care. Family members also were distressed when staff members were too busy to give needed care or too busy to make sure that their loved one was involved in resident activities.

Family caregivers also complained that staff caregivers viewed the job of caregiving as simply doing tasks for the residents, that they worked only to maintain the institutional routine and control, having little consideration for the needs of the patient. Families thought that staff members typecast them, avoided them, and disregarded their importance to the resident.

Whether all of this is true is less important than whether family members *believe* it is true. Family caregivers act on their beliefs; and family members' beliefs about the care of their relatives are based almost entirely on the quality of their own interactions with staff caregivers. Family members appear to assess quality of care by how well the staff protects the dignity and individuality of the resident.[8]

There are also some unpleasant realities in how staff members in many nursing homes interact with families. Most staff members are not well equipped to deal with the problems that families bring to the nursing home. Direct care staff often have little preparation for dealing with grieving families and little knowledge of the family history of each resident. They have a hard enough time getting to know each resident.

▶ **QUICK TIP SUMMARY**

Communication Problems of Staff Members That Cause Family Caregivers to Complain

1. Staff members fail to ask family members for help with the care of the resident.
2. Staff members appear too busy to provide adequate care.
3. Staff members do not know residents well and do not get them to appropriate activities.
4. Staff members work for the institution and not for the family. They ignore the family's needs.
5. Staff members "dump" too many resident care duties on them.
6. Staff members typecast families, avoid them, or disregard their importance to the patient.

SOLUTIONS TO CONFLICTS AND POSITIVE TECHNIQUES FOR COMMUNICATING WITH FAMILIES OF ALZHEIMER'S DISEASE PATIENTS

To reduce conflicts, both staff and family members have to make adjustments. Two things must happen: First, staff members must become sensitive to the family's anxiety; second, family members must be willing to relinquish the primary caregiver role. One of the best ways for direct care staff members to pay attention to the family's concerns and to ease tension is to practice empathic listening skills. As defined earlier in this in-service, empathic listening seeks to capture or validate the feelings of the speaker and to build rapport rather than to defend or argue a particular point. Empathic responses usually are effective in easing the level of emotional tension and helpful in allowing people to clarify their positions. Empathic responses encourage family members to solve their own problems (Recommendation Box 8-1). The following phrases will help you shape your own empathic responses with family members:

• "It sounds as if you're—"
• "You seem to be—"
• "What I'm hearing from you is—"

- "I sense that—"
- "You must have felt—"
- "Let me see if I understand—"
- "That does present a problem."

RECOMMENDATION BOX 8-1
Suggestions for Empathic Listening

- Convey a positive attitude through your nonverbal behavior: maintain eye contact, assume an interested facial expression, and use open, nonthreatening body postures and gestures, such as nods and light touch. Avoid body language that inadvertently intimidates: don't turn your back, cross your arms, frown, sigh, or roll your eyes. Reinforce your nonverbal behavior with encouraging verbal responses, such as "Oh," "Yes, I see," and "Um-hmm."
- Ask as few direct questions as possible. You do not want the person to have the feeling of being interrogated. You may be surprised to learn that your empathic listening responses and open body language are just as effective as direct questions for finding out what you need to know.
- Use open-ended requests to show your interest, such as the following:
  - "Can you give me an example?"
  - "Let's talk about this in private."
  - "Please tell me more."
  - "I'd like to hear what you have to say. Come back at about 2:00, when I can spend more time with you."
  - "I always value your opinion (observations)."

See if the complaining family caregiver can become part of the solution rather than one who only defines the problem. Try requests such as the following:
- "What have you already tried?"
- "Tell me some of your ideas for working this out."
- "Do you know other people who would be willing to help with this?"
- "Would you like to bring your questions (concerns) directly to the doctor (floor nurse, administrator)? I'd be happy to help (or to find someone else to help)."

Avoid:
- Jumping in with a quick solution or advice before you understand what the real problem is. The family member may be talking about one issue but actually be angry about another. Or the problem might not be as serious as initial complaints suggest.
- Interrupting
- Trying to distract the person by supplying unrelated information
- Using stereotyped "Band-Aid" statements (e.g., "I know just how you feel." "Isn't that just like a man (woman)?" "That's just the way it is. I can't change it." "Well, we all have our troubles." "Must be a full moon.")
- Becoming defensive (e.g., "You have no idea how hard our job is in this facility." "You can't talk to me that way." "He hit me first.")
- Criticizing or belittling the family member's feelings or the complaint (e.g., "You shouldn't let yourself get so upset." "I can't understand why this is bothering you." "Well, this isn't the first time [patient's name] has done that.").
- Spreading toxic talk (see In-Service 7) around the facility about relatives who are "troublemakers," "always complaining," or "impossible to deal with."

Before relatives can relinquish their primary caregiver status, they need reassurance that their loved ones are being cared for as well as, or better than, they are at home. You, the professional caregiver, must assume responsibility for communicating that reassurance (Recommendation Box 8-2).

RECOMMENDATION BOX 8-2

Suggestions for Reassuring Family Members That Their Relative is Receiving Good Care

- See the resident as a member of a family unit. View the family as an extension of the resident. Keep the family informed about the resident's likes, dislikes, and adjustment to life in the nursing home.
- Engage the family's participation in the resident's care from the beginning. Families can be a good source of information. For example, a family member can tell you much about a patient's eating habits—what foods he or she likes and dislikes, whether the big family meal is at midday or at night, whether the patient likes to snack, whether the patient prefers hot or cold food. Sometimes family members can help feed the patient. A husband or wife may take great pride in how well he or she is able to get the spouse to eat (Box 8-1).
- Provide support for the family during the difficult period of role transition.
- Encourage your facility to establish an orientation program for family caregivers, and participate in that program. When nursing homes do not provide clear guidelines for families regarding their roles and responsibilities, ambiguity and conflict are inevitable.
- Be willing to listen to families during the period of adjustment. You do not always have to stop what you are doing, just let them know you are listening while you work. Usually families do not expect you to give them advice; they just need to talk. Because most primary family caregivers have a restricted social life, you might be the only person available who understands their situation.
- Help them "learn the ropes" of the nursing home; empower them whenever possible. Families need to know, for example, to whom they should go with a complaint. Sometimes families take small complaints, such as lost laundry, toileting, or mistakes in the patient's diet, noisily to the administrator of the nursing home because they do not know who is directly responsible.
- Suggest things to do during family visits. Having observed successful visitors over time, you can suggest to family members activities such as brushing or grooming their relative's hair, watching a home video together, praying, or singing.
- Encourage families to attend support groups. Good support groups can reduce family members' isolation and help them realize that their relative is being cared for as well as or better than he or she would be at home.
- Visit a family support group meeting to better understand the self-help process.

BOX 8-1   Family Participation in Patient Care

Exasperated, the head nurse stands eye-to-eye with Morris, who sits confused on the side of his new nursing home bed. Holding a paper cup in one hand and two pills in the other, she looks helplessly over his shoulder as his wife, Shirley, enters the sun-filled room.

"We've tried everything," the nurse laments to the wife. "We cannot get him to take his medication. I don't know what we're going to do. How did you ever manage him at home?" "I didn't have a problem with that," Shirley responds calmly. She takes the cup and pills from the nurse and gets a paper cup of water for herself. Smiling, she caresses the side of Morris' face until he is looking directly at her. She lefts her cup in the air for a toast, shouts "Cheers!" pretends to put pills in her mouth, then drinks down the water.

"Cheers!" Morris declares, raising his cup. Down go the pills; down goes the water. He hands Shirley the cup with a satisfied smile and lies back down on the bed, untroubled.

From Santo Pietro MJ: Assessing the communicative styles of caregivers of patients with Alzheimer's disease, *Seminars in Speech and Language* 15:236, 1994.

BOX 8-2   Summary of Components of Partners in Caregiving

- Introduction to Partners in Caregiving (30 minutes). Statement of program goals and major activities. Includes a "warm-up" introduction exercise for group members.
- Sharing successful family-staff communication techniques (45 minutes). Brainstorming exercises in which participants generate examples of their efforts to encourage communication with the other group and their greatest challenges in dealing with the other group.
- Advanced listening skills (60 minutes). Training in active listening skills (e.g., encouraging others to talk, asking open-ended questions), avoiding communication blockers (e.g., labeling, moralizing, avoidance), and using feedback techniques. Role playing to practice the skills.
- Saying what you mean clearly and respectfully (45 minutes). Introduction to the concept of I-messages and practice using role plays based on participants' experiences.
- Cultural and ethnic differences (30 minutes). Small-group discussion of cultural and ethnic differences in the nursing home and how they interfere with good communication. Brainstorming how the communication techniques learned earlier can help in such situations.
- Handling blame, criticism, and conflict (60 minutes). Seven steps for dealing with the other group in situations of open conflict. Role play and discussion.
- Understanding differences in values (30 minutes). Guided exercise exploring differences in values in the nursing home. Participants rate importance of various values for families, staff, and administrators. Discussion of perceived differences in values and their effects on communication.
- Planning a joint session for families, staff, and administrators (30 minutes). Planning and organization of joint meeting by each group.
- Joint session (90 to 120 minutes). After completion of training, both groups meet with administrator to discuss concerns. Format helps identify, prioritize, and plan changes.

Modified from Pillemer K, and others: Building bridges between families and nursing home staff: the Partners in Caregiving program, *Gerontologist* 38:499, 1998.

JOINT TRAINING PROGRAM FOR FAMILY AND PROFESSIONAL CAREGIVERS

In 1998, Pillemer et al.[9] reported the successful implementation of a program called Partners in Caregiving. Partners in Caregiving consists of two parallel workshop series, one for nurses and nursing assistants in a long-term care facility and one for family members of residents in the same facility. The program acknowledges that many of the strains between professional caregivers and families arise owing to the structure, policies, and practices of the institution over which neither has control. The staff workshop is structured as a full in-service day. The family program includes three 2-hour sessions conducted weekly. This program has been shown effective not only in improving the communication skills of individual caregivers but also in building bridges between professional and family caregivers. A complete manual for conducting Partners in Caregiving can be obtained from Dr. Pillemer. A summary is presented in Box 8-2.

GOOD PRACTICE 8-1

Attitudes and Concerns of Family Members and Professional Caregivers

Directions: Indicate whether the following statements best describe family caregivers (FC), nursing home staff caregivers (SC), or both (B). What do your answers tell you about the differences or similarities between family and professional caregivers?

_____ 1. Most believe that nursing homes are places for old people who have no other place to live.

_____ 2. They are frequently overwhelmed by the responsibilities and stresses of the daily duties of caregiving.

_____ 3. They continue to feel responsible for the patient when they are no longer primary caregivers.

_____ 4. They tend to judge the quality of the patient's care by the way in which the caregiver interacts with and protects the dignity and individuality of the patient.

_____ 5. They generally have inadequate preparation for dealing with the communication problems of the person with Alzheimer's disease and of other caregivers.

_____ 6. If they feel they are not in control of the patient, they criticize the other caregivers.

_____ 7. They are sometimes reluctant to share knowledge about the patient's personal life and preferences with other caregivers.

_____ 8. They may know best how to communicate appropriately with the resident who has Alzheimer's disease.

_____ 9. Their efforts to spend time conversing with the person with Alzheimer's disease are important to the patient's well-being.

_____ 10. When a resident dies, memorial services at the nursing home might assist them in the grieving process.

GOOD PRACTICE 8-2

Role Play: Interactions with Family Members

Directions: Select two or three of the following role play scenarios and have the group read and discuss the communication problems they might encounter in each situation. Then select participants to play the roles. The roles of a family member and a staff person can be played by members of the group, or if role playing is a new experience for the group, the instructor can take the part of the family member.

1. *Keep the family informed about the patient's adjustment to the nursing home environment.* Since being placed in the nursing home, Harry has been extremely resistant and restless. A month has gone by, and he still has not settled into a routine. The staff has tried several things to ease his behavior, but you suspect that Harry is also feeling displaced and isolated. His son and other family members rarely visit, and then only for brief moments. You want to enlist the son's help in finding solutions. Now you see the son hurriedly entering Harry's room. How are you going to approach him? Given the son's constant rush, how much will you be able to say?

2. *Engage family participation in patient care from the beginning.* Peggy is willing to take time off from work 5 days a week to feed her mother at lunch. You are grateful until you see what Peggy's feeding skills are like. She feeds rapidly, puts too much food on the spoon, distracts her mother constantly instead of helping her to focus on safe chewing, swallowing, and meal completion, even occasionally gives her mother bites that are too hot. The mother is often in a state of acute distress by the end of a meal. Your options are to tell Peggy that she is no longer welcome to feed her mother, to refer her to your supervisor, or to offer some gentle instruction and demonstration about how to feed her mother safely and pleasantly. How can you use one of these options without offending Peggy in her role of family caregiver?

3. *Provide support for the family during role transition, be willing to listen to family members during the period of adjustment.* Mrs. Collister is wonderfully supportive of the staff but feels guilty about placing her husband in the home. She attends the nursing home support meetings but also wants to interact with the nursing assistants who care directly for her husband. What active listening techniques can you use to comfort Mrs. Collister as she speaks about her worries?

4. *Help family members learn the ropes. Let them know how they can help and to whom they can complain.* Mr. Robbins's daughter, Janice, is complaining loudly about how his television has been moved again, after she has repeatedly moved it to a spot in the room where he can see it best. You are the person who has been returning the set to its original spot because of safety regulations, which state that electrical wires cannot extend more than a certain number of feet from their source. You suspect that Janice's anger actually stems from no longer having control over her father's life and environment. Are you going to handle this interaction merely as a safety issue? If you are not the best person to handle the complaint, how can you guide Janice? Can you offer solutions that would not interfere with your routine but would give Janice some sense of control?

5. *Suggest things to do during family visits.* Mrs. Ames's two nieces are young, cheery, and a good antidote for their very confused aunt. Tell the girls about two or three activities that their aunt might enjoy attending. Describe the activities in a way that shows how the nieces could be of real help (e.g., transporting her to activities, staying with her so she will not wander, keeping her hands busy so that she does not pick, and reading to her at a time when she tends to nag the staff). How can you guide the girls to more productive use of the time with their aunt?

Continued

GOOD PRACTICE 8-2

Role Play: Interactions with Family Members — cont'd

6. *Encourage family members to attend family support groups.* Mr. Jones took care of his wife for years before finally placing her in the nursing home but has never joined a support group. When he visits Mrs. Jones, which is frequently, Mr. Jones expects busy staff members to listen while he talks endlessly about his wife and every caregiving mistake or victory he ever had. You are a good listener and are happy to have some of the information, but his lengthy monologues are beginning to intrude on your tight schedule. You recently attended a meeting of the nursing home's support group and were impressed by the participants' sharing of information. How would you encourage Mr. Jones to try it?

GOOD PRACTICE 8-3

Attending a Support Group Meeting

Directions: Attend one or two meetings of your nursing home's support group for family members of residents with Alzheimer's disease. Go with one of your coworkers if possible. Together, answer the following questions and report your insights to your supervisor at the next staff meeting or at the next in-service training session on communication skills.

1. What was the location like where the meeting was held? Was there a comfortable atmosphere (e.g., good lighting, comfortable seating, and good acoustics)? Was the place distraction-free (e.g., no paging system, television noise, or traffic through the room)?

   _____

   _____

   _____

2. Did you let the group know ahead of time that you were going to attend? Did you feel like an outsider or did you feel comfortably included? Were you personally introduced? Was there a general introduction when everyone said who they were or why they were attending, or did this seem to be a set group where people took it for granted that everyone knew everyone else?

   _____

   _____

   _____

3. Was the group facilitator a lay person, a professional healthcare worker from outside your nursing home, or an employee of your facility? Did the facilitator encourage people to vent, complain, and commiserate about the burdens of caregiving, or did the facilitator guide people toward finding and sharing solutions to their problems? _____

   _____

   _____

4. What observations did you make about the communication styles of certain group members? Refer to earlier sections of this in-service and to In-Service 5 for assistance in answering this question. Did anyone seem to have a communication disorder—hearing loss, dysarthria, Parkinson's disease—that caused speech problems?

Continued

GOOD PRACTICE 8-3

Attending a Support Group Meeting — cont'd

Did anyone have a communication style that was especially difficult for you to understand—foreign accent, rapid speech, mumbling, or overuse of complicated words?

_____

_____

_____

5. Was there a speaker? (Is there usually a speaker?) If so, what was the speaker's topic? How favorably was the information received by the other guests? As a caregiver, did you find the information useful or interesting?

_____

_____

_____

6. What do you think was the most valuable aspect of this support group meeting? Having attended a meeting, how do you now feel about recommending the support group to your patients' families? What changes or improvements would you make if you were in charge?

_____

_____

_____

REFERENCES

1. Richter J, Bottenberg D, Roberto K: Communication between formal caregivers and individuals with Alzheimer's disease, _Am J Alzheimer's Care Rel Dis Res_ 8:25, 1993.
2. Burley-Allen M: _Listening, the forgotten skill_, New York, 1982, Wiley.
3. Cafferata G, Stone R: Community caregivers' attitudes toward nursing homes, _J Long Term Care Adm_ 19:33, 1991-1992.
4. Rau M: Impact on families. In R Lubinski, editor. _Dementia and communication_, Philadelphia, 1991, BC Decker.
5. Lynch-Sauer J: When a family member has Alzheimer's disease: a phenomenological description of caregiving, _J Gerontol Nurs_ 16:9, 1989.
6. Paveza GJ, and others: Severe family violence and Alzheimer's disease: prevalence and risk factors, _Gerontologist_ 32:493, 1992.
7. Maas M, and others: Family members' perceptions: how they view care of Alzheimer's patients in a nursing home, _J Long Term Care Adm_ 19:21, 1991.
8. Johnson M: Daughter's responses to a parent's relocation to a nursing home. Presented at the 42nd Annual Scientific Meeting of the Gerontological Society of America, Minneapolis, 1989.
9. Pillemer K, and others: Building bridges between families and nursing home staff: the Partners in Caregiving program, _Gerontologist_ 38:499, 1998.

PART IV

Face to Face: Finding Communication Opportunities with Persons Who Have Alzheimer's Disease

Creating Successful Conversations

IN-SERVICE OUTLINE

PREMISE

No one has ever found a better therapeutic technique than conversation. Persons with Alzheimer's disease often are so impaired that any social conversation with them is difficult and may seem useless. "What can I say? He's not going to answer anyway." "He doesn't make any sense." "She can't understand me, so why try?" Why indeed?

First, given the right support, many people with Alzheimer's disease are still capable of having brief but meaningful conversations. These opportunities to maintain social abilities should not be lost. To keep residents in the "conversation game," you must encourage them to communicate to the best of their abilities whenever and however they can. Second, despite massive impairments, residents' attempts to communicate deserve to be treated with respect. Caregivers who respond to a patient's efforts in a positive manner do much to protect the patient from feelings of worthlessness and despair.

Third, fewer abusive incidents or catastrophic reactions are reported in work settings in which caregivers provide liberal amounts of social communication along with the necessary task-oriented communication. Residents with Alzheimer's disease tend to be less disruptive when their social as well as their medical and custodial needs are met. This in-service describes a number of techniques that can help you develop successful conversations with residents who have Alzheimer's disease.

LEARNING OBJECTIVES

- Describe the differences between "social conversation," "task talk," and "institutional talk," and explain the appropriateness of each.
- List the five attitude adjustments likely to be the greatest help to staff members who want to have a successful conversational moment with residents who have Alzheimer's disease.
- Define and give specific examples of the conversational techniques of choice questions, matching comments, closure, and repair.
- Explain four conversational techniques that are not effective in facilitating good communication with persons who have Alzheimer's disease.
- Identify five dos or don'ts for successful conversation with persons who have Alzheimer's disease that can be implemented in the participant's daily interactions.

DEFINITIONS

Conversation   Interaction in which two or more people talk to one another on a subject of mutual interest. It is only one avenue of communication, but it is the one with which we are most familiar.

Task talk   The type of communication that caregivers use to get patients to do something. The underlying agenda is to maintain efficient caregiving. "Turn over now." "Here's your lunch. Sit up." "Move your arm." The language is basic and functional. The tone of voice may be warm and friendly, but task talk works best if it is short and uncluttered by detail, especially with a person who has Alzheimer's disease. Studies show that at least 67% of all talk directed at nursing home residents by caregivers is task-oriented.[1] The disadvantage of task talk is that it limits the patient's incentive to practice social conversational skills. Task talk invites patients to respond in one of two ways: complain or comply. As important as task talk is for getting a job done, if used to excess it casts the patient into a passive role and fosters dependency and learned helplessness.

Institutional talk   A style of communication defined by attitude and tone of voice. The speaker's voice or words come across as false and exaggerated, as when humoring a small child. The underlying agenda is to maintain a parent-child relationship. Institutional talk uses "we" and "our" instead of "you" and "I," as in "It's time for our medicine." Take, for example, the voice of a staff person gushing loudly over the patient's pureed diet: "Look at those delicious carrots! Better eat them all. Our cook will feel real bad if you don't. My, don't we love that smell! Mmmmm. Yummy-yum." Institutional talk is meant to be friendly, teasing, and cheerful, but actually it distances the caregiver from the patient.

   Like task talk, institutional talk discourages two-way conversation. Most people, even those with dementia, feel bored, embarrassed, and demeaned when they have to endure institutional talk. Because persons with Alzheimer's disease can sense emotional intent and body language long after they cease to understand words, institutional talk does little to raise their self-esteem.

Social conversation   Communication that establishes relationships and nourishes self-esteem. The underlying agenda is to maintain adult-to-adult communication. "Bella, how's your sister?" "We saw the best movie last night!" "Where did you get your hair cut? I love it." As the abilities of persons with Alzheimer's disease decline, the language of caregivers often becomes stereotypic and dull. Caregivers stop sharing tidbits from their personal lives. They no longer look for new topics to interest their patients. Their interactions become solely task talk or institutional talk. Residents seldom make an effort to respond genuinely to anything except social conversation.[2]

Conversational success   True spoken interaction between adults that lasts for as little as 5 seconds. Communication does not depend on eloquent speech or serious subject matter. What counts is that two people have shared or connected with each other for a moment. Conversational success with a person with Alzheimer's disease is achieved through support of the patient's efforts to function as a sociable human being. You will

---

BOX 9-1 What is Conversational Success?

Anita, a volunteer at Merryhart Nursing Home, is distressed by Maude's insistence that the two women once were neighbors. Every time Anita passes Maude's wheelchair, Maude reminds her of events and people they once knew. To Anita's embarrassment, Maude scolds her about not coming to visit more often, complaining and crying all the while. Protests Anita, "I was never her neighbor! I never heard of any of those people. I try to tell her that, but she won't listen." "Does it matter so much that Maude is mistaken about who you are?" chides the nursing supervisor gently, "We're just so pleased that she wants to talk to you."

---

be more successful in your conversations with a resident with Alzheimer's disease if you do the following:

- Watch carefully for signs that the patient wishes to communicate.
- Accept responsibility for keeping the conversation alive by using helpful prompts and phrases.
- Introduce topics that the patient enjoys and that are at his or her level of understanding.
- Accept even brief exchanges as being worthwhile.
- Stop worrying about the "correctness" or "logic" of the patient's utterances.

Bohling[3] found that when eight human service workers in an adult day care center conversed with clients, the workers seldom attempted to listen or speak in the frame of reference of the person with Alzheimer's disease. In general, the workers spoke only of their own interests and did not listen to the residents. The residents with Alzheimer's disease expressed frustration with caregivers who controlled conversations and ignored residents' attempts to join in (Box 9-1).

TALKING WITH PERSONS WHO HAVE ALZHEIMER'S DISEASE: FOUR CONVERSATIONAL TECHNIQUES THAT WORK

Four techniques helpful in conversing more successfully with persons with Alzheimer's disease are *choice questions, matching comments, closure,* and *repair.* There is no special magic about these techniques. Most people use these techniques every day to keep conversations going, but research has shown that these four techniques are especially powerful in helping persons with Alzheimer's disease stay with a conversation.[4]

1. *Choice question.* A choice question is a request phrased so that the listener has a choice between two acceptable alternatives, which can be objects, words, actions, or opinions. Someone asking a choice question presents two pieces of information in the hope that the resident will recognize the best choice and be encouraged to respond. "Elsa, were you married in Scranton or in Pittsburgh?" "Harry, would you rather wear the blue shirt or the one with the brown stripes?"

Persons with Alzheimer's disease, as do those without Alzheimer's disease, respond better to questions requiring recognition memory than to those requiring recall or episodic memory.[5] For example, an anatomy quiz that has open-ended questions such as "To which system does the small intestine belong?" seems more difficult than a test that has a choice of possible answers: "The small intestine is part of (a) the respiratory system or (b) the digestive system?" In a true or false or recognition-type test, even students who have not studied have a 50% chance of answering correctly. Questions that are too open-ended or nonspecific are especially difficult to answer for persons with Alzheimer's disease. These types of questions do not offer enough information for the person to respond (e.g., "What did you do today?" or "Tell me about your children"). Persons with Alzheimer's disease are unable to give the elaborative answers that most open-ended questions require, so they say nothing. Conversation finished.

Choice questions have other benefits for communication with persons with Alzheimer's disease. They are an excellent vehicle for managing behavior and avoiding confrontation. Rather than saying, "Mr. Johnson, put your socks on now." Try, "Mr. Johnson, do you want help with your socks, or can you put them on yourself?" When residents feel they have some choice, some control over events, they are less likely to refuse and resist.

2. *Matching comment or association.* Caregivers often remark that residents with Alzheimer's disease cannot maintain a topic in conversation. "She makes a comment," a nursing assistant remarks, "but when I ask a follow-up question, she has nothing more to say." One way to help the resident maintain the conversation is to offer a matching comment rather than a follow-up question. A matching comment or an association is a technique in which you offer your own opinion or some information about your personal experience as a follow-up to the resident's remark. This natural response gives the person with Alzheimer's disease additional information to build on. If a resident muses "I love red roses," you could reply, "You love red roses? My favorite flowers are pansies. I plant pansies every spring." This might enable the resident to respond, "Roses—lotsa work," or "Pansies come out first thing in the spring," or even, "I had a garden, but I never had pansies."

3. *Closure.* Closure is a technique that omits the last word or two from a sentence to let the listener "fill in the blanks." You might say to a resident with Alzheimer's disease, "Let me see, your daughter's name is _____?" Some residents will not notice the cue, but even persons with severe Alzheimer's disease sometimes respond when the ritual is a familiar one. Closure is also a good technique to use when you simply are looking for a way to help a resident practice the vocabulary he or she has left. For instance, you might gesture with the coffee pot and say, "How about a cup of _____?" Practicing vocabulary is important because the more often a word is used, the longer it remains available to the patient.

4. *Repair.* A repair is a word or statement that corrects the patient's utterance or fills in a missing piece of information in a patient's utterance. A repair allows you to correct the patient's mistakes without insulting the person or discouraging a rare attempt to communicate. For example, the person says, "Boy, is it snowing!" Instead of replying, "No, Josh, that's not snow, that's rain. It's raining, see?" you could make a repair by saying, "Yes, it's pouring rain. I really got wet from that rain this morning." With a repair, you affirm the resident's desire to communicate and respond to his intent. The exchange becomes a brief successful conversation rather than an instructional "put-down."

A repair can be made by substituting a specific word for a vague term used by a resident. Opportunities to try the technique of repair are frequent because people with Alzheimer's disease use many "fuzzy," nonspecific words, such as "it," "that thing," "over there," and "the other one." This kind of empty speech (see In-Service 1) is so characteristic of Alzheimer's disease that listeners tend to dismiss it as lacking meaning and importance. However, if you observe the context closely, think about the patient's personal history, and guess at the resident's intent, you can often interpret an empty speech statement and make a successful repair.

Listen for words that do not carry much meaning, then fill in the words you think your resident meant. For example, if the person says, "It's over there," you might repair by answering, "Yes, your robe is in the closet." If you have guessed incorrectly, the patient may even correct you. For example, you may say, "James, I understand you grew up in Cleveland." James may respond, "Pittsburgh." In this instance, the resident has repaired your speech! In any case, your conscious use of the repair technique has succeeded in increasing active participation in conversation by a person with Alzheimer's disease.

TALKING WITH PERSONS WHO HAVE ALZHEIMER'S DISEASE: FOUR TECHNIQUES THAT DO *NOT* WORK

1. *Direct orders.* Many times a caregiver wants a resident to do one thing while the resident is determined to do another. In this situation, the caregiver might instinctively respond with a direct order. For instance, while you are helping her put on her house slippers, the resident stands up abruptly and prepares to leave. You say, "Sit down. I'm not finished." The resident leaves anyway. Direct orders are all too often ineffective. You feel ineffectual and frustrated.

Direct orders are "bossy" in tone and intention. Research has shown that the more commanding or demanding a caregiver is, the more resistant persons with dementia become.[6] Like all human beings, persons with Alzheimer's disease become defensive when they are ordered about. They do not like to be told what to do. A direct order not only is a poor behavior management technique but also is destructive to a resident's self-esteem and a poor technique for maintaining social conversation skills.

Direct orders are not the same as task talk. Task talk does not have to be commanding to be effective. You can choose to give instructions in a pleasing tone of voice, softened with reassurance, sprinkled with praise, and personalized with the individual's name. The more you improve your other communication skills, the less often you will need to resort to direct orders (Recommendation Box 9-1).

2. *Affirmations.* Affirmations are short responses such as "Yes," "Um-hum," "I know," and "Oh." As listeners, we use affirmations to show interest in what our companions are saying and to keep them talking. Social workers and members of the clergy use affirmations frequently to encourage people to share information. However, to stay on topic, persons with dementia need to hear many concrete words—words that remind them of the names of things. They need encouragement, and affirmations alone are not encouragement enough. Like open-ended questions, repeated affirmations do not carry enough information to help people with Alzheimer's disease develop responses. Conversation quickly dies (Recommendation Box 9-2).

3. *Insistence on "the truth."* If a resident is able to enjoy a conversation with you about lunch or the weather, does it matter whether she thinks you are a friend from the old neighborhood and not the nursing assistant? Does it matter whether she believes it is May when it is really June? Studies have shown that reality orientation as a treatment of patients with Alzheimer's disease is ineffective at restoring memory. Insisting on reality in conversation, constantly correcting a resident's errors, and repeatedly insisting the resident accurately report personal information result only in frustration for both you and the resident.

RECOMMENDATION BOX 9-1
Recommendations for Avoiding Direct Orders

- Do not argue when you and the resident have opposite goals.
- Offer choice questions instead of commands.
- Enlist the resident's help. "Hey, I'm on my way to the cafeteria. Let's head down and be the first to the dessert table."
- Use words that describe and call attention to the resident's behavior. For example, the resident tries to leave, but you have not finished dressing her. You might say, "Feeling pretty restless today, hmm?"
- Redirect the resident's attention to another activity or topic. For example, "Let's walk for a moment. My, look at that snow! Remember those winters when we were kids?" After a few steps or a few moments of chatting, the patient may be persuaded to resume dressing.

> **RECOMMENDATION BOX 9-2**
> **Recommendations for Using Affirmations**
>
> - Use affirmations only occasionally by themselves.
> - Use affirmations in combination with requests or directives to soften the impact and to reassure the resident that all is going well. For example, a resident keeps pulling his foot away and complaining. You might say, "I know, I know, you don't like to have your toenails clipped. OK, please let me hold your foot. Um-hmm. That's it. Almost done with your toenails. Good job."

4. *Yes-or-no questions.* Questions that can be answered with a simple "yes" or "no" can stop conversation (e.g., "Did you have a good time?" "Have you met Hannah's new boyfriend?" "Do you want some more ice cream?"). People with Alzheimer's disease tend to respond in the shortest, easiest way possible. Yes-or-no questions allow them to answer without making any effort to add information. Stay away from yes-or-no questions if you want to experience conversational success.

► **QUICK TIP SUMMARY**

Techniques for Successful Conversations with Persons Who Have Alzheimer's Disease

Use the following:
- Choice question: a question that contains the word "or" and gives the person two choices
- Matching comment or association: a response that draws from the caregiver's personal experience or opinion
- Closure: an unfinished sentence that the resident is encouraged to complete
- Repair: a word or statement that corrects the resident's error, fills in missing information, or replaces a vague term with a concrete one

Avoid the following:
- Direct order: meeting a resident's resistance with a command
- Affirmation: brief, agreeable responses that do not give enough information to help the resident think of an answer
- Insistence on the truth: correcting a resident's errors, insisting on accuracy of reporting, often combined with the phrase, "Don't you remember?"
- Yes-or-no questions: making inquiries that require only a simple "yes" or "no" response. Persons with Alzheimer's disease seldom respond to yes-or-no questions with more than one word.

DEVELOPING INTERVENTION TECHNIQUES FOR EFFECTIVE COMMUNICATION WITH ALZHEIMER'S DISEASE PATIENTS IN ALL SITUATIONS

The following is a list of 20 additional general dos and don'ts to help you achieve successful conversation with residents who have Alzheimer's disease.

1. *Use adult language.* You are communicating with adult residents. Patients are apt to respond negatively when you address them as children, no matter how kind you intend to be. To help the resident maintain self-respect, use an adult communication style.

2. *Maintain eye contact.* Alzheimer's disease patients need as many nonverbal cues as possible. Eye contact is vital for maximum communication. If the person is not looking at you, establish eye contact by calling his or her name or gently touching the patient's arm. Always stand face to face with an Alzheimer's disease patient when speaking. If the person is in a wheelchair, bring yourself to that person's eye level.

3. *Use visual cues whenever possible.* Evidence shows that Alzheimer's disease patients continue to respond appropriately to visual communication longer than they do to spoken communication. Written words, pictures, gestures, and facial expressions help to get information across to patients with Alzheimer's disease.

4. *Use simple words and short sentences.* Simple words remain available to Alzheimer's disease patients longer than do complex ones, and short sentences are easier to comprehend than are long ones.

5. *Keep your explanations short.* Alzheimer's disease patients are more likely to complete longer tasks if the tasks are broken into single-step directions. For example: "Pick up the spoon. Put the spoon in the bowl."

6. *Paraphrase, do not just repeat.* If the resident has difficulty understanding a message, find a different way to say it rather than repeating the original words over and over. Other words might be more meaningful.

7. *Avoid saying, "Don't you remember?"* Chances are, the resident does not. Constant reminders that the person's memory is failing can be very distressing for both patient and caregiver. You would not ask a blind person, "Don't you see?" Constant quizzing does not bring memories back.

8. *Use touch.* Guidance, reassurance, affection, and humor can be communicated to a person with Alzheimer's disease through touch even in the later stages of the disease.

9. *Do not shout.* If hearing is not a problem, your tone of voice may frighten the resident or put the person in a defensive mood. If hearing is a problem, shouting distorts your message. Many hearing-impaired elderly patients also suffer from *tinnitus* (ringing in the ears) or *recruitment* (an inability to hear soft noises while loud noises are perceived at their actual level of loudness). Shouting at persons with tinnitus or recruitment makes the problems worse and stresses the patient.

10. *Do not interrupt.* Try not to interrupt unless necessary. If you interrupt a resident with Alzheimer's disease in the middle of an attempt to communicate or in the middle of a task, it is likely that the person will forget what he or she was saying or doing. Persons with Alzheimer's disease are easily distracted, even when they are speaking or acting with firm intent.

11. *Avoid competition.* Avoid competing signals, such as television, radio, or other conversations. If you have something important to tell a person who has Alzheimer's disease, speak to the person face to face in a quiet place.

12. *Use a calm, reassuring tone of voice.* If your voice is warm and pleasant, the patient may want to listen to your message. Alzheimer's disease patients respond to emotional tone. Your voice should communicate support and reassurance, not anger and annoyance, well into the late stages of the disease.

13. *Do not talk negatively about a patient in his or her presence.* Even persons in the late stage of Alzheimer's disease have moments of lucidity. Be careful not to talk negatively about a resident to another patient or colleague. Overhearing criticism or sarcastic comments may account for at least some of a patient's negative behavior.

14. *Be realistic in your expectations.* If you are expecting normal, rapid responses, you will always be disappointed. Know the person's weaknesses, address his or her communication strengths, and be justifiably pleased with patients' honest efforts.

15. *Allow extra time for a resident to respond.* Persons with Alzheimer's disease process information slowly. If you wait for the patient to respond, you will sometimes be rewarded with an appropriate answer.

16. *Pay attention to nonverbal communication.* Often Alzheimer's disease patients cannot tell you what they mean in words, but their nonverbal communication may be very meaningful. Observe their gestures, nods, smiles, and frowns.

17. *Realize that catastrophic reactions are not meant to be manipulative.* Catastrophic reactions on the part of Alzheimer's disease patients are generally the result of frustration, cognitive overload, or the inability to communicate needs or to perform tasks. They seldom are a conscious effort of a patient to "get back at" caregivers. When a catastrophic reaction occurs, look for the cause. Examine your own communicative behavior to see whether you might have contributed to the reaction (see In-Service 10).

18. *Listen carefully to "rambling."* Do not assume that a resident's rambling has no meaning. If the person is talking, he or she is trying to communicate. Listen for hints of meaning in the rambling (see In-Service 1 for communication changes characteristic of Alzheimer's disease.)

19. *Be willing to talk about "old times."* Relate current topics to stored knowledge. Persons with Alzheimer's disease remember more about the distant past than they do about the present. Do not be afraid to spend time in the past with a resident. The person will enjoy reminiscing, and it might help him or her to perform better in the present.

20. *Continue to enjoy life.* If you feel only sad, burdened, and exasperated in dealing with residents who have Alzheimer's disease, you will have difficulty communicating with them. Persons with Alzheimer's disease are still capable of enjoying many happy moments in life. If you can enjoy some of the remaining moments with them, communication will be worthwhile for you both.

GOOD PRACTICE 9-1

Describing Your Interactions with Residents Who Have Alzheimer's Disease

Directions. During the first 3 hours of your next shift, pay attention to how many instances of task talk, institutional talk, and social conversation you use with the residents.

- Was more than half of your talk with residents task oriented?
- How often did you hear yourself speaking in institutional talk?
- How many truly social conversations did you have or attempt to have with your residents?

GOOD PRACTICE 9-2

Identifying Conversational Techniques

Directions: Write down the conversational technique that the staff member is using in each example (choice question, matching comment, closure, repair, direct order, affirmation, insistence on truth, yes-or-no question). Then circle "E" or "I" to indicate whether the technique is usually effective or ineffective for fostering social conversation with persons who have Alzheimer's disease.

- How about some more- (showing patient a piece of pie).
  _____ E/I
- We have a guitar player coming. Would you like to stay in your room or go hear the music? _____ E/I
- You're from Ireland? The necklace I'm wearing came from Ireland.
  _____ E/I
- Oh. Um-hum. That's so. I know. Well. _____ E/I
- Mary, it's not June, it's May. Don't you remember? We just had Mother's Day.
  _____ E/I
- The resident says, "Cold out. I need a coal." You reply, "Yes, it is cold. Wear the blue coat. You need a coat." _____ E/I
- Sit down right now! _____ E/I
- You're right, Pete. It's a sunny day. The kind of day I like to work in my garden.
  _____ E/I
- So your daughter is visiting. Is this Marissa or Claire?
  _____ E/I
- Hurry up, finish this. _____ E/I
- The resident says, "I want that thing." You say, "Here's your wallet, the wallet with your pictures in it." _____ E/I
- "Did you enjoy the music program, Maggie?"
  _____ E/I

GOOD PRACTICE 9-3

Specific Techniques for Maintaining Effective Communication with Alzheimer's Disease Patients

Directions: Rewrite the final statement in each of the following scenarios, or state an action you would take to use the technique named. In each case, how could the nursing assistant respond to or communicate more effectively with the resident with Alzheimer's disease?

Or: Use these scenarios as a role-play activity to give students an opportunity to practice and build their communication skills with Alzheimer's patients.

1. *Use adult language.* A resident needs his toenails clipped but has his legs folded under the chair.
   Nursing assistant: Hey, cutie, how about giving Mama Lou your little tootsies so I can clip 'em just a smidge?
2. *Keep your explanations short.* A resident refuses to get up to walk and moans softly.
   Nursing assistant: Zelda, I know you're sad that your husband didn't get here, but he called this morning, or maybe last night, to let you know that he had to go to your daughter's house this morning and he'll be late. He wants you to call

Continued

GOOD PRACTICE 9-3

Specific Techniques for Maintaining Effective Communication with Alzheimer's Disease Patients — cont'd

over to your daughter's and tell them what time you finish therapy and what time lunch is served today. Okay?"

3. *Paraphrase, do not just repeat.* The nurses' station receives a call from a resident's daughter asking whether a package of family photographs has arrived. The nurse sends the nursing assistant to check whether Mr. Miller received them. Mr. Miller does not seem to know what she's talking about.
Nursing assistant: Mr. Miller, your daughter wants to know whether you have your wife's photograph up on your bulletin board.
Patient: What?
Nursing assistant: Your daughter wants to know whether you have your wife's photograph up on your bulletin board.

4. *Be realistic in your expectations.* A patient unexpectedly vomits after he has had an apparently routine day.
Nursing assistant: George, you have to tell me where you were and exactly what you ate this afternoon. Tell me right now!

5. *Realize that catastrophic reactions and crying out might not be manipulative.* In her room down at the end of the hall, a patient cries and cries.
Patient: Please help me. Where's the doctor? Please call the doctor. I'm in pain. I need help. Please help me.
Nursing assistant [attempting to ignore this endless, annoying monologue]: Miriam, just quiet down now. You're driving everybody crazy.

6. *Be willing to talk about old times.* As a staff member attempts to help a patient finish his lunch, the patient begins a familiar story.
Patient: You know, life was not easy in the Depression. Tough. Very tough. My brother and I sold apples. Apples. Don't eat apples. Can't no more.
Nursing assistant: I know, Jack, I know. Pay attention here. Are you going to eat this applesauce or not?

7. *Listen carefully to rambling.* As the nursing assistant prepares the patient for bed, Harry rambles on and on.
Patient: You know Mary is such a pain in the neck. Pain in the neck. Never could do anything right. Always was, always will be. Wasn't my fault, and it was over. Just like that. Mary, Mary, Mary.
Nursing assistant: Quiet down, Harry. You don't know what you're talking about. Everything is okay.

8. *Use touch.* A patient is clearly agitated and fidgets in his wheelchair.
Patient: Where are you taking me, you bastard? What's going on here? I'm not supposed to be going anywhere! Leave me alone, dammit!
Nursing assistant: Now you just calm down, Mr. Peters, nobody talks to me that way! There are no yelling and no cursing on this floor!

9. *Pay attention to nonverbal communication.* A patient is bent limply forward over his food tray. So far, he has resisted all attempts by the nursing assistant to feed him. He shakes his head and occasionally raises a weak finger to his left cheek.
Nursing assistant [ignoring patient's poor eating posture and hand movement]: Come on, Joe. Eat your peas. Try some of this tasty meat loaf. I've got lots of work to do today.

10. *Use simple words and short sentences.* A patient is dawdling over his occupational therapy project in the day room.
Nursing assistant: Lawrence, the basic requirement here is that you complete this art project, do what you have to do in the lavatory, and get yourself down to the dining room as punctually as possible.

REFERENCES
1. Seers C: Talking to the elderly and its relevance to care, *Nursing Times* 82:51, 1986.
2. Lubinski R: Why so little interest in whether or not old people talk? A review of recent research on verbal communication among the elderly, *International Journal of Aging and Human Development* 9:237, 1978.
3. Bohling H: Communication with Alzheimer's patients: an analysis of caregiver listening patterns, *International Journal of Aging and Human Development* 33:249, 1991.
4. Santo Pietro MJ, and others: Conversations in Alzheimer's disease: implications of semantic and pragmatic breakdowns. Presented at the annual convention of the American Speech-Language-Hearing Association, Seattle, 1990.
5. Wilson B, Moffat N: *Clinical management of memory problems*, Rockwell, MD, 1984, Aspen.
6. Hamel M, Gold D, Andres D: Predictors of consequences of aggressive behavior by community-based dementia patients, *Gerontologist* 30:206, 1990.

Handling Difficult Communication Situations

IN-SERVICE OUTLINE	Premise
	Learning Objectives
	Definitions
	Communicating Effectively with Persons Who Have Catastrophic Reactions or Exhibit Sustained Levels of High Anxiety
	Effective Communication Techniques to Use When Coping with a Resident's Inappropriate Repetitive Behaviors
	► QUICK TIP SUMMARY: Difficult Communication Situations
	GOOD PRACTICE 10-1: Role Playing Difficult Communication Situations
	GOOD PRACTICE 10-2: Difficult Communication Situations: What Can You Do?

PREMISE

"Although new staff receive training on the technical aspects of providing care, they generally receive no training in ways to handle interpersonal problems that arise with patients."[1]

Even the most experienced caregiver finds it difficult to communicate successfully with a person with Alzheimer's disease who is having a catastrophic reaction or who is in a mode of stubborn resistance. Caregivers grow weary of offering supportive communication when their patients display the irritating repetitive behaviors characteristic of dementia. Staff members need reliable communication techniques in such difficult moments. Central to the effectiveness of communication techniques is a communication style that is calm and flexible rather than rigid and demanding.

LEARNING OBJECTIVES

- Give examples of catastrophic outbursts of Alzheimer's residents that have been observed or experienced and describe the communication of all persons involved.
- List the communication goals for coping with a resident who is having (or is about to have) a catastrophic reaction. Work out a method of alerting other staff when assistance with an emotionally overwrought resident is needed.
- Demonstrate the ideal body language, tone of voice, and communication style that caregivers should adopt with a person who is in the midst of a catastrophic reaction.
- Describe how caregivers might interact with a resident who is hallucinating.
- Describe two reasons why a resident persists in saying the same things over and over and explain how memory devices, way-finding cues, and attention focus can reduce repetition.

- Demonstrate recommended techniques for reducing resident resistance or refusal.
- Describe at least two communication techniques that direct-care staff could use with residents who frequently wander or pilfer the belongings of others.
- Explain why a paranoid resident's claims always should be taken seriously.

DEFINITIONS   **Inappropriate and repetitive behaviors**   Persistent behaviors, such as primitive outbursts of emotion, habitual hostile resistance despite caregiver assurance, hallucinations, unfounded paranoia, repeated questions, incessant wandering, and pilfering, in the middle and later stages of Alzheimer's disease are caused by the failure of neurons in certain areas of the brain to connect properly. When a resident exhibits one of these behaviors, the usual flow of social interaction and routine is disrupted. Caregivers need additional communication skills for coping successfully with persistent and troublesome behaviors.

Catastrophic reaction   An emotional response inappropriate or out of proportion to a situation that reflects the extreme anxiety of a person with Alzheimer's disease who is trying to cope with real or imagined events. The reaction can be triggered by an event in the present or in the distant past. Persons with Alzheimer's disease also are prone to extended periods of high anxiety and agitation. Communication between residents and caregivers is liable to break down in the midst of these critical moments.

COMMUNICATING EFFECTIVELY WITH PERSONS WHO HAVE CATASTROPHIC REACTIONS OR EXHIBIT SUSTAINED LEVELS OF HIGH ANXIETY

When a resident is already out of control, caregivers need to exhibit a cool, firm, yet flexible communication style. Later, but always, the staff should try to identify antecedent events that might have triggered the outburst. Because the goal is to avoid further emotional outbursts from an anxious resident, all possible sources of the problem should be evaluated. The staff must consider the resident's physical, emotional, and cognitive status and make necessary adjustments in medication and routine care. But that is only the first step. To attribute a resident's high anxiety, agitation, or disruptive reactions solely to the fact that "he (or she) has Alzheimer's disease" is not fair, nor is Alzheimer's disease likely to be the entire explanation.

Physical and psychosocial environments constantly operate to support or weaken the resident's fragile defenses and communication skills. Staff should use the environment to minimize disruptive behaviors by maintaining a comfortable temperature and adequate light, providing appropriate activities, and seeking a delicate balance of stimulation and social contact.[2,3]

The caregiver's style of communication is critical in the prevention of emotionally volatile situations and in calming residents. How much attention is being paid to residents' repeated requests? How much control do the residents have over their own situations? How tactful, or demanding, are staff in their requests to get routine tasks completed? How "correct" or "unacceptable" are residents' behaviors in the context of their own living quarters?

Goals for dealing with catastrophic reactions through effective communication are as follows (Recommendation Box 10-1):

- To ensure the safety of the patient, yourself, and nearby persons
- To keep the situation from escalating
- To restore the patient to calm and routine behavior
- To understand the meaning of the patient's message

> ### RECOMMENDATION BOX 10-1
> **Recommendations for Effective Communication When Coping with Catastrophic Reactions**
>
> - Arrange a set of signals with other staff members or wear a beeper to use when you need help. Set up your signal system before a crisis occurs so that you can act quickly.
> - Eliminate distractions immediately. Distractions include blaring televisions, people moving around, and glaring lights.
> - Notice the body language and tone of voice of the patient. Can you differentiate fear, anger, frustration, confusion, or sadness?
> - Use the following communication techniques to avoid triggering the person's physically defensive reaction:
>   - Observe your own body language: move slowly, keep your arms down and hands open.
>   - Establish eye contact. Keep your facial expression open, warm, and friendly.
>   - Use a gentle reassuring touch, but only if you think the resident can tolerate touch in this moment.
>   - Speak slowly in a calm, firm, low-pitched voice. Remember that you are speaking to an adult, not to a child. Do not let a sing-song or patronizing tone enter your voice; avoid sounding either too authoritarian or overly jolly.
>   - Use the person's name as an alerting cue, and use your own name as orientation: "John. It's me, Nancy."
>   - Provide frequent verbal reassurances: "I'm here to help you."
>   - Speak in short sentences.
>   - Try humming or singing softly to distract or soothe.

EFFECTIVE COMMUNICATION TECHNIQUES TO USE WHEN COPING WITH A RESIDENT'S INAPPROPRIATE REPETITIVE BEHAVIORS

Five behaviors are typical of patients with Alzheimer's disease: hallucinations, inappropriate repetitive speech, resistance or refusal, wandering and pilfering, and paranoia. When working with persons who exhibit any of these irritating repetitive behaviors, your communication goals are to

- Reduce staff and patient frustration
- Understand the resident's underlying message
- Reshape the resident's repetitive behaviors into useful communication
- Reshape caregiver responses to match the resident's behavior

1. *Hallucinations.* The word hallucination is taken from a Latin word that means to "wander in the mind." Persons who hallucinate subjectively perceive visual, auditory, olfactory, tactile, and taste sensations. *Subjective* means that the sensations are very real to the person but have no basis in external stimuli.[4] Hallucinations are not uncommon in the middle and later stages of Alzheimer's disease (Box 10-1, Recommendation Box 10-2).

  2. *Repetitive requests or statements.* A common verbal symptom of persons with Alzheimer's disease is the frequent repetition of questions, requests, or statements. Repetition, as annoying as it may be for caregivers, has a basis in reality for the resident. First, repetition can result from the resident's failing memory; the person cannot recall recent events. If damaged short-term memory is at the root of the

---

BOX 10-1   Miriam's "Guests"

Miriam sat in her room nodding cheerfully and speaking first to one "guest" and then to another. "Ah Bernice, nice. Nice you're here. The purple is nice." "Homer, sit on the bed. Sit, sit. Comfortable, yes? Good." I loved dropping in on those occasions. I always sat down too for a moment, enjoying the "tea" Miriam had prepared, the pleasantries, and sometimes an introduction: "Josephine, have you met —?" And to me: "Now what was your name again, dear?" It tickled me that she remembered so well all those lovely friends who inhabited her gentle hallucinations yet still did not have a clue about my name. Me, Sharon, who has been caring for her every day for 2 years!

RECOMMENDATION BOX 10-2

Recommendations for Responding to Hallucinatory Behavior

If a resident is neither upsetting nor harming herself or himself or others:
- Do not waste time and energy arguing over whether the perceptions are "true" or "real."
- Use the occasion to create a conversation with the person. You can be attentive and responsive without actually denying or agreeing with what the resident says.
- Listen carefully to what the person is saying and how he or she is reacting to the hallucination. You will certainly learn something that helps you understand the resident better.

If the person is frightened by the hallucination or is upsetting others:
- Refer to the communication techniques suggested for coping with catastrophic reactions (see Recommendation Box 10-1).
- Be empathic: "I know. This is very scary for you." "I'm right here with you." "Mary, don't be afraid."
- Shift the resident's sensory focus. Keep in your pocket an object that has an interesting texture, color, or scent, such as a pretty scented scarf, for just this purpose. Turn on soothing music, an audiocassette of nature sounds, or a videotape of beautiful scenery that creates different visual images for the person. A startling taste sensation such as cold lemonade (use a covered cup) may alter the intense feelings of a resident in the grip of a frightening hallucination.

---

problem, caregivers should devise ways to address the memory deficit directly (Recommendation Box 10-3).

Annoying repetition can be a sign of loneliness or boredom. A patient who makes constant bids for attention soon begins to annoy a busy staff, and caregivers feel they cannot stop and chat. Both residents and staff pay a high price for work demands and schedules that are so crammed there is no time left for the people who live in the facility. If loneliness and boredom are the cause of the problem, staff priorities and resident activities need to be reevaluated and changed. In either case—memory problems or need for attention—the resident's repeated verbalizations have meaning. The person is trying to communicate something, even though the meaning is not at first apparent (Recommendation Box 10-4).

Another instance of repetitive statements is the endless crying out of a person who suffers from late-stage dementia. These severely impaired residents can have

RECOMMENDATION BOX 10-3

Recommendations for Coping with Inappropriate Repetitive Speech Caused by Memory Problems

- Capitalize on the resident's ability to comprehend single words, short phrases, or visual aids, such as familiar pictures, to stimulate memory.[5] For example, if the person wants to know whether it is time for lunch.
- Make a small folder of strong material that can be attached to the person's wrist or belt.
- Print a short list of words that explain the day's activities. Use a black marker and print in lower-case letters.
- Arrange the words in a column.
- Include simple line drawings beside each word or phrase, if you wish.
- Give this "schedule" or "appointment book" to the resident.
- Each time the resident asks about lunch, staff members or volunteers point to the words on the appointment book and say "Harvey look at your book." Even patients who have fairly advanced dementia have been able to learn to refer independently to their schedule (Figure 10-1).[5]
- See In-Service 11 for interventions that address memory deficits, including memory wallets and books and the spaced retrieval program.

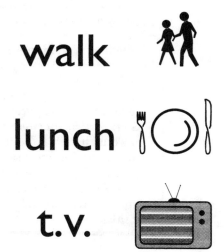

FIGURE 10-1   Simplified daily schedule of patient's activities.

unmet needs about which they are trying to communicate. This type of repetitive disruptive vocalization is specifically addressed in In-Service 12.

3. *Resistance or refusal.* It is widely reported that resistance and refusal are characteristic among persons with Alzheimer's disease; but why are they such a problem? Like all human beings, persons with Alzheimer's disease find it irritating to be ordered around. Elderly persons with dementia are especially touchy. Even when caregivers do not intend to act like "sergeants," these patients are likely to interpret the simplest request as a demand.[7] And a particular caregiver's style of communication (tone of voice, attitude, body language, manner, choice of words) actually may be authoritarian. The resident's perception in this case is correct, and he or she does not like it (Box 10-2)!

RECOMMENDATION BOX 10-4
If Repetition Is the Result of Loneliness or Boredom

- Ask every caregiver on a shift to spend 1 to 2 minutes every hour exclusively with the resident. Residents depend on their familiar "home" caregivers for companionship. The importance of your accessibility and the comfort of your personal attention should never be underestimated.
- Initiate a Communication Partners program (see In-Service 11) as another means of easing the patient's sense of isolation in a organized and ongoing way. The program involves volunteers or fellow residents who are trained to be communication companions with Alzheimer's disease patients.[6]
- Review the resident's access to and interest, attendance, and participation in activities. Look for signs that the resident's cognitive ability no longer matches the level or type of activities (e.g., the resident is being scheduled for activities that are not challenging enough or, because of cognitive decline, are no longer appropriate). Rearrange the schedule accordingly and notice whether the resident is less persistent with requests for attention.

BOX 10-2 Effects of Resistance and Refusal

Throughout a recent in-service session at a large nursing facility, we emphasized how Alzheimer's disease patients, more than the rest of us, dislike being ordered about and how they strenuously resist this communication approach. Several alternative communication techniques were explained and modeled. Then it was time for practical application.

Staff participants were given a tough communication situation and asked how they would handle it. A nursing assistant in the first row quickly replied, "Here's what I say to this one resident that I take care of: 'Mr. Jones, you have to get dressed now. The minister is coming, and you *must* have your clothes on. Put those pants on, *now*!'" Later, this same nursing assistant complained: "Mr. Jones never does what I tell him to." Without realizing it, she had illustrated our point perfectly.

A patient's resistance and refusal could be caused by poor comprehension: the patient does not understand what he or she is supposed to do. In places other than a special unit for Alzheimer's disease residents, refusing to do something until we understand what is going on is not considered a *pathological* response. In the context of an institutional regime, however, resistance is seldom *acceptable*.

If the struggle is chronic and has become a generalized response to every little thing, the resident is probably communicating the anger and frustration of feeling lack of control over everything. Change, no matter how small, is particularly difficult for Alzheimer's disease patients. Change is scary for all of us, but most of the time we are able to reason and work our way through it. Persons with Alzheimer's disease no longer have their protective cognitive and emotional defenses intact, so change represents fearful insecurity for them. Their instinctive, anxiety-ridden response is to resist (Recommendation Boxes 10-5 and 10-6).

4. *Wandering and pilfering.* Wandering and pilfering are characteristic of many persons with impaired memory, cognition, and perception. Some wandering residents are compulsive "walkers," intent on moving forward no matter what. They follow a set path but one that may take them one direction in the morning

RECOMMENDATION BOX 10-5

Recommendations for Determining Reasons for Resistance or Refusal Behaviors

- Assess the resident's pattern of resistance. Determine whether the behavior is attached to specific persons, events, or time of day. Is it before or after medication administration; is it to everyone and everything? Analyze the resident's behavior, so that you can adapt your style to the person rather than escalating the problem by "resisting resistance."
- Develop a treatment plan:
  - Change the style of communication that is being used with this resident to a friendlier, less brusque manner that supports better comprehension, allows the resident control over how the task is done, and reduces fear of the unknown (see Recommendation Box 10-6).
  - Search for ways that the resident can feel in control of some aspects of nursing home life (e.g., choice of clothing, of activities, of flowers to plant or pick in the garden, of times to rise or go to bed, of early morning coffee routine), even though certain routines must be followed.
  - Take the resident's fear of change seriously even if the event seems trivial or has been recently faced without fear. Interview the family about the person's earlier fear reactions ("Did she always startle when she saw a spider? Is she 'seeing' something now that triggers the same response?").
  - Find ways to reduce the fears. Change the sequence of tasks; break tasks into smaller steps and rest between each one; search for a staff member whom the frightened resident trusts to perform a particularly difficult task with him or her.

RECOMMENDATION BOX 10-6

Recommendations for Effective Communication Techniques That Avoid or Reduce the Resident's Refusal to Cooperate

- Begin the task in a quiet spot; eliminate visual and auditory distractions before giving directions.
- Speak to the person at eye level. Be aware that standing above the person suggests "authority," such as that of a boss or a parent.
- Offer choices that enlist the patient's cooperation rather than demand compliance ("Socks first or undershirt?" "Will you walk to the garden or use the wheelchair?" "It's cold today. I'm glad I have on my warm jacket. Do you want to wear your blue sweater or the gray jacket?") (see In-Service 9).
- Talk about interim steps. "Do you want to use the lavender soap or the liquid suds today?" "How are you going down the hall today, walking or wheelchair?" "Walking? OK, can I walk to music with you?" rather than "Time to take your bath!" or "You have to go to music *now.*"
- Simplify and shorten your requests; give only one direction at a time. ("Hold the toothbrush for me. Toothpaste in the other hand. Now squeeze. Squeeze the toothpaste. Good. Didn't spill a bit. Arm up. Now brush. That's it. Brush. Nice work.")
- Combine verbal with nonverbal directions ("Please move your foot." Then point to or touch the person's foot).

Continued

and another in the afternoon. Other residents are curiously tolerant of the wanderer's incessant strolls through their rooms (no matter that the door is closed), across their pathways, or in front of the large activity room television set, as long as the intruder does not pilfer. When a resident wanders into neighbors' rooms and begins to rummage through their possessions, that is another story. The resident companions become frustrated and angry and verbally nasty. They feel their private territory has been invaded, and it has.

The nature of institutional environments and routines can intensify this common symptom of Alzheimer's disease. The more rigid the schedule and the personnel, the more intense and anxious the walker may become. Persons with Alzheimer's disease are easily confused when all doorways look alike, when nameplates with small print are placed above eye level, and when their seats in the dining hall have no familiar identification. Constant changes in roommates, staff, visitors, volunteers, and physicians add more confusion. The more severe the dementia, the more difficulty patients have remembering the names and roles of all these people.

It is difficult to reason with a wandering or rummaging resident. Instead, reframe the problem; look at it from a different point of view. The way we label people and behaviors influences our mindset and our methods of interaction. For example, in an institution we may "manage" patients; in a nursing facility or special care unit, we may "take care" of residents; in a setting with a homelike environment, we provide "assistance and service" to the people who live there. In this light, renaming the behavior, reshaping staff responses, and rearranging the environment may help "normalize" many "inappropriate" behaviors. Developing socially thoughtful and humane solutions to problems that arise with residents who wander and pilfer also is a means of protecting the security and privacy of the facility. This is not a small issue for families or security inspectors (Recommendation Box 10-7).

At the Jewish Home and Hospital, Bronx, New York, for example, a huge oak wall unit dominates one end of the third floor activity area. This creative piece of furniture houses compartments, drawers, and cubbyholes of all sizes and shapes. Each opening is invitingly accessible to the residents by latch, large (attached) key,

---

RECOMMENDATION BOX 10-6

Recommendations for Effective Communication Techniques That Avoid or Reduce the Resident's Refusal to Cooperate — Cont'd

- Use verbal positive reinforcement after every two or three statements, letting the person know you are pleased even if she or he does not understand. Say the same key words over and over to remind the person of the task. "I like to brush my teeth after lunch. Ah, I found your toothbrush. You can brush here at the sink. Brushing teeth keeps that smile lookin' good. That's it, brush away."
- Rephrase if the person does not know what you mean. Saying the same thing in different words sometimes helps an Alzheimer's disease patient understand ("Time for the music program." Then: "We're singing some oldies but goodies in music." Finally, "Let's get warmed up for music: 'By the light . . . of the silvery moon . . .'").
- Use a firm voice but one that is quiet and friendly. If your communication style becomes brusque and demanding, the patient is likely to become more fearful and resistant.
- Keep goals small and flexible so that the two of you can take delight in many small accomplishments rather than fume over one big failure.

sliding frames, pull knobs, chains, and slide bolts. It is filled with scarves, socks, stuffed toys, and other harmless objects just waiting to be pilfered or sorted.

5. *Paranoia.* Another behavior characteristic of persons with Alzheimer's disease is paranoia, that is, the belief that someone is trying to steal from or hurt them. As a professional caregiver, you understand that the resident's suspiciousness is part of the disease pattern and typical of brain deterioration. However, at a psychological level, the paranoia can be understood as a manifestation of the patient's deep-seated fear that his or her most valuable possessions (cognition, memory, health, family, friends) are lost, as indeed they are, and with terrible finality. The resident must at times feel extremely vulnerable and bereft without the familiar identities and supports that have defined his or her whole life.

But what of the unsuspecting fellow resident who is being accused of stealing from or trying to kill the paranoid patient? That resident is likely to react with predictable defensiveness, hurt, or anger. You need to avoid or intervene tactfully in the heated argument (Recommendation Box 10-8).

RECOMMENDATION BOX 10-7

Recommendations for Reframing Language Use with Wandering and Pilfering Residents

- Make residents' way finding a priority on your unit (see In-Service 3).
- Attach distinguishing marks or pictures (e.g., a bluebird) or first names to places where the resident likes to sit (e.g., "her" dining room chair, at her favorite planting station in the garden, or her usual seat at the craft table). Laminate a card that has the same mark, picture, or name. Attach it to the resident's wrist or waistband with elastic banding. Guide the resident by matching the card at her place so she can find her place independently.
- Choose room and area names that are unique, attractive, and decorated in an appealing mode: "Rose's Garden Room," "Coffee Klatch Corner," "The Pub," "Celebrity Lounge." (Hotels, restaurants, and cruise lines know that customers are attracted and soothed by labels and decor that set a pleasant, welcoming tone. Such creative and inexpensive "de-institutionalization" appeals to visitors too.)
- Develop kinder terms for wandering or intrusive behavior, such as "shopping," "sight-seeing," "taking a vacation," or "finding the best restaurant in town," and always use them in the presence of residents.
- Find socially acceptable areas where the wanderers are welcome to rummage to their hearts' content: a "shopping" area where they can pick up anything they like, such as books, plastic containers, clothing, especially clothes that suggest "vacation," "sight-seeing" materials, and "tours" to other acceptable places in the nursing home.

RECOMMENDATION BOX 10-8

Recommendations for Coping with an Alzheimer's Disease Patient's Paranoid Accusations

- Restore order; this is your first goal. This is not the time to get caught up in an argument over who is right or wrong or whether anything happened at all.
- Read the underlying meaning of the accusing resident's complaint: "You stole my rosary!" This could mean, "I've lost something precious." Another interpretation: "My God, why have You forsaken me?" The emotional issue for this person is "loss" or "feelings of abandonment."

Continued

RECOMMENDATION BOX 10-8

Recommendations for Coping with an Alzheimer's Disease Patient's Paranoid Accusations — cont'd

- Avoid taking sides with words or attitude, even if in your heart you feel more sympathetic to one person than the other. "Joe, I know you're angry that Alice is accusing you." "Alice, you can't find that lovely rosary? You look pretty unhappy right now."
- Be a communication model: quiet tone, sensible and firm words, quiet body language. One or both persons might sense your style, imitate your controlled tone of voice, and become calm. At the very least, this approach should save the situation from getting worse.
- Lead the more agitated person to a quiet area or distract that person as quickly as possible, and talk comfortingly about the safety and protection of the nursing home: "We're here. We want to take good care of you. We'll help you find your rosary."
- Return to the other resident. Do not leave him or her hanging in the midst of emotional turmoil. Reassure and praise the resident for any restraint or tact that was shown during the incident: "Joe, I was impressed with your patience. I know I can rely on your good judgment when things get scary."

▶ **QUICK TIP SUMMARY**

Difficult Communication Situations

Nonverbal and verbal communication skills are critical in reducing catastrophic reactions of Alzheimer's disease patients. A flexible and calm communication style is the key to dealing effectively with five difficult behaviors exhibited by residents who have Alzheimer's disease.

- Hallucinations: If the patient is doing no harm to himself or herself or to others, turn hallucinatory incidents into short conversations.
- Repetitive speech: Be sympathetic to memory problems, boredom, and loneliness. Devise simple memory aids. Schedule moments at regular intervals when you can talk with the resident.
- Resistance or refusal: Assess all possible reasons for refusal to cooperate. Respond sensitively to a strong dislike of being "bossed around," to a patient's poor comprehension of what is expected, and to a patient's generalized feeling of lack of control or fear of change.
- Wandering and pilfering: Take a hard look at how well the facility's environment supports residents in finding their way about and whether creative approaches could offer new solutions to wandering and pilfering.
- Paranoia: Paranoia is to be expected. Your primary communication responsibility as a mediator is to diffuse strong emotions of both pilferer and victim. Restore order and reassure all parties involved that their rights and safety are being protected.

GOOD PRACTICE 10-1

Role Playing Difficult Communication Situations

Preparation time: 10 minutes. Includes selection and assignment of team members; selection of resident who exhibits representative behavior; and review of appropriate recommendations.
Role Play time: 3-4 minutes
Discussion: 5-10 minutes

Directions: Select two teams of three players each. Each team decides who will play caregiver, resident, and recorder. (If the role play calls for three players, the instructor should ask someone from the audience to observe and record notes on the role play for later discussion.) The instructor assigns a different difficult communication situation to each team. Each team thinks of a resident who is known to them or is in their care and who exhibits the target behavior (e.g., hallucination, routine resistance of a task). In preparing for the role play, each team must consult the set of recommendations from In-Service 10 (or other in-services in this book) that pertain to each one's assigned difficult situation. The team recorder tells the audience which set of recommendations applies to the team's role play.

Role Play 1: Catastrophic reaction: two caregivers and one resident
Role Play 2: Hallucinations: one caregiver and one resident
Role Play 3: Repetitive speech: two caregivers and one resident
Role Play 4: Resistance and refusal: one caregiver and one resident
Role Play 5: Wandering and pilfering: one caregiver and two residents
Role Play 6: Paranoia: one caregiver and one resident

Observation Sheet For Recorder
The difficult communication situation was _____.
Recommendations for this difficult situation are on page _____ of the text.

_____The resident accurately demonstrated behaviors typical of this difficult communication situation.
_____The caregiver's communication techniques were well matched to the difficult communication situation.
_____The caregiver's communication was effective in preventing escalation of the resident's behavior.
_____The caregiver's communication style was calm and clear.
_____The caregiver was able to adjust communication style to the resident's changes in mood or movement.
_____The caregiver made a believable attempt to understand or was able to interpret the resident's needs.
_____The caregiver was able to meet the resident's needs.
_____The caregiver's communication style was helpful in restoring order to the situation.

Reflection for the Entire Class
• What did the players do that was realistic during the role play?
• What was the most effective communication technique the caregiver used?
• What else could have been done or said that would be effective?
• What did the role players learn from this experience? What did the audience learn?

GOOD PRACTICE 10-2

Difficult Communication Situations: What Can You Do?

Directions: Discuss several ways to improve each of the following difficult communication situations between caregivers and resident.

1. Paul was admitted to the nursing home soon after his wife died. He is in the middle stages of Alzheimer's disease. Paul wanders restlessly from room to room asking about Doris. "Have you seen Doris? Do you know where she is?" Some of the residents become very angry or agitated by his intrusions. Paul is oblivious to the commotion he causes. In what way could communication play an important role in managing Paul's behavior?

2. Antonio moved to the United States when he was 12 years old. He speaks excellent English and was a research scientist at a nearby university. As his disease has progressed, Tony has begun to revert to his native Italian. He has also become strongly resistant, refusing to dress, to be led to the toilet, to eat with other residents, to do anything cooperatively. He is not combative—yet. There is a church nearby whose pastor is Italian, but Tony's intake sheet declares he has "no religion." What strategies might caregivers use to reduce Tony's resistant behaviors?

3. Bridget accuses staff of stealing or hiding her possessions. She has recently begun to accuse one of the nursing assistants from Manilla. The assistant is a very skilled caregiver but also has great national pride. She thinks Bridget is making ethnic slurs. How could this aide use communication to preserve her pride and her job and at the same time appropriately manage Bridget's paranoia?

REFERENCES

1. Pillemer K, Bachman-Prehn R: Helping and hurting: predictors of maltreatment of patients in nursing homes, *Research in Aging* 13:74, 1991.
2. Cohen-Mansfield WP: Environmental influences on agitation: an integrative summary of an observational study, *American Journal of Alzheimer's Disease and Other Dementias* 10: 32, 1995.
3. Cohen-Mansfield WP: Managing agitation in elderly patients with dementia, *Geriatric Times* May-June: 3, 2001.
4. Stedman's *Pocket medical dictionary*, Baltimore, 1987, Williams & Wilkins.
5. Bourgeois MS: Evaluating memory wallets in conversations with persons with dementia, *Journal of Speech and Hearing Research*, 35:1344, 1992.
6. Lyon J: Communication partners: their value in reestablishing communication with aphasic adults. In T Prescott, editor: *Clinical aphasiology*, Boston: 1989, College-Hill.
7. Smith C, Ventis D: Cooperative and supportive behavior of female Alzheimer's patients. Presented at the annual meeting of the Gerontological Society of America, Boston, 1990.

Direct Intervention Programs: Increasing Communication Opportunities for Residents with Alzheimer's Disease in the Nursing Home

PREMISE

Good clinical practice is always based on sound research principles. It is well known that Alzheimer's disease patients respond best when they reside in a safe and predictable physical environment and are cared for by calm, supportive personnel. This management philosophy has been discovered through clinical experience and through the rigorous research of health care investigators.[1]

Communication skills are like most other human abilities—you must use them or lose them. For persons with Alzheimer's disease, the adage should read "use them or lose them faster." If patients with Alzheimer's disease have few or no opportunities to use retained communication skills, the relative strengths described in In-Service 1 (e.g., procedural memories and social rituals) diminish from disuse at a quicker rate. Instead of learning to maintain function with the skills remaining, residents learn helplessness (see In-Service 1 for a definition of learned helplessness.) Out of genuine concern for the patient's safety and well-being, caregivers and family members prevent them from engaging in activities that would allow them to exercise their remaining skills.

This in-service acquaints you with a number of research-tested methods for offering residents with Alzheimer's disease opportunities for maintaining their communication skills. All have been tested and used in the nursing home setting.

LEARNING OBJECTIVES

- List at least 10 techniques for maintaining successful communication with residents with Alzheimer's disease.
- Identify and differentiate informal opportunities that allow for spontaneous supportive communication and formal communication intervention programs that require specific responses and document specific communication changes in the resident.
- Describe in detail three formal communication programs. Discuss the possible benefits and limitations of implementing one of the formal programs.

DEFINITIONS

Communication opportunity Any encounter that offers the possibility for good communication between two persons. A communication opportunity can be a passing moment of contact in the hallway, a Sunday afternoon visit, or a planned group social activity.

Direct communication intervention program Specific, defined approaches that provide encouraging communication opportunities for persons with Alzheimer's disease.

COMMUNICATION OPPORTUNITIES: WHAT IS COMMUNICATION INTERVENTION AND WHY SHOULD WE PROVIDE IT?

Increased attention is being paid to direct intervention programs that help patients maintain or even improve their levels of communication. Although research on the topic is new, several treatment techniques appear to show positive results. Successful intervention has the following goals:

1. Maintain as many of an Alzheimer's disease patient's residual functional communication strengths as possible.
2. Prevent caregivers' overreaction to disability and residents' learned helplessness.
3. Relieve the burden of caregiving; maintain the health and integrity of the caregiver.
4. Improve the quality of life and maintain the human dignity of both patient and caregiver.
5. Establish harmonious functioning within the nursing home setting.

Many caregivers believe there is no point in trying to work with residents who have Alzheimer's disease through formal intervention programs: "They are only going to get worse." "They don't remember anything you teach them." "They're confused." But Alzheimer's disease patients are living longer and longer, and we are living with them. We need to communicate with them, and they have a great need to communicate with us. Direct intervention programs offer caregivers specific guidelines for implementing and then carefully evaluating the results of particular ways to communicate. As long as there are persons with Alzheimer's disease, there will be a need to seek formal and informal methods of improving communication between patient and caregiver.

COMMUNICATION INTERVENTIONS THAT HAVE PROVED EFFECTIVE IN NURSING HOME SETTINGS

Several promising, new communication treatments can be implemented by direct care staff with guidance from speech-language pathologists. Of the six treatment plans discussed here, four target the resident's communication skills directly, and two seek to enhance the caregiver's communication skills.

1. Spaced retrieval training[2]
2. Communication notebooks or wallets[3, 4]
3. Communication Partners[5]
4. The conversation group[6]
5. The Breakfast Club[7, 8]
6. The FOCUSED program for caregivers[9]

All six treatment protocols were developed according to the following guidelines. For detailed information about each treatment and for directions on how to conduct each, consult the references at the end of this in-service.

In choosing a communication intervention for *residents*, keep the following advice in mind:

- Choose activities for practicing everyday communication skills, ones that recur in the patient's daily life and that the environment will support.
- Choose activities that match the everyday routines of the nursing home (e.g., do not rely on a single caregiver to provide the activities if there is a large turnover of personnel, do not work on singing if residents are required to keep quiet).
- Choose activities that capitalize on the resident's remaining abilities.
- Reduce demands on episodic and working memory and rely more on recognition memory and long-term memory.
- Choose activities that entail *action* and *emotion*. Persons with Alzheimer's disease respond best if they are actively (hands-on) engaged in the treatment and personally and emotionally involved.

In choosing a communication intervention for *caregivers*, keep the following advice in mind:

- Target communication behaviors that are likely to occur in the everyday repertoire of the caregiver and the resident.
- Target communication behaviors that are achievable and have tangible results.
- Match the goals of the program to the level of the patient with whom the caregiver is communicating.

Spaced Retrieval Training
Spaced retrieval training (SRT) is a method for teaching persons with Alzheimer's disease new information and helpful behaviors.[2] It has been successful in helping patients retain simple information such as staff names, lunch times, and room numbers. SRT also can be used to teach functional behaviors such as getting out of bed safely and walking with a quad cane. In SRT, a patient is told a piece of information in the course of an engaging activity (card game, conversation) and then is asked to recall that information repeatedly and systematically over time. Intervals between requests for recall are gradually increased from 1 minute to 10 minutes to the point at which the information is retained for weeks or months. SRT requires little cognitive effort and can occur without the patient's having explicit recall of the training situation. SRT strengthens automatic associations in the brain and reduces the patient's reliance on episodic and working memory, both of which are impaired in Alzheimer's disease

Memory Books or Wallets

Many speech-language pathologists working in nursing homes have found that making a memory notebook as described by Mateer and Sohlberg[3] or a memory wallet as described by Bourgeois[4] is extremely helpful in providing communication opportunities for persons with Alzheimer's disease.

The *memory notebook* involves the assembly of current, pertinent information about the resident and his or her present surroundings: name, room number, schedule, roommate, and family pictures with names. The book also includes references to events and pictures from the past: information about who the person was before becoming ill. Information is printed in simple, declarative sentences; pictures are captioned with simple, identifying sentences.

The memory notebook serves many purposes. It takes advantage of the patient's retained ability to read single words. It helps to strengthen the person's present orientation and to maintain early life memories. Caregivers can use the notebook (1) as a daily review with the patient, (2) as a source of the patient's history, (3) as a tool for informal conversation, or (4) as a means of encouraging interaction between patients. If visitors pause to comment on the book, the resident has additional opportunities to communicate (Figure 11-1).

The *memory wallet* is a more portable form of the memory notebook. It includes personal information and photographs but is easier for the resident to keep at hand. Bourgeois taught professional nursing home caregivers to train patients with middle-stage Alzheimer's disease in the use of memory wallets. At regularly timed intervals, caregivers asked patients simple questions that could be answered with information in the wallet. Within 3 months, the residents learned that when they could not answer questions, they should reach for their memory wallets. Bourgeois found that although the deterioration caused by Alzheimer's disease continued, these patients began to use more statements of fact and more "novel utterances" and sought conversation more frequently after they learned to use their wallets.

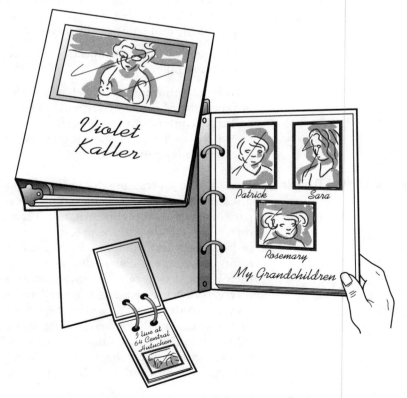

FIGURE 11-1   Example of a Memory Book.

Conversation Groups

Conversation groups give Alzheimer's disease patients "a means to establish an interpersonal situation in which meaningful, motivating, and reinforcing communication can occur."[10] Being present in a group stimulates the resident's verbalizations, increases interactions, and renews the skills of group members as independent participants. Group sessions can take many forms. *Reminiscence groups* are particularly valuable in stimulating the long-term memories and preserved skills of persons with Alzheimer's disease. *Current events discussions and cognitive stimulation groups* have been shown to help maintain the mental and language functions of residents with Alzheimer's disease. Games, projects, and free exchanges of ideas, experiences, and feelings (validation therapy)[11] also have been described (Recommendation Box 11-1).

RECOMMENDATION BOX 11-1

Conducting Conversation Groups with Residents with Alzheimer's Disease

- Therapeutic groups for persons with Alzheimer's disease work best with four or five participants and should have no more than seven participants with an aide.
- Participants should be seated around a table, and some food should be served. This physical arrangement helps maintain focus and attention.
- The table should be in the corner of the room. The walls give residents a feeling of stability and security. Wanderers can be seated in the corner so that leaving is less inviting.
- A "crier" should be removed from a conversation group if the activity does not have a quieting effect on the person after the second session.
- Large-print name tags should be provided for each member. Members should be referred to frequently by name.
- Speak slowly, loudly, and clearly.
- Use stimuli that are tangible and of real interest to the group. Have things (pictures, objects, words) on the table to look at, to touch, and to pass around.
- Provide rewards and positive feedback. Every member's effort to speak should be supported and reinforced.
- Do not force or correct responses. The resident is at least attempting to communicate, and his or her effort should be greeted positively.
- Progress from simple to complex in all activities. (Example: Pass around a pot of flowers, touch, smell, and name the parts. Then pass and comment on items for planting. Finally, plant some flowers in a new pot.)
- Encourage group members to do most of the talking, especially to each other. Avoid a classroom question and answer format whenever possible.
- Develop a theme (holidays, hearing aids, wedding anniversaries, child-rearing practices) but allow the residents' responses to dictate the course of the conversation.
- Summarize and restate points frequently. Help keep the participants on topic.
- Offer opportunities to each member to join in the group at his or her own level of communication ability.

Modified from Clark L, Witte K: Nature and efficacy of communication management in Alzheimer's disease. In Lubinski R, editor: *Dementia and communication*, Philadelphia, 1991, BC Decker.

The Breakfast Club

The Breakfast Club is a group communication intervention that incorporates everything known about effective communication with nursing home patients with Alzheimer's disease. Developed by Boczko and Santo Pietro,[8] the breakfast club is a directed activity in which a small group of residents with Alzheimer's disease prepares, serves, and eats breakfast and cleans up afterward. Ideally, the 45-minute meetings are held five mornings a week in a homelike kitchen setting that is carefully controlled for visual and auditory distractions. Five residents who have not yet had breakfast are seated around a rectangular table with the facilitator at one end.

To avoid sensory overload and confusion, the program's food choices are limited and include only those items the participants are capable of preparing. Tasks progress from simple ones (e.g., choosing butter or jam for toast) to more complex ones (e.g., actually making French toast or pancakes and flipping them on the griddle) as the program progresses.

The breakfast club seeks to provide residents with the following specific benefits:
- Maintenance of organizational, decision-making skills
- Maintenance of conversational and social skills
- Maintenance of early life memories
- Maintenance of interest and involvement
- Facilitation of retained procedural memories
- Facilitation of retained language abilities and reading skills
- Stimulation of hearing, vision, smell, taste, and touch
- Stimulation of positive emotions
- Prevention of learned helplessness
- Prevention of isolation and premature deterioration of communication skills

The Breakfast Club follows a structured format from beginning to end with a 10-step protocol that includes greetings, choices of juices and breakfast foods, joint preparation of coffee and breakfast, serving of coffee and breakfast entree, cleanup, conversation over coffee, and leave taking. In the beginning, residents do only as much of the preparation and cleanup as they are able, but greater levels of independence are encouraged over time.

Throughout the Breakfast Club sessions, the group leader uses generous amounts of feedback and positive reinforcement and incorporates language stimulation strategies, such as choice questions and closure (see In-Service 9). The leader's language style encourages, inspires, and animates the residents with words that convey warmth and acceptance, yet the style definitely reflects an adult attitude. The leader does not try to control every interaction. By being a good listener, the leader encourages patients to initiate conversation and to talk to one another as well as to the leader.

Results of research on the effectiveness of the Breakfast Club are impressive. Over a 12-week period, Breakfast Club participants in the Jewish Home and Hospital for Aged in Bronx, New York, not only improved in the use of language and communication skills but also showed renewed use of procedural memories for preparing, sharing, and eating a meal and significantly more independence and calmness in their everyday lives. Their social ritual abilities resurfaced, and they began to show genuine social concern for one another[8] (Box 11-1).

Communication Partners

Communication Partners is a communication intervention program initially developed by Lyon for use with poststroke patients.[5] In this program a volunteer is trained to communicate more successfully with communication-impaired residents. For the program to work for an Alzheimer's disease patient, the volunteer should master techniques such as those presented in In-Services 8 and 9.

Volunteers are first sought from among the resident's acquaintances. A second source might be the nursing home's volunteer service or the members of a local

---

BOX 11-1   Gertrude and the Breakfast Club

Week 1. Nursing staff expressed reservations about Gertrude's participation in the experimental group. She was isolated and uncooperative on the floor. In the early sessions, Gertrude appeared frightened and frustrated and remained silent most of the time. She refused to try to crack her egg. She could not spread jelly on toast even with coaching from the leader.

Week 2. Gertrude became so upset one day at the prospect of participating, she left the room.

Week 3. Gertrude smiled and independently cracked her egg. When the facilitator asked her to help Miriam, Gertrude responded, "No. Mine's okay, hers is something else." But at the end of the session, she said to Miriam, "Come on, Miriam, are you ready to go?"

Week 7. Gertrude held the door open for other members and told everyone it was her job. Then she walked in and pointed to her chair and said, "That's my chair." She commented on Jack's cracking of his egg, "He's cracking it right, but it's taking him a long time."

Week 8. When Mildred passed out utensils, Gertrude commented, "That's a girl. You're doing a great job!"

Week 10. Gertrude showed her name tag to everyone and crowed, "This is my name and it's a good one."

Week 12. At a meeting of the nursing staff on the floor, a nursing assistant remarked, "Gertrude is so much more cooperative. She can really follow directions now."

---

senior center or church. Fellow residents who are cognitively intact also make excellent and available volunteers. Family members or regular professional caregivers cannot play this role. Once the volunteer is comfortable communicating with the patient, a regular program of communication opportunities is planned. Activities might include in-room visits or games, walks, gardening, or trips outside the nursing home. Whenever possible, the activities should cater to the resident's preferences and reinforce the person's remaining independence and communication skills. Volunteer visits might be once a day or once a week, but they must occur on a regular basis.

Although spaced retrieval, memory books, the Breakfast Club, and other group therapies are most helpful for patients who are in the middle stages of Alzheimer's disease, programs that include pets, stuffed animals, music, and communication partners can serve residents who have Alzheimer's disease up through their final hours. Sitting in quiet companionship with a patient who has late-stage disease, stroking the patient's hair, singing softly or humming, and helping to feed or calm the patient during the last days are wonderfully human ways of extending a communication partners project (see In-Service 12). If a Communication Partners program is begun early enough in the stay of an Alzheimer's disease patient, the patient can have a familiar companion throughout the ordeal of decline.

The FOCUSED Program for Caregivers

The FOCUSED program, developed by Ripich,[9] is a caregiver intervention program that has proved effective in fostering positive communication exchanges between nursing home staff members and patients with Alzheimer's disease. It entails nonverbal and verbal communication strategies and, like the Communication Partners program, can be used throughout the course of the disease. Directed at family and professional caregivers, the FOCUSED program incorporates seven general communication strategies into a framework that can be recalled and applied by the use of the acronym FOCUSED: *f*ace the person, *o*rient to the topic,

TABLE 11-1	**FOCUSED Program for Alzheimer's Disease Caregivers**		
F	**Functional** and **Face** to attract attention	• Face persons directly and check lighting • Call persons by their name or use gentle touch • Gain and maintain eye contact at eye level	
O	**Orientation** to topic of conversation	• Repeat the topic, key words, and sentences • Repeat sentences exactly as spoken • Use specific nouns, names of persons, and places • Give person time to comprehend what you say	
C	**Continuity**, or maintenance of the topic (**Concrete** topics)	• Continue same topic of conversation for as long as possible • Prepare person for when a new topic is being introduced	
U	**Unsticking** for overcoming communication blocks	• Use questions to seek clarification (e.g., "Do you mean . . . ?") • Repeat the person's sentences using the correct word • Indirectly suggest the word for which you think the person is searching	
S	**Structure** of questions	• Use choice rather than open-ended questions • Provide only two options at a time	
E	**Exchange** of ideas, needs, and feelings during conversation and **Encourage** interaction	• Keep the conversational exchange of ideas going • Begin conversations with pleasant, normal topics • Give the person clues as to how to answer	
D	**Direct** types of verbal messages	• Use simple, short sentences • Use sentences with the active rather than passive voice • Use specific, concrete nouns and avoid pronouns • Communicate verbally and nonverbally in as many modalities as possible	

From Ripich D: A communication strategies program for caregivers of Alzheimer's disease patients. In Clark L (editor): *Communication disorders of the older adult: a practical handbook for health care professionals*, New York, 1993, Hunter/Mt. Sinai Geriatric Education Center.

continue the topic, *u*nstick communication blocks, *s*tructure with questions, *e*xchange conversation, and use *d*irect statements.

Each of the FOCUSED strategies represents a set of techniques that must be mastered to put the program into effect. The techniques can be learned from a caregiver manual developed by Ripich and Wykle[9] (Table 11-1).

Additional Programs

Additional direct communication interventions have appeared in the research literature. Camp and Brush have developed a multicomponent treatment program for Alzheimer's disease patients that is based on Montessori activities.[11] In one study elderly residents with Alzheimer's disease were paired with children at similar cognitive levels. The researchers found that the elderly not only provided good procedural models for the children but also became more engaged in their surroundings and more adept at the tasks in the process. Some facilities have successfully used Validation therapy,[10] an approach to supporting Alzheimer's disease patients' strong feelings of frustration, anger, and fear without affirming the reality of their complaints in order to reduce ongoing anxiety and outbursts. Pet therapy, the provision of dolls and stuffed animals, music therapy, and the use of therapeutic audiotapes also have been shown effective in calming Alzheimer's disease patients and engaging them in the communication process.

Bell and Troxel[12] have developed a comprehensive approach to the care of persons with Alzheimer's disease that is based on a "best friends" model. These authors suggest a number of communication techniques based on a framework of friendship (Recommendation Box 11-2).

RECOMMENDATION BOX 11-2

Elements of Friendship and Alzheimer's Disease Care

Friends Know Each Other's History and Personality

In Alzheimer's care, a Best Friend

- Becomes the person's memory
- Is sensitive to the person's traditions
- Learns the person's personality, moods, and problem-solving style

Friends Do Things Together

In Alzheimer's care, a Best Friend

- Involves the person in daily activities and chores
- Initiates activities
- Ties activities into the person's past skills and interests
- Encourages the person to enjoy the simpler things in life
- Remembers to celebrate special occasions

Friends Communicate

In Alzheimer's care a Best Friend

- Listens skillfully
- Speaks skillfully
- Asks questions skillfully
- Speaks using body language
- Gently encourages participation in conversations

Friends Build Self-esteem

In Alzheimer's care a Best Friend

- Gives compliments often
- Carefully asks for advice or opinions
- Always offers encouragement
- Offers congratulations

Friends Laugh Often

In Alzheimer's care, a Best Friend

- Tells jokes and funny stories
- Takes advantage of spontaneous fun
- Uses self-deprecating humor often

Friends are Equal

In Alzheimer's care, a Best Friend

- Does not talk down to the person
- Always works to protect the dignity of the person, to "save face"
- Does not assume a supervisory role
- Recognizes that learning is a two-way street

Friends Work at the Relationship

In Alzheimer's care, a Best Friend

- Is not overly sensitive
- Does more than 50% of the work
- Builds a trusting relationship
- Shows affection often

From Bell V, Troxel D: *The best friends approach to Alzheimer's care*, Baltimore, 1997, Health Professions Press.

DEVELOPING INTERVENTION TECHNIQUES FOR EFFECTIVE COMMUNICATION WITH ALZHEIMER'S DISEASE PATIENTS IN ALL SITUATIONS

Dos and Don'ts for Maintaining Successful Communication with Alzheimer's Disease Patients

Once you have a clear understanding of the communication problems and strengths of Alzheimer's disease patients as well as your own communication problems and strengths, you can work to create your own mini-interventions with elderly patients with dementia. Below is a list of 21 general "dos and don'ts" to help you achieve successful communication with your Alzheimer's disease patients.

1. *Use adult language.* You are communicating with adult patients. Patients are apt to respond negatively when you address them as children, no matter how kindly you intend to be. To help the patient maintain self-respect, use an adult communication style.

2. *Maintain eye contact.* Alzheimer's disease patients need as many nonverbal cues as possible. Eye contact is vital for maximum communication. If the patient is not looking at you, establish eye contact by calling his or her name or gently touching the patient's arm. Always stand face-to-face with an Alzheimer's disease patient when speaking. If the patient is in a wheelchair, bring yourself down to the patient at eye level.

3. *Use visual cues whenever possible.* There is evidence to show that Alzheimer's disease patients continue to respond appropriately to visual communication longer than spoken communication. Written words, pictures, gestures, and facial expressions all help to get information across to patients with Alzheimer's disease.

4. *Use simple words and short sentences.* Simple words remain available to Alzheimer's disease patients longer than difficult ones, and short sentences are easier to comprehend than complex ones.

5. *Keep your explanations short.* Alzheimer's disease patients are more likely to complete some longer tasks if the tasks are broken into single-step directions. For example: "Pick up the spoon. Put the spoon in the bowl."

6. *Paraphrase, do not just repeat.* If the patient has difficulty understanding a message, find a different way to say it rather than repeating the original words over and over. Other words might be more meaningful.

7. *Avoid saying, "Don't you remember?"* Chances are, the patient does not. Constant reminders that the patient's memory is failing can be very distressing for both patient and caregiver.

8. *Do not insist on "the truth".* If a patient can walk to the dining room, feed himself a meal, and enjoy it, does it matter if he thinks that breakfast is lunch? Or that April is June? Insistence on correctness stifles attempts at communication and corrections are soon forgotten anyway.

9. *Use touch.* Guidance, reassurance, affection, and humor can be communicated to an Alzheimer's disease patient through touch even in the later stages of the disease.

10. *Do not shout.* If hearing is not a problem, your tone of voice may frighten the patient or put the patient in a defensive mood. If hearing is a problem, shouting distorts your message. Many hearing-impaired elderly patients also suffer from tinnitus (ringing in the ears) or recruitment (an inability to hear soft noises while loud noises are perceived at their actual level of loudness). Shouting at persons with tinnitus or recruitment makes the problems worse and stresses the patient.

11. *Do not interrupt.* Try not to interrupt unless it is absolutely necessary. If you interrupt an Alzheimer's disease patient in the middle of an attempt to communicate or in the middle of a task, it is likely that the patient will forget what he or she was saying or doing. Alzheimer's disease patients are easily distracted, even when they are speaking or acting with firm intent.

12. *Avoid competition.* Avoid competing signals, such as television, radio, or other conversations. If you have something really important to tell an Alzheimer's disease patient, speak to the person face-to-face in a quiet place.

13. *Use a calm, reassuring tone of voice.* If your voice is warm and pleasant, the patient may want to listen to your message. Alzheimer's disease patients respond to emotional tone. Your voice should communicate support and reassurance, not anger and annoyance well into the late stages of the disease.

14. *Do not talk about the patient in his or her presence.* Even late-stage Alzheimer's disease patients have moments of lucidity. Be careful not to talk negatively about a patient to another patient or colleague. Overhearing criticism or sarcastic comments may account for at least some of a patient's negative behavior.

15. *Be realistic in your expectations.* If you are expecting normal, rapid responses, you will always be disappointed. Know their weaknesses, address their communication strengths, and be justifiably pleased with patients' honest efforts.

16. *Allow extra time for a patient to respond.* Patients with Alzheimer's disease process information slowly. If you wait for the patient to respond, you will sometimes be rewarded with an appropriate answer.

17. *Pay attention to patients' nonverbal communication.* Often, Alzheimer's disease patients cannot tell you what they mean in words, but their nonverbal communication may be very meaningful. Observe their gestures, nods, smiles, and frowns.

18. *Realize that catastrophic reactions are not necessarily manipulative.* (See Unit 10 for a definition of catastrophic reactions.) Catastrophic reactions in Alzheimer's disease patients are generally the result of frustration, cognitive overload, or the inability to communicate needs or to perform tasks. They are seldom a conscious effort of a patient to "get back at" caregivers. When a catastrophic reaction occurs, look for the cause. Examine your own communicative behavior to see whether you might have contributed to its occurrence.

19. *Listen carefully to "rambling."* Do not assume that the patient's rambling has no meaning. If the patient is talking, he or she is trying to communicate. Listen for hints of meaning in the patient's rambling. (See In-service One for communication changes characteristic of Alzheimer's disease.)

20. *Be willing to talk about "old times."* Relate current topics to old stored knowledge. Alzheimer's disease patients remember more about the distant past than the present. Do not be afraid to spend time there with the patient. The patient will enjoy reminiscing, and it might help him or her to perform better in the present.

21. *Continue to enjoy life.* If you feel only sad, burdened, and exasperated in dealing with Alzheimer's disease patients, you will have difficulty communicating with them. Alzheimer's disease patients are still people, and they are still capable of enjoying many happy moments in life. If you can enjoy some of the remaining moments with them, communication will be worthwhile for you both.

GOOD PRACTICE 11-1

Implementing a Direct Intervention Program: Group Discussion

Directions: Select one program from this list of direct communication intervention programs for Alzheimer's disease patients and answer at least four of the following questions, including Question 1. Share your answers with the rest of the persons in the group.

- Spaced retrieval
- A memory book or wallet
- Communication program
- Breakfast club

1. Program: The direct communication intervention program that I have selected is
   _____
   _____

2. Candidates: Which patients might be good candidates for this program?
   _____
   _____

3. Location: Where would be a good location for the program? (Think of convenience of transportation, proximity of toilet facilities, noise and traffic distractions, lighting.) _____
   _____

4. Scheduling: How many times per week should the program be held? _____
   _____

   How long could each session be (exclusive of transport time)? _____
   _____

   What would be a good time of day to hold the sessions? _____
   _____

   How many weeks should the program run altogether? _____
   _____

5. Personnel: Who could organize and coordinate the program? _____
   _____

   Who could facilitate the sessions? _____
   _____

   Where or from whom might you be able to learn the actual procedures to conduct such a program? _____
   _____

   Would you have assistants? How would you use them? _____
   _____
   _____

6. Training: Would any special training be necessary for the facilitator or assistants?
   _____

   How or where could this training be obtained? _____
   _____

7. Your role: How could you personally contribute to the success of the intervention program? _____

   What did you learn from this activity? _____
   _____

GOOD PRACTICE 11-2

Specific Techniques for Maintaining Effective Communication with Alzheimer's Disease Patients

Directions: Rewrite the final statement of each of the scenarios below or state an action you would take to use the technique named. In each case, how could the nursing assistant respond to communicate more effectively with the Alzheimer's disease patient?

Or: Use these scenarios as a role-play activity to give students an opportunity to practice and build their communication skills with Alzheimer's disease patients.

1. *Use adult language.* A patient needs his toenails clipped but has his legs folded under the chair.
   Nursing assistant: Hey, cutie, how about giving Mama Lou your little tootsies so I can clip 'em just a smidge?

2. *Keep your explanations short.* The patient refuses to get up to walk and moans softly.
   Nursing assistant: Zelda, I know you're sad that your husband didn't get here, but he called this morning, or maybe last night, to let you know that he had to go to your daughter's house this morning and he'll be late. He wants you to call over to your daughter's and tell them what time you finish therapy and what time lunch is served today. Okay?

3. *Paraphrase, do not just repeat.* The nurses' station receives a call from the patient's daughter asking whether a package of family photographs has arrived. The nurse sends the nursing assistant to check whether Mr. Miller received them. Mr. Miller does not seem to know what she's talking about.
   Nursing assistant: Mr. Miller, your daughter wants to know whether you have your wife's photograph up on your bulletin board.
   Patient: What?
   Nursing assistant: Your daughter wants to know whether you have your wife's photograph up on your bulletin board.

4. *Be realistic in your expectations.* A patient unexpectedly vomits after he has had an apparently routine day.
   Nursing assistant: George, you have to tell me where you were and exactly what you ate this afternoon. Tell me right now!

5. *Realize that catastrophic reactions and crying out might not be manipulative.* From her room down at the end of the hall, the patient cries and cries.
   Patient: Please help me. Where's the doctor? Please call the doctor. I'm in pain. I need help. Please help me.
   Nursing assistant [attempting to ignore this endless, annoying monologue]: Miriam, just quiet down now. You're driving everybody crazy.

6. *Be willing to talk about old times.* As the staff member attempts to help the patient finish his lunch, the patient begins a familiar story.
   Patient: You know, life was not easy in the Depression. Tough. Very tough. My brother and I sold apples. Apples. Don't eat apples. Can't no more.
   Nursing assistant: I know, Jack, I know. Pay attention here. Are you going to eat this applesauce or not?

7. *Listen carefully to rambling.* As the nursing assistant prepares the patient for bed, Harry rambles on and on.
   Patient: You know Mary is such a pain in the neck. Pain in the neck. Never could do anything right. Always was, always will be. Wasn't my fault and it was over. Just like that. Mary, Mary, Mary.

Continued

GOOD PRACTICE 11-2

Specific Techniques for Maintaining Effective Communication with Alzheimer's Disease Patients—cont'd

Nursing assistant: Quiet down, Harry. You don't know what you're talking about. Everything is okay.

8. *Use touch.* The patient is clearly agitated and fidgets in his wheelchair.

Patient: Where are you taking me, you bastard? What's going on here? I'm not supposed to be going anywhere! Leave me alone, dammit!

Nursing assistant: Now you just calm down, Mr. Peters, nobody talks to me that way! There is no yelling and no cursing on this floor!

9. *Pay attention to nonverbal communication.* The patient is bent limply forward over his food tray. So far, he has resisted all attempts by the nursing assistant to feed him, shaking his head and occasionally raising a weak finger to his left cheek.

Nursing assistant [ignoring patient's poor eating posture and hand movement]: Come on, Joe. Eat your peas. Try some of this tasty meat loaf. I've got lots of work to do today.

10. *Use simple words and short sentences.* The patient is dawdling over his occupational therapy project in the day room.

Nursing assistant: Lawrence, the basic requirement here is that you complete this art project, do what you have to do in the lavatory, and get yourself down to the dining room as punctually as possible.

REFERENCES

1. Dwyer B: *Focus on geriatric care and rehabilitation,* Frederick, MD, 1987, Aspen Publications.
2. Brush J, Camp C: *A therapy technique for improving memory: spaced retrieval,* Beachwood, OH, 1998, Menorah Park Center for the Aging.
3. Mateer C, Sohlberg M: A paradigm shift in memory rehabilitation. In H Whitaker, editor: *Neuropsychological studies of non-focal brain injury: dementia and closed head injury,* New York, 1988, Springer.
4. Bourgeois MS: Evaluating memory wallets in conversations with persons with dementia, *J Speech Hear Res* 35:1344, 1992.
5. Lyon J: Communication partners: their value in reestablishing communication with aphasic adults. In T Prescott, editor: *Clinical aphasiology,* Boston, 1989, College-Hill.
6. Clark L, Witte K: Nature and efficacy of communication management in Alzheimer's disease. In R Lubinski, editor: *Dementia and communication,* Philadelphia, 1991, BC Decker.
7. Santo Pietro MJ, Boczko F: The Breakfast Club: results of a study examining the effectiveness of a multi-modality group communication treatment, *Am J Alzheimers Dis* 13:146, 1998.
8. Boczko F, Santo Pietro MJ: Nursing home settings and residents with Alzheimer's disease: the Breakfast Club and related programs. In B Shaddon and M Toner, editors: *Aging and communication, by clinicians for clinicians,* Austin, TX, 1997, Pro-Ed.
9. Ripich D, Wykle M: *Alzheimer's disease communication guide: the FOCUSED program for caregivers,* San Antonio, TX, 1996, The Psychological Corporation.
10. Feil N: Validation therapy, *Geriatr Nurs* 3:129, 1992.
11. Camp C, and others: An intergenerational program for persons on dementia using Montessori methods, *Gerontologist* 37: 688, 1997.
12. Bell V, Troxel D: *The best friends approach to Alzheimer's care,* Baltimore, 1997, Health Professions Press.

Last Things: When a Person with Alzheimer's Disease is Dying

PREMISE   A direct care staff is dedicated not only to "caring for" but also to actively communicating with residents who have Alzheimer's disease through the final stages of illness. Complementary, or integrative, therapies provide important opportunities for caregivers to convey nonverbal messages of compassion, support, and dignity to residents. Attention to the spiritual aspects of death and dying eases the burden of caring for residents with late-stage Alzheimer's disease and strengthens communication between nursing home staff, families, and faith communities.

LEARNING OBJECTIVES
- Explain the difference between perfunctory "tending to" and genuine "communicating with" a resident in the final stages of Alzheimer's disease.
- Describe at least two complementary or nontraditional therapies that convey nonverbal assurance of compassion and peace to the patient.
- Explain why nontraditional approaches might increase the patient's feelings of comfort and safety.
- Develop a personal style and comfort level for offering appropriate verbal and nonverbal means of spiritual support to residents in the final stages of Alzheimer's disease and to their family members.

DEFINITIONS   **Alternative therapy, complementary or integrative therapy**   Nontraditional interventions used in place of Western medical practices are *alternative therapies*. The term *complementary* or *integrative therapy* embraces a variety of interventions that integrate with or are accepted as enhancing traditional Western medical practices. Today the credibility of countless integrative therapies is being documented with increasing frequency in respected medical journals. Whether complementary or alternative, one culture's nontraditional approach may be another culture's mainstream option. Acupuncture and homeopathic remedies are considered either complementary or alternative in Western medical practice but have long been central to respected medical care in other countries.

Disruptive vocalizations   Inappropriate, repetitive, inconsolable, and very loud noises or words shouted by residents in the late stages of Alzheimer's disease. Fewer than 15% of persons with dementia exhibit this behavior,[1] but the sound of even one screaming resident on a unit makes the meaning of *disruptive* distressingly clear to anyone within earshot.

Palliative care   The active total care of patients who are dying, whose disease is considered incurable, and for whom life-prolonging procedures are no longer viable. The precepts of palliative care are

- Ethical decision-making that respects patient autonomy and the role of family or legal surrogates
- Interdisciplinary team approach to care
- Treatment of patient and family as a single unit
- Intensive symptom management
- Improved quality of life as a primary goal
- Recognition of the importance of the inner life of patients
- Bereavement support to the family during the initial period of grieving[2]

THE CHALLENGES OF COMMUNICATING WITH RESIDENTS WHO HAVE SEVERE DEMENTIA

As residents enter the final stages of cognitive decline, the professional caregiver's goals appear to be more concrete. A patient for whom "nothing more can be done" is basically one who must be kept quiet, comfortable (e.g., pain free), clean, and safe. But for a busy caregiver, a resident in the final stages of Alzheimer's disease can also mean no more coaxing to activities, no rushing with the lunch tray, no dallying to answer endless questions, and no wasting precious time with reassurances during routine tasks. One might think, "If she gets lonely (does she even have emotions like loneliness anymore?), we'll turn on the television and leave it on all day. It will keep her company."

The process of dying accompanied by severe cognitive deficits can be horribly isolating. The decline of sensory acuity naturally widens the gulf between a person and his or her environment. Caregivers may experience a subtle shift in their own attitudes. It is not that they care less, it is just that other residents rapidly take up the creative attention and energy that the dying person used to take. A conscientious nursing home staff must guard against detaching too quickly, thus adding emotional abandonment to the dying patient's sensory isolation. Caregivers have both an ethical and a professional mandate to continue to address social and emotional needs through communication and to care for the physical needs of residents with late-stage Alzheimer's disease. The caregiver's own turmoil is not an insignificant issue in this circumstance and must be addressed along with that of the dying resident.

Table 12-1 illustrates six situations that can occur when a resident has severe dementia and staff members begin to let the lines of communication slip away.

TABLE 12-1	Communication Decline in Severely Demented Patients and Ineffective Caregiver Responses	
CONDITION	**INEFFECTIVE RESPONSE**
1. Patient is mute or constantly cries out.	1. Caregiver isolates patient physically or emotionally, stops communicating socially, is less sensitive to cries as genuine requests for help or signals of pain or illness.
2. Patient can no longer draw or use information from environment owing to severe perceptual and cognitive impairments.	2. Caregiver speaks carelessly in the presence of the patient about the patient's condition or other confidential information or makes less effort to offer purely sensory information and comfort.
3. Patient is no longer independently mobile or is totally bedridden.	3. Caregiver is less inclined to make patient and activities accessible to each other, does not leave routines and normal work paths to say hello.
4. Patient may have rare windows of lucidity, that is, he or she understands and responds fully to the situation.	4. Caregiver interprets these incidents to mean that the patient "really understands more than he or she lets on for a moment" or is just being stubborn the rest of the time.
5. Patient no longer self-feeds and is at risk of dysphagia and aspiration.	5. Caregiver loses patience with time-consuming feeding; feeds resident as quickly as possible, risking aspiration; delays trays and feeding assistance until more intact residents are cared for.
6. Patient is very near death, although this condition may last for weeks or months.	6. Caregiver avoids interactions with family members because "there is nothing new to report" or fears "saying the wrong thing." Is unable to communicate empathy or consolation to either family or patient.

These scenarios are not merely resident care problems but are premature breakdowns in the relationship between caregiver and care recipient. How can caregivers cope more effectively in these difficult situations?

THE RESIDENT WHO CONTINUALLY CRIES OUT: A SPECIAL PROBLEM

Caregivers need to muster their most creative communication skills when patients with late-stage disease engage in continuous crying out or disruptive vocalization. Disruptive vocalization takes many forms: loud or repetitive verbal utterances ("Help me! Help, help, help me!"), nonsense or animal-like sounds, screaming, or moaning. There are several possible explanations for the endless stream of cries. Residents may be sick or in pain, and wailing is the only way left for them to seek help. They may be suffering from anxiety due to overstimulation. If a resident has visual and hearing impairment, sensory deprivation (under-stimulation) or depression may be the root cause. Whatever the reason, the noise constitutes a major environmental management problem.[1]

The problems caused by constant crying out are not endured by the patient alone. This disturbance affects the communication of everyone in the vicinity. The staff's communication styles are deeply affected by the disruption. Continual moaning raises the noise level of a unit and increases stress on the staff. People talk louder or turn up their radios and televisions. Other patients are awakened from their rest or become distracted and agitated. To visitors and potential clients, such wailing typifies the institutional atmosphere of a nursing home.

In the late stages of dementia, crying out is a response that can no longer be shaped into meaningful speech. In some cases at least, the cries can be interpreted. Then staff can perhaps revise responses and adjust environments. Box 12-1

BOX 12-1   Ten Questions to Help Determine Best Care Practices for Residents Who Have Disruptive Vocalization

Rule Out Physical Causes

1. Has the medical chart been thoroughly reviewed and the resident thoroughly examined to rule out causes of a painful medical nature?
2. Does the crying decrease even a little if the staff consistently tends to the resident's physical needs sooner rather than later: repositioning, hydrating, feeding, changing clothing and protective garments, and attending to oral hygiene?

Determine a Pattern, Reallocating Staff or Volunteers

3. Is there a time pattern to the patient's crying behavior? This information can be obtained by charting the times and extent of the cries for 5 to 7 days during the shifts when crying is most pervasive.
   NOTE: This charting project would be an excellent project for students of speech-language pathology or geriatric nursing or a participant in the communication in-service certificate program (see Notes to the Instructor).
4. If there is a pattern, could a volunteer or family member plan to be with the resident during times when the resident is expected to cry out? Even in the absence of a perceptible pattern, could staff or volunteers establish their own pattern of visits to the resident (Box 12-2)?
5. Are there staff members or volunteers who are better at quieting patients in distress? Could more of their time be allocated to these severely demented patients?

Make Environmental and Logistical Adaptations

6. Could certain areas be especially prepared for patients who cry out (e.g., carpeting on the floor and walls, heavier curtains, shades, plants)?
7. Could sound buffers be used to protect other residents from the noise (e.g., sound-proofing or dividers, assistive listening devices such as earphones for nearby patients for effective focusing of their hearing and attention)?
8. Could the crying residents be placed closer to the hub of activity where they would receive more attention? Have they been placed too far away, becoming isolated from vital caregiving time, attention, and visibility? If the cause appears to be overstimulation, should these residents be placed in a less busy room down the hall?

Provide Direct Intervention

9. Have you tried behavior modification, that is, giving attention to the resident during his or her quiet times rather than during the noisy hours?
10. Have other types of sensory stimulation been used *consistently* (not just once or twice) with residents who exercise disruptive vocalization? Such stimuli include lotions; audiocassettes of white noise such as hissing, familiar voices, music or church services; specific auditory, tactile, or olfactory therapies; light or temperature variations; and multimedia environmental systems (see In-Service 3). Have any of these techniques been even slightly effective, that is, worth experimenting with further?

---

contains 10 questions to help you assess each person and situation to find an intervention that will quiet a resident whose outbursts are grating on everyone's nerves. The approach suggested is an individualized one. What works for one resident may not be suitable for another. Keep trying!

BOX 12-2 Scheduled Visits

During one of our recent workshops on communication with patients who have Alzheimer's disease, a participant shared her experience: "Harold was an outgoing talkative guy while he was still up walking around. When he went into major decline, all he did was lie in bed and yell: 'Hey! Come 'ere. Hey! Come 'ere.' We checked but he didn't seem to need anything. He was making us crazy. Then someone suggested we take turns visiting him on a regular basis. We made a rotating schedule. Each person on a shift agreed to spend 1 minute out of every hour with Harold unless he was asleep. This was in addition to his regular care routine. We'd comb his hair or hold his hand and hum a tune or say a 'Hail Mary'—he was Catholic. His yelling out decreased to almost nothing in 3 days. He died 5 weeks later, and he definitely seemed to be more at peace. I know we were, and it cost each of us just 8 minutes a shift."

COMPLEMENTARY THERAPIES AND MEETING THE COMMUNICATION NEEDS OF RESIDENTS WITH LATE-STAGE COGNITIVE IMPAIRMENT

Ira Byock, MD, a leader in the hospice movement, suggests that the deepest communication needs of the dying can be described simply but elegantly in only five phrases: "Forgive me"; "I forgive you"; "Thank you"; "I love you"; and "Goodbye."[3] Residents in the final stages of Alzheimer's disease need to receive similar messages of love, peace, reassurance, respect, and forgiveness. As emphasized throughout this book, even patients with dementia so severe that they no longer understand deserve to hear these sentiments from their caregivers frequently and by whatever means possible. The caregiver-care receiver bond is one to be nurtured until the very end.

In recent years, caregivers' efforts to stay in a close and comforting relationship with dying patients has led to interest in a number of nontraditional therapies referred to as *complementary* or *alternative* depending on their function in the treatment plan. The acronym for complementary and alternative medicine is CAM. Advocates contend that CAM therapies are particularly valuable for easing the discomfort of certain health problems among the aged, such as dementia.[4]

As a way of bridging a communication gap between needs of patients with end-stage Alzheimer's disease and their caregivers, the four therapies described herein—music therapy, healing touch, massage, and aromatherapy—involve techniques for caregivers to stay in touch with Alzheimer's disease residents when words no longer work. Positive results are most frequently described as reduced anxiety, a state of deep relaxation, and improved ability to accept and cope with problems. Results seem to be independent of cognition, memory, or language, and only the passive presence or cooperation of the resident is required.[4] These four therapies specialize in stimulating the senses, offering a sensory experience that cradles the recipient in a message of peace, tenderness, and reassurance.

Training programs for these four complementary therapies educate practitioners to become licensed or certified (or for music therapy, obtain a master's degree) in a certain specialty, but training is not restricted to health care professionals. Lay persons are generally welcome, a fact that may appeal to family members who are looking for ways to add meaning and purpose to their visits. The complementary therapies presented in this in-service are low risk and noninvasive. Except for full body massage, treatments do not require a doctor's orders. *Nevertheless, the staff must have a policy of checking with the attending physician and asking permission of the nearest relative.* The therapies are portable, requiring very little equipment. This flexibility

---

BOX 12-3   Serving the Nursing Home Holistically

A bright and imaginatively lettered sign hung on the door to the treatment room shared by the massage therapist and the healing touch therapist:

TO THE STAFF AT ST. BERNARD'S NURSING HOME:

COMPLIMENTARY TREATMENTS
FROM YOUR COMPLEMENTARY FRIENDS

Stop in for a free 10-minute trial session
And enjoy today . . .
what our residents have known about
for a long time

---

allows the therapist to come to the resident's bedside, making treatments accessible to all patients and protecting the patient's privacy. Treatments are much less expensive than chemical restraints and pain relievers and infinitely more humane than physical restraints. Last but not least, these treatments are very calming for the person who provides the therapy, another advantage for family members or direct care staff who become involved.[5] Integrative therapy treatments also can be a wonderful perquisite for staff members who want to work on their own stress management (Box 12-3).

► **QUICK TIP SUMMARY**

Advantages of Four Complementary Therapies: Music Therapy, Healing Touch, Massage, and Aromatherapy

- Treatments provide techniques for caregivers to stay in touch when words no longer work.
- Treatments may benefit patients after other interventions have ceased to be effective.
- Treatments may be successful means of reducing resident anxiety and inducing a peaceful and relaxed state.
- Treatment success is independent of active participation of the patient.
- Treatments are noninvasive, do not require a physician's order, except for full body massage, which must be conducted by a certified, and in some states licensed, massage therapist.
- Treatments are low risk for physical or emotional damage or abuse.
- Treatments are at the resident's bedside and thus both accessible and private. The therapist's equipment is portable, allowing for greater flexibility in scheduling.
- Treatments can be as comforting to the giver as they are to the receiver.
- Treatments are inexpensive compared with chemical restraints and are more humane than physical restraints.
- Training programs are not restricted to health care professionals, so it is possible for family members to learn the techniques.

1. *Music therapy.* Music therapy is the systematic use of music with goals to actively engage and stimulate the person and to support life processes. The effectiveness of music therapy among persons with dementia has been demonstrated by an impressive array of well-researched programs.[6] Many investigators believe that music serves as a supportive stimulus for speech and provides pathways to memories and associations that cannot be retrieved through other memory avenues.[4] Music therapy is prescriptive in nature; musical selections are based on the needs and preferences of the resident (or the resident's family). In a nursing home setting, the music therapist designs multipurpose programs for residents that not only passively entertain but also relax, stir memories, encourage movement and singing, and bring smiles and laughter to the participants. Therapists also plan tailor-made music menus for residents, choosing particular songs and renditions, scheduling times of day to play or perform the music, and making decisions about who should implement the program (e.g., the therapist or someone supervised by the therapist).[7,8]

Music thanatology is a type of therapy in which the dying, even comatose, patient passively receives the music. Music thanatology is palliative therapy, meaning that the therapist seeks to calm and comfort the dying person after traditional interventions have been exhausted. The music is specialized, consisting of either soft chanting or harp music.[9]

We only have to look to ourselves to understand that positive or negative responses to music are closely tied to our personal experience and to the culture and time in which we grew up. One generation's symphony is another generation's cacophony, and even within these parameters, tastes vary widely. Selecting music that is insensitive to the needs and enjoyment of a patient, such as leaving a radio on for hours at a time, is not music therapy. Noxious music can drive a person with dementia into deeper states of restlessness, boredom, agitation, and depression. Music as a complementary therapy, whether intended to engage, soothe, or usher the person through dying, is best initiated and monitored by a student or graduate of an authorized music education program.

2. *Energy bodywork therapies.* Energy bodywork therapies include healing touch, therapeutic touch, reiki, and massage therapy. In the early 1980s, the nursing profession led in the research and development of two complementary therapy programs, healing touch[10] and therapeutic touch.[11] Now international in scope, both programs train therapists who serve in a variety of health care facilities and private practice offices. Reiki emerged from the ancient Japanese healing arts and is growing in popularity in the United States.[12] All three (and other touch therapies not covered in this discussion) are characterized as "energy bodywork."

When a person is ill, the healthy energy that normally flows through and around the body becomes blocked. For the touch therapist, *healing* is not synonymous with *curing*, that is, the disappearance of the illness. Touch therapy promotes a state of deep relaxation so that the person's immune system is reenergized and the body's resources for combating disease are optimized (Figure 12-1). The goal of touch therapy is to bring the whole person into balance or harmony—body, mind, spirit, and emotions—so that conditions are most favorable for what needs to occur next. For the dying, touch treatments can bring the person to a state of peace so that he or she is ready to move through the final phase of living with less anxiety or resistance.[13]

In touch therapy, the hands or fingertips rest quietly and lightly on or just above a specific anatomical point of the body for 1 to 3 minutes then move on to the next placement point. The therapist does not rub or stroke the body, although the technique may call for mild hand movement *over* an area. Treatments take 5 to 30 minutes and must be conducted in a quiet environment. The therapist's attention is focused into an intentional attitude of listening and responding to the resident's every move and breath.

We conducted a study of the effects of healing touch on nursing home residents who had middle- to late-stage Alzheimer's disease. Each resident underwent 10 treatments over 5 weeks. The direct care staff provided twice-weekly scores on a set of 10 resident behaviors. These scores were compared with those of a control group who had received no treatments. The experimental group showed a significant

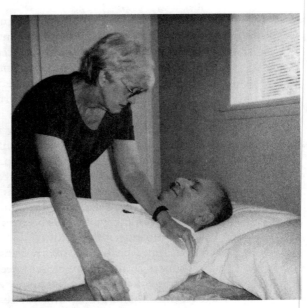

FIGURE 12-1   Example of healing touch.

decrease in incidents of anxious behavior and in reports of pain and discomfort. Among the eight other behaviors measured, significantly more remained stable, and more showed a positive if statistically insignificant trend within the experimental group than within the control group, among whom a greater number of behaviors deteriorated. We concluded that healing touch is a promising therapy for nursing home patients with dementia of the Alzheimer's type.[5]

3. *Massage therapy*. Massage therapy is a familiar type of energy bodywork to many people. Massage therapy may sound a little too vigorous to use as treatment of dying residents. If used judiciously, however, massage provides caregiver and patient opportunities to build mutual trust and for the caregiver to communicate nonverbally in a meaningful yet nonauthoritarian manner. Massage soothes, invigorates, and relaxes the patient and reduces agitation. For a bedridden patient in a constantly contracted position, massage therapy eases tightened muscles, releases the antistress hormones cortisol and norepinephrine, and boosts immune function while decreasing pain and skin breakdown. In sum, massage therapy protects residents, already orphaned by dementia, from feeling totally untouchable.[14]

A massage therapist brings specialized knowledge and training far beyond the gentle hand-and-lotion massage that caregivers often give to their residents.[15] Because of the extreme vulnerability of all systems of an aging, dying body, physician's orders and treatment-oriented goals are required for massage therapists to provide full body massage. Massage is rarely deep for elderly or dying residents. Massaging breasts or genitalia, open areas, abrasions, wounds, or areas that are inflamed is always contraindicated, and massage is never applied to the lower legs of inactive elders or to very fragile skin.[14]

4. *Aromatherapy*. Human beings are literally led around by our noses. Just as we cannot *not* communicate, we cannot *not* smell! We smell always and with every breath, and according to some experts, we can differentiate more than 10,000 scents.[16] We cannot shut our noses to the fact that some scents are exceedingly pleasant and calming to the emotions. Rigorous research is now showing what practitioners of the ancient healing arts knew long ago, that certain aromas can likewise be curative for some bodily ailments.[17] The olfactory sense offers direct and immediate entry into the person's consciousness, often bringing rapid yet safe relief from physical and emotional distress.

Aromatherapy uses the scents of certain natural, pure, or essential oils derived from a highly select group of plants. As with touch therapies, aromatherapy seeks to balance the flow of energy in a person's body and to dissolve energy blocks caused by illness or emotional distress. The aromatherapist applies a drop or two of the diluted oil to, for example, the sole of the foot, the palm of the hand, or the abdomen and gently rubs it in so that the healing properties will circulate throughout the desired area.[18]

Aromatherapy is never used to disguise unpleasant odors or to overwhelm those present with strong application. Although an aromatherapist will agree that a warm, sweet-smelling bubble bath or a scented candle is pleasant, the essential oils used in aromatherapy are room temperature, never warmed or heated. Other precautions govern the use of essential oils: They must be carefully stored away from resident access, tested to make sure the receiver's skin is not sensitive to the selection, rotated in use to reduce cumulative or decreased effect, and diluted according to precise formulae. Essential oils are not to be ingested by mouth and should be used only as recommended by a knowledgeable and experienced clinician.[14,17] The proper study of aromatherapy is complex, and educational requirements and certification standards are still developing. Nevertheless, as a means of palliative care for severely demented and dying residents, this complementary therapy is gaining credibility and acceptance.

In In-Service 4, we encourage professional caregivers to support residents' spiritual yearnings as one critical means of maintaining communication with persons in their care. Review those pages because the information and recommendations that bring spiritual solace to living residents apply to those who are dying. Dying residents even marginally aware of being cared for are comforted by a caregiver's tactful but genuine spiritual attentions. When a resident is unresponsive, the caregiver's role is even more critical. It entails not only spiritual solace but also acting along with family members as speaker and advocate for the dying person. The precepts of palliative care presented in "Definitions" provide a rationale for changing the psychosocial environments of residents and for performing certain final tasks (Recommendation Box 12-1).

LAST THINGS

Last things are no more than a summary of the highest goals that this book espouses, the essential issues that bond caregiver to care receiver:

- The importance of social communication and relationships
- The commitment to quality of service and care
- Respect for the dignity of the person with Alzheimer's disease no matter what the stage of disease or the condition of the patient
- The right of both direct care staff and the residents to environments, procedures, and policies that encourage and support their best efforts
- The acknowledgment of human values that include body, mind, and spirit

We applaud you as professional caregivers in a career that has a unique blend of challenges and rewards. May these last things that have so engaged us as speech-language pathologists, speakers, and writers for the past 3 decades become the cornerstone first things of your own special journey.

M. J. S. P.
E. J. O.

RECOMMENDATION BOX 12-1

Recommendations for the Spiritual Support of Dying Residents and Their Families

- Ask about the availability of complementary therapy treatments if none has yet been tried.
- Have on file lists of local religious establishments, phone numbers, addresses and directions, up-to-date pastors' names, and their expected visiting times to assist families from different geographic areas who do not have easy access to this information.
- Be familiar with the systems of interdepartmental communication regarding the exchange of information on dying residents.
- Request an in-service from your chaplain or a member of the local clergy regarding spiritual practices that he or she has found helpful with the dying and their families.
- Hold memorial services for residents on your unit who have died. Closure is important for residents who experience loss of one of their community. Closure also is important for staff and between staff and familiar visitors. Some of these relationships are long-standing and will come to an end as well. It is nice but not necessary to have memorial services conducted by a member of the clergy.
- Remember that the more cognitively aware residents may be affected by a death in their unit's "family," especially a roommate. Resist the impulse to decide that "they do not notice." Treat residents as you would treat any family member who has just lost a relative: Communicate your own steadfastness to their care, reassure them if they fear their own deaths, and share feelings of grief, however they may be expressed.

GOOD PRACTICE 12-1

Role Play Between Family Members of a Dying Resident with Alzheimer's Disease and a Professional Caregiver

Directions: Divide the class into groups of three. Participants decide who will play the professional caregiver and who will be the two family members. Have the family members decide the relationships they want to assume (e.g., sister, husband).

Scenario: The family members visit their dying relative once a week. They can see for themselves a gradual decline but want reassurance of good care and specifics of the status of the patient. They also want advice about how to make their visits more meaningful. Their concern and their need to stay in contact with the staff are their last and only avenue to be loving caregivers for their relative. You are the professional staff member they approach every week. Why do they prefer to come to you? What is it about your manner and your information that feeds their yearning so effectively?

The role play will simulate three separate visits from the family members. Each time, they ask the same questions: "How has he been over the past week?" "Is there anything more we could be doing?" The questions are general, but the family members want specifics. The challenge to the caregiver is to stay interested enough in the family members and the dying resident to respond in a different but caring manner after the visit. Each of the three scenes begins with the caregiver greeting the family members after they have just been to visit their relative. The activity should last for approximately 5 minutes and include hellos and good-byes before and after each conference.

Continued

GOOD PRACTICE 12-1

Role Play Between Family Members of a Dying Resident with Alzheimer's Disease and a Professional Caregiver—cont'd

REFLECTION QUESTIONS FOR THE ENTIRE CLASS

To the family members: How did you feel about the caregiver's responses to your questions? Were the responses as helpful and reassuring one time as another?

To the caregiver: How was it trying to come up with a variety of responses that would demonstrate your sincere and care-filled monitoring of their relative's condition? Did you want to "duck and run" by the third time?

To the class: What were your observations? Did the interactions differ in any way? What did you think of the caregiver's responses? How would you have responded differently?

GOOD PRACTICE 12-2

Speaking of Dying: Role Play Between a Resident in the Final Stages of Alzheimer's Disease and a Caregiver

Directions: Before In-Service 12, assign class participants to fill out a Resident Social Communication Profile (see In-Service 4, Good Practice 4-1) on themselves (myself as a dying resident). As they complete the questionnaire, participants are to imagine themselves as an actual resident who is in the final stages of Alzheimer's disease.

Divide the class into pairs. Each couple designates one person to play herself or himself as a dying resident and one to play caregiver. The caregiver interviews his or her partner as if the partner were really a resident in the facility who wants to have as many physical, emotional, sensory, communication, spiritual, and psychosocial needs met as possible during this final phase of life. In preparation for the role, the participant who is dying should consider: How do I want to be treated when I am ill? What consolations do I prefer? What will be extremely important to me? For greater realism, have the "dying resident" lie down. The "caregiver" should pose each question slowly and thoughtfully, giving the resident time to reflect and respond from the heart.

Call time after 5 minutes of role play and ask the partners to switch roles.

INTERVIEW QUESTIONS

- How can I make you more comfortable? What about the bedclothes? The temperature of the room? The noise level? How well are you able to tolerate your pain (arthritis, broken bones, cancer)?
- How do you feel about being touched, stroked, massaged with lotion? What, or whose voice, do you want to hear? Whom do you want to see? What do you want to touch? To smell? To feel? To taste?
- What foods make you feel better? What are some foods you would never tolerate even in the best of health? How are we doing with feeding you? Too fast? Bites too big? Food cold? Would you rather not eat? Would a gastric tube be acceptable?
- When you experience brief moments of understanding, how do you feel? Are you frightened? Angry? Puzzled? Eager to have everything over with?
- How do you feel about attention and visitors? Do you wish more people would stop by or that more would leave you alone? Do you like having a roommate, or do you prefer to be alone? Is there anything you are trying to say?

Continued

GOOD PRACTICE 12-2

Speaking of Dying: Role Play Between a Resident in the Final Stages of Alzheimer's Disease and a Caregiver—cont'd

REFLECTION QUESTIONS FOR THE ENTIRE CLASS

Take approximately 10 minutes.

- *Dying resident:* What was it like being asked questions about yourself and your preferences as if you were the one who was dying? Specifically, what communication needs did you feel were most important?
- *Caregiver/interviewer:* Did the emotional impact of the interview questions change as you played each role? Did you have any thoughts you had not had before about addressing the needs, especially the communication needs, of the person in the final stages of Alzheimer's disease?
- What was the most important aspect of the exercise for you?

REFERENCES

1. Sloan P: Managing the patient with disruptive vocalization. Presented at *Shaping Alzheimer Care: The Power to Change*, the 5th National Alzheimer's Disease Educational Annual Conference, part II, session C-4, Chicago, 1996.
2. Byock I, Caplan A, Snyder JD: Beyond symptom management: physician roles and responsibility in palliative care. In Snyder L, Quill TE, editors: *Physician's guide to end-of-life care*, Philadelphia, 2001, American College of Physicians.
3. Byock I: *Dying well: the prospect for growth at the end of life*, New York, 1997, Riverhead.
4. Adams L, Gatchel R, Gentry C: Complementary and alternative medicine: applications and implications for cognitive functioning in elderly populations, *Altern Ther Health Med* 7:52, 2001.
5. Ostuni E, Santo Pietro MJ: Effects of healing touch on nursing home residents in later stages of Alzheimer's disease. Presented at the World Alzheimer's Congress, Washington, DC, 2000.
6. Hanser S: Music therapy in dementia care. Presented at World Alzheimer's Congress, Washington DC, 2000.
7. Brotons M, Pickett-Cooper P: The effects of music therapy intervention on agitation behaviors of Alzheimer's disease patients, *J Music Ther* 33:2, 1996.
8. Brotons M, Pickett-Cooper P: Preferences of Alzheimer's patients for music activities: singing, instruments, dance/movement, games, and composition/improvisation, *J Music Ther* 31:220, 1994.
9. Schroeder-Sheker T: *Chalice of repose: a contemplative musician's approach to death and dying* [videotape], Louisville, CO, 1998, Sounds True.
10. Mentgen J, Bulbrook MJ: *Healing touch notebooks*, ed 2, levels I and II. Lakewood CO, 1996, Colorado Center for Healing Touch.
11. Krieger D: *Therapeutic touch inner workbook*, Santa Fe, 1997, Bear & Company.
12. Stein D: *Essential reiki: a complete guide to an ancient healing art*, Freedom, CA, 1996, Crossing Press.
13. Graham R, Litt F, Irwin W: *Healing from the heart: a guide to Christian healing for individuals and groups*, Winfield, BC, Canada, 1998, Wood Lake Books.
14. Canarius M: Massage and aromatherapy: understanding, initiating and modifying programs for all levels of care. Presented at the World Alzheimer's Congress, Washington DC, 2000.
15. Snyder M, Egan E, Burns K: Efficacy of hand massage in decreasing agitation behaviors associated with care activities in persons with dementia, *Geriatr Nurs* 16:60, 1995.
16. Ackerman D: *A natural history of the senses*, New York, 1990, Random House.
17. *Essential oils desk reference*, ed 2, Orem, UT, 2000, Essential Science Publishing.
18. Flanagan N: The clinical use of aromatherapy in Alzheimer's patients, *Altern Complement Ther* 378:377, 1995.

APPENDIX I

Quizzes

INTRODUCTION QUIZ

Directions: Circle all the possible correct answers to each question.

1. Most people communicate
   a. Without saying words.
   b. Much less through words than through expressiveness and body language.
   c. Both as senders and as receivers of messages.
   d. Best when using words alone to convey important messages.

2. Good ways to communicate nonverbally might be to
   a. Touch your daughter's shoulder.
   b. Write your dad a letter.
   c. Hum a song while you bathe a resident.
   d. Have a heart-to-heart conversation with your best friend.

3. Nonverbal styles of communication are
   a. Pretty much universal for all people.
   b. An excellent means of enhancing any message.
   c. Unnecessary when working with residents with Alzheimer's disease.
   d. Largely determined by the culture in which a person was raised.

4. Some of the reasons we need to communicate are
   a. To get an education.
   b. To show love and acknowledge love from others.
   c. To hold down a job.
   d. To get others to do what we want.

5. Effective communication
   a. Takes place when the message you intend is accurately understood by another who then responds appropriately.
   b. Saves time and money in the nursing home.
   c. Prevents residents' catastrophic behaviors and reduces the potential for abusive incidents.
   d. Is possible between coworkers but not between staff and residents with Alzheimer's disease.

6. When we refer to a "common frame of reference" in communication, we mean
   a. We should place photos of the residents' relatives in contrasting frames within their line of vision.
   b. We have had experiences that are very similar to those of the person we are talking to.
   c. We share many ideas and ways of looking at things with the people with whom we were raised.
   d. The two people speaking are in similar good or bad frames of mind.

7. Which of the following statements is true about the set of mental abilities necessary to communicate effectively?
   a. Two people must be able to see or hear each other. (This means that two deaf persons or two blind persons are incapable of effective communication.)

160

b. Both people in a conversation must be able to pay attention to one another. If one or both have poor listening habits, communication breaks down.

c. Two people must be able to understand each other's ideas; you cannot explain your thoughts to persons who cannot grasp them.

d Short-term memory is essential to the ability to stay on topic or add details to a story.

8. Qualities that both parties must bring with them to ensure a good communication situation are

a. Respect and trust.

b. Financial independence.

c. A common language.

d. An open attitude.

9. Openness in communication means that

a. The door to your office is always open.

b. Your mouth is always open when you speak.

c. You are willing to say anything that the other person wants to hear in order to make him or her feel better.

d. You are willing to listen to what someone has to say even though you may not agree.

10. Being an effective communicator means that

a. You will never have an argument.

b. You have worked on developing healthy attitudes toward yourself and others.

c. You know that no one else can "make" you say anything you don't want to say.

d. You must have mastered all the requirements for effective communication listed in the Introduction or it is not worth the effort.

IN-SERVICE 1 QUIZ:
Communication Problems and Strengths of Patients with Alzheimer's Disease and Related Disorders

Directions: Circle one correct answer for each question.

1. In the early stages of Alzheimer's disease, residents
   a. Lose orientation to time, place, and person.
   b. Seldom self-correct.
   c. Cannot remember phone numbers.
   d. Lose apparent desire to communicate.

2. In the middle stages of dementia, residents typically
   a. Do not seem to know when someone is speaking to them.
   b. Ask fewer questions, and start fewer conversations.
   c. May lose speech altogether and become mute.
   d. Lose time orientation only.

3. Patients in the final stages of Alzheimer's disease
   a. Lose grammar and diction and speak in jargon.
   b. Lose the ability to understand what is read, although reading mechanics are preserved.
   c. Can pay attention to a speaker for a few minutes but are easily distracted.
   d. Use related words, such as "horse" for "cow."

4. Empty speech is very common among persons with Alzheimer's disease and means that
   a. They are apt to say the same things over and over.
   b. They talk only when their stomachs are empty.
   c. They are depressed and have little to say.
   d. They use vague terms, such as "it," "those," and "over there" in place of specific names such as "Doris" or "the coffee."

5. If a resident stops conversation by swearing, walking away, crying, or making rude statements, we call that behavior
   a. A window of lucidity.
   b. A violation of conversational rules.
   c. Stereotypic language.
   d. Empty speech.

6. "Learned helplessness" is most apt to result from
   a. Resident's loss of career or social role.
   b. Resident's becoming less physically attractive with old age.

c. Caregivers' showing a resident that his or her actions have little effect on the outcome of any situation.

d. Residents no longer being able to walk to activities by themselves.

7. The most difficult-to-resolve situation preventing elderly persons from communicating is
   a. They cannot find their false teeth.
   b. They are involved in watching TV.
   c. Their favorite companions and family members—the persons with whom they most enjoy talking—have moved or passed away.
   d. Their hearing aids are not functioning.

8. Which statement is true concerning the course of decline of persons with Alzheimer's disease?
   a. Memories of long-ago events disappear early in the disease.
   b. Procedural memory, or the knowledge of how to perform familiar tasks, is lost very early in the course of Alzheimer's disease.
   c. Persons with Alzheimer's disease quickly lose their need for human contact; the loss of desire for communication is an early warning sign of Alzheimer's disease.
   d. Despite their annoying behavior, residents with Alzheimer's disease continue to expect to be treated as adults and in fact perform better when handled with adult respect.

9. Residents with Alzheimer's disease who exhibit a desire for interpersonal interaction
   a. Are really just trying to manipulate the staff and upset them.
   b. Are liable to "tell on" the staff members who are mean to them.
   c. Will always speak and behave well with staff members who are good to them.
   d. Benefit from caregivers who try as many ways as possible to capitalize on this desire.

10. All of the following are procedural memories except
    a. Driving a car.
    b. Buttoning a button.
    c. Playing the piano.
    d. Telling details about the neighborhood where you grew up.

IN-SERVICE 2 QUIZ:
Additional Communication Disorders Frequently Found in Older Residents with Alzheimer's Disease

Directions: Circle one correct answer for each question.

1. Elderly nursing home residents with Alzheimer's disease are likely to have
   a. Many more pleasant days than those without Alzheimer's disease because they are less prone to other illnesses.
   b. Additional communication problems from causes other than Alzheimer's disease.
   c. So many communication problems that there is no use trying to treat each one individually.
   d. A hearing loss that does not interfere with communication.

2. Speech, language, and voice
   a. Are three unique aspects of communication.
   b. Are all names for the same thing: talking.
   c. Are each different aspects of communication, and in persons with Alzheimer's disease, voice is the most likely to deteriorate quickly.
   d. Are each different aspects of communication; language encompasses how the words sound when we talk; speech includes vocabulary and grammar; and voice is measured by how well we sing.

3. Which of the following are sensory impairments leading to breakdowns in communication?
   a. Dysphagia and dysarthria.
   b. Stroke and hemiplegia.
   c. Hearing loss and vision disorders.
   d. Loss of common sense.

4. Aphasia is primarily
   a. An inability to chew and swallow food safely.
   b. A disorder which requires patients to breathe with a respirator.
   c. An illness that causes patients to hallucinate.
   d. A language impairment caused by stroke or head injury that disrupts understanding and expressive communication.

5. Which of the following statements is not true?
   a. Persons with Alzheimer's disease are at higher risk of hearing loss than is the general population.
   b. There is nothing that can be done for Alzheimer's patients who suffer from hearing loss.

c. Even an otherwise healthy person with a hearing loss finds listening stressful and exhausting.

d. Many persons with sensorineural hearing loss also have tinnitus. Tinnitus gets worse in the presence of noise.

6. If one of your residents with Alzheimer's disease has a hearing loss, you should
   a. Keep the neurologist informed about the patient's progress.
   b. Be aware that a sensorineural hearing loss can be caused by drugs and monitor the patient's reaction to sound and voice over time.
   c. Always stand behind the patient when you speak and use a high-pitched loud voice.
   d. Stand with your back against the window glare.

7. Xerostomia refers to
   a. Difficulty with chewing and swallowing food safely.
   b. A hole in Xeroxed materials.
   c. A language problem often caused by stroke.
   d. A chronically dry mouth, often a reaction to drugs, that causes soreness and bleeding of gums.

8. The most common drug-related changes in the patient's ability to communicate are
   a. Slurred speech, difficulty opening the jaw to eat or speak.
   b. A tendency to speak in short, quick rushes of speech.
   c. The use of an extremely loud voice.
   d. An improved ability to read fine print and detailed information.

9. Dysphagia, or swallowing problems, may be signaled by
   a. A wet, gurgly voice.
   b. An extended period of chewing followed by difficulty triggering the swallow.
   c. A low-grade fever.
   d. All of the above symptoms.

10. Persons with Alzheimer's disease
    a. Seldom experience depression, because they have so little idea of what is happening.
    b. Often have movement and balance problems that require them to pay more attention to where they are going than to what someone is saying to them.
    c. Can be "jollied" out of depression easily.
    d. Are pretty agile up until the last stages of the disease and therefore should be responsible for their own grooming.

IN-SERVICE 3 QUIZ:
Making Changes in the Physical Environment That Support Communication

Directions: Select all of the possible correct answers to each question.

1. "The less competent the individual, the greater the impact of environmental factors on that individual." This implies that
   a. A resident with Alzheimer's disease might react negatively to even the smallest obstacle or distraction in the environment.
   b. The environment plays an active part in what Alzheimer's disease patients do and how well they do it.
   c. Environments can be arranged to reduce learned helplessness for individuals with cognition, memory, and language problems.
   d. New staff members, people with disabilities, family members, and volunteers will all function better in a nursing home that has a user-friendly environment.

2. Which of the following examples are physical barriers to communication?
   a. Long distances between the activities room and the resident's room.
   b. A minister or counselor who rarely visits the facility.
   c. Signs, notices, and nameplates that are written in small print, placed above eye level, or cluttered with too much information.
   d. An unwritten policy that staff may enter residents' rooms without notice or knocking.

3. Rearranging physical environments to better accommodate the communication problems of persons with Alzheimer's disease
   a. Takes administrative time and is not worth the effort.
   b. Is sometimes costly, but many good solutions are inexpensive.
   c. Is more effective if the ideas come from direct care staff.
   d. Is convenient because once a change has been implemented, further monitoring is rarely necessary.

4. Some good reasons to print all identifying labels in large block print are that
   a. This practice will help residents gauge distances and depth as they walk from place to place.
   b. The words can been seen more easily even when lighting is less than adequate.
   c. This practice supports residents' ability to read single words until late in the disease.
   d. It gives the residents a good opportunity to practice their penmanship.

5. Residents with Alzheimer's disease who suffer from visual defects will also have the following communication problems:
   a. Difficulty reading the facial cues of their speaking partners.
   b. Inattention to another's speech when they are trying to walk, find their forks, or read signs.
   c. Getting as much enjoyment out of mealtimes as previously.
   d. Remembering childhood memories.

6. If you are working with a person who has Alzheimer's disease who also has a hearing loss, you should not
   a. Use a low-pitched voice.
   b. Work near noisy areas, such as the floor waxing machine or the tray cart.
   c. Lower the volume of televisions, radios, and paging systems.
   d. Lower yourself to the resident's eye level when you speak.

7. Poorly controlled odors and unappetizing food presentation
   a. Can be countered by releasing enjoyable aromas in the residents' vicinity just before mealtimes.
   b. Make it useless for nursing assistants to alternate flavors, textures, and temperatures of the food when feeding the residents.
   c. Are part of being in a nursing home and cannot be changed.
   d. Can have a great impact on the Alzheimer's disease resident's interest in eating.

8. Some ways to overcome a resident's lack of interest in food might be to
   a. Use pleasant words, such as "crunchy," "juicy," "smooth," or "delicious" to prepare the resident for taste and texture differences.
   b. Heighten the resident's anticipation with comforting parental phrases such as "Let's eat our yummy carrots," or "Ooooh, that's just too hot for our little tongue."
   c. Feed the resident rapidly so that he or she will not notice the bland taste or the lumpy texture of the food.
   d. Spruce up the dining room with pretty plants and napkins, look through books of beautiful food pictures before lunch, encourage family members to bring in treats from home.

9. Living environments designed especially for residents with Alzheimer's disease such as the Eden Alternative and the Heritage Woods programs
   a. Are built deep in the forest so that wandering residents are not a danger to themselves or others.
   b. Reflect a home-like neighborhood atmosphere.
   c. May include children, animals, birds, and plants.
   d. Focus on greater freedom of movement and choices for the residents.

10. Gardening and sharing sensory experiences are therapeutic activities for the resident with Alzheimer's disease because
    a. They keep the resident occupied while the staff is on break.
    b. They can be adapted to the level of functioning of the resident.
    c. They appeal to individual sensory preferences that tend to remain intact longer than specific memories or language skills.
    d. Residents with Alzheimer's disease can be included in the design and construction of the landscaping or the installation of the Snoezelen therapy rooms.

IN-SERVICE 4 QUIZ:
Making Changes That Support Communication in the Psychosocial Environment

Directions: Select all of the possible correct answers for each question.

1. Which of the following are examples of psychosocial barriers to communication?
   a. A long narrow hallway with a line of women in wheelchairs.
   b. A noisy paging system.
   c. A high rate of staff turnover and absenteeism.
   d. No opportunities for residents and family members to have private discussions.

2. Circle the good ideas for reducing psychosocial barriers and making residents feel less isolated.
   a. Make a photograph album of direct care staff members that is clearly marked with names and shifts.
   b. Learn about a resident's personal history and refer to it frequently.
   c. Knock or call out your name or the resident's name before entering the person's room.
   d. Complain about the resident to your colleagues so that they, too, are familiar with his or her shortcomings.

3. Examples of what can happen when the remaining cognitive skills of a person with Alzheimer's disease are not fully supported by staff are:
   a. Family members quickly assume the responsibility for keeping the resident active.
   b. The resident becomes increasingly isolated.
   c. The person's communication skills decline faster because of lack of practice.
   d. The resident is at higher risk of becoming more dependent on staff members (learned helplessness).

4. The Resident Social Communication Profile
   a. Is used to assess how social the person is with other residents.
   b. Is against the law because it pries into confidential information about the resident.
   c. Serves as a useful resource for conversations between resident and caregiver.
   d. Can never be used with any person who has Alzheimer's disease because the information must be obtained directly from the resident.

5. When you assemble a photo album of the staff to share with your residents with Alzheimer's disease
   a. It is best to take group shots—that is, everyone together.

b. Take a picture of every single person who comes onto the unit.

c. Exclude the family from this activity.

d. Collect head shots of staff members, volunteers, or visitors who spend the most time with the resident.

6. Absenteeism and staff turnover can be a major source of confusion and a psychosocial communication barrier for Alzheimer's disease patients because

a. Residents do not have a consistent person with whom to communicate or bond.

b. Severe memory problems interfere with the person's ability to remember so many people.

c. Residents have difficulty getting used to new styles of touch, speaking, and being cared for.

d. Staff members often fail to say good-bye or to leave a memento before going; the resident is seldom afforded a ritual closing to the relationship.

7. The concept of privacy and personal space for persons who have Alzheimer's disease

a. Is ridiculous and impractical in a setting such as a nursing home.

b. Can be supported by remembering to knock, identifying yourself before entering, and allowing the resident a moment to process your presence.

c. Can be honored by remembering to say, "Excuse me" when interrupting an activity or conversation, even if the resident is in the last stages of the illness.

d. Can be enhanced by reserving private places for residents to be alone with their companions.

8. Some topics that staff members might wish to avoid but persons with Alzheimer's disease need to talk about are:

a. Their true feelings about the food, certain staff members, the institutional routine, or their bothersome roommate.

b. The confusing ending to last night's television show.

c. Their fear of death and dying.

d. The design of the nursing home and the layout of the grounds.

9. Professional caregivers can share spiritual needs with persons who have Alzheimer's disease by

a. Learning about their religious history.

b. Holding a resident's hand and saying a prayer for the person's final comfort and peace of mind.

c. Learning to conduct religious services for residents who are dying.

d. Avoiding the priest, minister, or rabbi whenever he or she visits the unit.

10. A caregiver's attention to spiritual comfort of the residents may serve as

a. An opportunity to show honor and respect for the resident's struggle and courage.

b. A chance to examine one's own spiritual needs and values.

c. A means of maintaining caring and sensitivity for the residents who are often messy and difficult to care for.

d. All of the above.

IN-SERVICE 5 QUIZ:
Communication Strengths and Problems of Professionals Who Care for Persons with Alzheimer's Disease

Directions: Circle one correct answer for each question.

1. One often-overlooked reason for communication breakdowns between a professional caregiver and a patient with Alzheimer's disease is that
   a. The patient feels hopeless and does not attempt to understand anything.
   b. The family has probably interfered with the communication process repeatedly.
   c. The caregiver has poor communication skills.
   d. The previous shift got everyone upset.

2. The following statement is the least realistic communication strategy for professional caregivers:
   a. Work until you attain such good communication skills that you can handle all tough communication situations by yourself.
   b. Know when to ease up on yourself and take a break.
   c. Spend a little time learning about each patient's likes and dislikes.
   d. Believe that good communication encourages better cooperation from your residents with Alzheimer's disease.

3. Certified nursing assistants provide ____% of direct care to residents and incur ____% of violence by patients against staff:
   a. 25, 25.
   b. 50, 50.
   c. 75, 75.
   d. 90, 90.

4. If you suspect that you have a hearing loss, you should
   a. Act normal so no one will notice.
   b. See a neurologist.
   c. Wait and see if it gets worse.
   d. See a licensed audiologist.

5. Humor is healthy in the workplace; it relieves stress and builds relationships. Therefore, it is OK to
   a. Tell the patients funny or embarrassing things you did as a teenager.
   b. Keep coworkers laughing with ethnic jokes as long as you are sure the patients cannot hear you or can no longer understand.
   c. Laugh politely when residents make ethnic jokes.
   d. Share with your coworkers, in delightful detail, the embarrassing things that residents with dementia or their relatives have done.

6. If you are a foreign-born employee of the nursing home, you should
   a. Realize that your communication problems with residents would be eliminated if you did not have difficulty with English.
   b. Make a special effort to advocate for diversity training in your facility.
   c. Make fun of the way you were raised so that everyone will see that you are a "regular" person.
   d. Assume that the other people on your shift are going to be sincerely interested in your culture.

7. Caregivers who are extremely extroverted
   a. Are likely to be the best listeners.
   b. Can make a patient feel overwhelmed.
   c. Should be counted on to inject excitement and unpredictability to an otherwise dull job; if they do all the talking, you don't have to.
   d. Are best suited to work with Alzheimer's disease patients under any conditions.

8. Continuing education programs
   a. Can help you integrate your daily experience with new ideas.
   b. Are the perfect answer; you cannot get enough of the new information about recent developments that might solve all of your problems.
   c. Are nonsense; you've had 20 years of experience and can usually tell the instructor a thing or two.
   d. Are a bore; how can anyone sit through that stuff?

9. An example of communicating responsibly in a sensitive situation is
   a. The time Mabel fell out of bed and you didn't tell the supervisor about what happened.
   b. The day Benny died and you told his roommate he had gone back to his wife.
   c. The time Adele was really agitated, and you adopted a very slow, low-key way of speaking.
   d. Using a consistent communication style no matter what happens.

10. The felt burden of professional caregiving is always related to
   a. The number of elderly patients you have in your care at one time.
   b. How demanding your situation is at home: finances, kids, alcoholic husband, personal ambitions, whatever.
   c. Your supervisor's mood.
   d. How overwhelmed or confident you are feeling at the moment.

IN-SERVICE 6 QUIZ:
Multicultural Issues in Nursing Homes

Directions: Circle one answer for each question.

1. Cultural differences in communication
   a. Are permanent; with great effort we can reduce the barriers they create between people but never completely erase them.
   b. Rarely create communication problems between residents and employees in a nursing home.
   c. Have no place in a nursing home. The human resources or hiring department should carefully screen applicants so that everyone speaks standard English.
   d. Are not necessary and will not happen if we just try to love one another.

2. The term culture has a very broad meaning and can refer to
   a. Family ritual, "in" jokes, and child-rearing practices.
   b. A particular corporate or workplace environment.
   c. People from a different country or religion.
   d. All of the above.

3. If an employee "goes against the company culture," this means
   a. That person is looking for another job.
   b. That person does not follow the manner of dress, sense of humor, or other behaviors that are accepted and encouraged by fellow employees.
   c. That person works in a place where there is no "company culture."
   d. That employee is a hostile, suspicious person who never likes to have any fun.

4. Conflict between staff members and residents that is rooted in cultural differences
   a. Often arises because staff members have had little training in how to communicate with residents who have Alzheimer's disease.
   b. Is more likely to occur where staff members whose language and cultural practices vary widely with those of the residents.
   c. Will never happen in nursing homes that have diversity training classes.
   d. Is a sure sign that the nursing home is going to fail financially. Time to look for another job.

5. Misunderstandings among staff who represent diverse cultural backgrounds
   a. Only occur between individuals who do not speak the same language.
   b. Could be avoided if the nursing home regulations required all persons from one culture to work the same shift together.
   c. Are a sufficient reason to complain to the news media about unfair hiring practices in the nursing home.
   d. Have the potential to disrupt the quiet routine required by Alzhiemer's disease patients.

6. If you speak English as a second language, cultural differences in communication probably pose the least problem when
   a. Your supervisor gives you clear instructions, sometimes supplemented with pictures or demonstrations for carrying out procedures.
   b. You are speaking on the phone.
   c. You are from a different culture than one of your residents, and that person corrects your behavior every time you are with him or her.
   d. You are interacting with a resident's family.

7. Which of the following statements is true?
   a. Cultural differences in communication do not usually affect how a person uses touch or eye contact to convey messages.
   b. Persons from all cultures use about the same amount of space between themselves and their speaking partners.
   c. Discussion of some topics is taboo in some cultures but quite acceptable in others (e.g., income, age, personal illness or discomfort, or sex.)
   d. People from the same culture rarely, if ever, have difficulty communicating with one another.

8. Persons with Alzheimer's disease from culturally different backgrounds
   a. Are typically too old and infirm to express their biases regarding religion, politics, or race.
   b. Mellow out and seldom find it offensive to live closely with persons who look, sound, or behave differently from themselves.
   c. Need caregivers with special tolerance, tact, and an appreciation of the resident's personal social history.
   d. Can be taught through a direct communication intervention program to inhibit any hurtful communication behaviors.

9. Some ways to foster good communication in a multicultural setting are to
   a. "Americanize" a foreigner's name so that the person feels more at home and remind the person often about "how we do things here."
   b. Be watchful of a foreigner's manner of communication, especially if the person is from a country that has opposed the United States.
   c. Say that you understand a person even when you do not in order to avoid embarrassment.
   d. Advocate for diversity training in your facility. Attend workshops about the cultures and communication styles of people with whom you work.

10. The most important point to remember when working in a culturally diverse setting is that
    a. You are always responsible for controlling a resident's offensive remarks.
    b. It is in your best interest to erase as much evidence of your cultural background as possible when working in a nursing home.
    c. You can always control your own responses to the culturally biased behavior of others.
    d. Residents who have Alzheimer's disease become increasingly rude if they are allowed to get away with ethnic slurs.

IN-SERVICE 7 QUIZ:
The Toxic Effects of Verbal Abuse and Communication Neglect

Directions: Circle one answer for each question.

1. Acts of psychological abuse, including verbal abuse and communication, occur in nursing homes
   a. As much as physical abuse.
   b. Rarely.
   c. Approximately 10 times more frequently than acts of physical abuse.
   d. At least four times more than acts of physical abuse.

2. Verbal abuse
   a. Is against the law so should be used with caution.
   b. Is just a way of speaking to people in this day and age. No one means anything by it.
   c. Attempts to control a patient's behavior with violent words and actions as well as with physical force.
   d. Attempts to control a resident's behavior with violent words and gestures but without physical force.

3. Communication neglect
   a. Is necessary when the staff is busy. You do not have time to talk or to be pleasant.
   b. Dehumanizes the caregiver as well as the resident.
   c. Is necessary because it keeps you from getting too attached to residents and feeling bad when they die or are moved.
   d. Should never be a reason for firing an efficient employee.

4. Toxic talk
   a. Is irresponsible conversation about nursing home patients, events, or procedures.
   b. Is healthy because overworked staff needs to vent occasionally.
   c. Is OK as long as the wrong people do not hear what you are saying.
   d. Is a ridiculous concept. It is seldom "destructive" or "reflective of poor professionalism."

5. Which of the following statements is not true? Verbal abuse and communication neglect occur more readily in work settings where
   a. The acoustics are poor.
   b. Staff members are less experienced.
   c. The staff is poorly trained in the causes and prevention of abuse and neglect.
   d. Employees harbor negative attitudes toward the residents.

6. A high rate of aggression toward staff members by confused or demented residents may be a sign that
   a. The nursing home needs to hire a first-rate interior decorator.
   b. Most of the residents are from lower social and economic levels.
   c. The staff has gotten into habits of speaking and behaving that are insensitive to the needs and feelings of the residents.
   d. The staff is not being strict enough with the residents.

7. The possibility that you would ever commit an act of verbal abuse is reduced if
   a. You are a nice person.
   b. You had a decent upbringing; therefore, you know better.
   c. You rarely speak to the residents other than to tell them what to do.
   d. You are in tune with your emotions. You know when to back off from an especially irritating or volatile situation and ask for help.

8. If you suspected a case of ongoing communication neglect of a resident by one or more coworkers, you would be justified in
   a. Speaking confidentially to your supervisor or to the proper administrator.
   b. Keeping quiet and taking responsibility for being especially nice to the resident yourself.
   c. Asking other coworkers if they have noticed the same behavior.
   d. Going directly and immediately to state authorities.

9. Select the statement that is incorrect.
   a. Company cultures can harbor strong self-protective attitudes that discourage employees from reporting incidents of abuse or neglect.
   b. Failure to report suspected abuse could result in an increase of the incidents.
   c. Determination that abuse has actually occurred will be made by those who turn in the initial report of the incident.
   d. There are federal regulations, state laws, and organizational resources to support those who report and those who are victims of abuse and neglect in nursing homes.

10. The final point made in this in-service is that
    a. Abuse and neglect are at least as common in business and engineering as they are in the healthcare professions.
    b. Illegal practices decline where workers know that reporting abusive incidents is a fair way to deal with the problem.
    c. Many workers transfer into business and engineering because they are dissatisfied with the way verbal abuse and communication neglect are handled in nursing homes.
    d. Illegal practices disappear when everyone is afraid someone will "blow the whistle."

IN-SERVICE 8 QUIZ:
Communicating with Families:
Same Goals, Different Goals

Directions: Circle one correct answer for each question.

1. Rather than viewing families as a resource, nursing home personnel most commonly see them
   a. Primarily as volunteers for the nursing home's fund-raising activities.
   b. As an additional source of stress.
   c. As a great way to make new social contacts.
   d. As additional patients who must be nurtured, loved, and cared for.

2. Family members most often view nursing home personnel as
   a. Potential members for their church or synagogue.
   b. Incompetent, uncaring, or uneducated.
   c. The most valued persons in the facility.
   d. People who care greatly for the well-being of their relatives.

3. Most family members bring many personal biases to the nursing home. These generally include
   a. The conviction that placement in a nursing home is absolutely the best solution to their caregiving problems.
   b. The idea that they no longer need to control their relative's life and environment.
   c. The guilty feeling that people go to a nursing home only when there is no other place to live.
   d. The notion that placement in the nursing home is the most inexpensive means of caring for their loved one.

4. Before being placed in a nursing home, the patient and his or her primary family caregiver have often had severe communication problems leading to
   a. Either patient-to-caregiver or caregiver-to-patient violence.
   b. Vast improvement in the social life of the caregiver, who has typically learned to find fun and relieve stress outside the home.
   c. A higher rate of caregiver enrollment in psychotherapeutic counseling with a professional.
   d. A helpful change in the time that the two people communicate best with one another, usually from late evening to midday.

5. Families of Alzheimer's disease patients must make many emotional and spiritual adjustments. Which statement is most likely to be true?
   a. Typically, the person who has made the hard decision to place a relative in the nursing home is praised and supported by family members.
   b. The search for meaning in the disease is resolved by the time placement

occurs; caregivers are at peace with the thought that this was "God's will" or "meant to be."

   c. Caregivers have little need to grieve further over the loss of their loved one after nursing home placement; that is why nursing home memorial services are a waste of time and money.

   d. The feelings of guilt, anger, and mourning often resurface after the primary family caregiver has released a relative to the nursing home; this is why staff members see so much need for reassurance, denial of earlier problems, and defensiveness among family members.

6. Which of the following statements is true?

   a. The personal communication problems between family caregivers and their relatives dissolve quickly once the patient comes to live in the nursing home.

   b. Communication problems between family caregivers and patients are seldom the result of clinical communication impairments, such as hearing loss, depression, and other problems associated with aging.

   c. Family caregivers' personal communication impairments can often be the source of communication problems with the staff as well as with the patient.

   d. Because family members are generally so relieved when they discover their relatives are receiving superior care, it is easy and fun to work with them.

7. Family members' perceptions of the care their relatives receive is based almost entirely on

   a. The quality of their own interactions with staff caregivers.

   b. The quality of food in the nursing home.

   c. The level of training and education of the staff.

   d. How much they are left alone with their relative when they come to visit; privacy with the patients becomes very important to them.

8. According to studies, family members tend to be most sensitive to

   a. How clean, neat, and efficient the staff appears to be.

   b. How many activities their relatives are taken to in a day.

   c. The degree to which the nursing home environment is sunny, light, and attractive.

   d. How well the staff protects the dignity and individuality of the patient.

9. Which of the following statements is not true?

   a. Family members believe that their perceptions are true and they act on those beliefs whether or not they are accurate.

   b. You, the professional caregiver, cannot be responsible for reassuring family members or listening to their troubles and complaints; your role is to get your job done for the patients in your care.

   c. Most staff members do not feel prepared to deal with the problems that families perceive and bring to the nursing home.

   d. You might reduce conflicts with the family if you provide them with clear guidelines for how they can assist in caregiving, how they should direct their complaints, and how they might take advantage of a support group.

10. Families usually do not expect you to give them advice; they just need to talk. This means that as you listen, you should

   a. Interrupt frequently to keep them on topic.

   b. Ask a lot of questions so you will get information that is useful to you.

   c. Use empathetic statements that lead people to say how they feel.

   d. Immediately report any complaint to your supervisor and other staff members so that together you can plan ways to head off troublemakers.

IN-SERVICE 9 QUIZ:
Creating Successful Conversations

Directions: Circle all of the possible correct answers to each question.

1. You should frequently engage your Alzheimer's disease patients in social conversation because
   a. The patient's family will think you are a nice person.
   b. Many of these patients are still capable of meaningful communication.
   c. Responding to the social needs of the patient reduces the likelihood of catastrophic reactions.
   d. It forces you to practice good English.

2. Task talk
   a. Is abrupt and rude; it should seldom be used with Alzheimer's disease patients.
   b. Is any command that tells a patient what to do.
   c. Places the patient into a passive role and fosters dependency.
   d. Is the communication style used most often by direct-care staff members with their patients.

3. Social conversation
   a. Is a healthy, natural way to nourish another person's self-esteem.
   b. Tends to be fruitless with persons with Alzheimer's disease.
   c. Becomes more difficult with residents with Alzheimer's disease as their cognitive abilities decline.
   d. Is a type of communication that encourages persons with Alzheimer's disease to interact more genuinely.

4. Taking responsibility for social conversation with a resident with Alzheimer's disease means
   a. Giving the resident enough time to respond before going on to your next utterance.
   b. Understanding that the resident may not use the correct words or have the facts straight.
   c. Opening a conversation instead of waiting for the resident to begin.
   d. Bringing up topics of specific interest to the resident.

5. You know you have had a successful conversation with a resident with Alzheimer's disease when
   a. The resident eats a better lunch afterward.
   b. The resident answers you with a complete sentence.
   c. You see signs that the two of you have shared a thought or a feeling, eye contact, a nod or smile, a phrase or two in reply.
   d. A patient who has not spoken in a long while gives you an answer.

6. Choice questions
   a. Allow residents to recognize a possible correct answer.
   b. Demean patients because they make things too simple.
   c. Are often an excellent way to manage behavior and reduce refusal and resistance.
   d. Are not as helpful as open-ended questions, which allow patients to elaborate in any way they wish.

7. If you want to have a successful conversational exchange with a resident with Alzheimer's disease, you should never
   a. Bring up your own opinions or experience.
   b. Laugh at what they say.
   c. Rely on a series of friendly affirmations ("yes," "um hmm," "you don't say") to keep the conversation going.
   d. Use only task talk.

8. The following responses are examples of repair techniques:
   a. (Patient: "I need that. Hand it to me.") "The cup is hard for you to reach; here's your cup, Sarah."
   b. (Patient: "There aren't enough towels.") "Those aren't pillows, Jesse. That's toilet paper. Toi-let pa-per, see?"
   c. (Patient: "Abby came.") "I thought I saw Dolores in the hallway. Dolores, your daughter? Dolores has lost a little weight, hasn't she?"
   d. (Patient: "Hi, Ellen.") "It's not Ellen, honey. Don't you remember me? I'm here on the weekends. Good ole Helen, every Saturday just for you."

9. Direct orders should be used with residents who have Alzheimer's disease
   a. Because they make residents feel most secure when they are told what to do in no uncertain terms.
   b. Because they are just about the only way to get some patients to cooperate.
   c. Because they take less time.
   d. As little as possible because they invite resistance and refusal.

10. Recent research shows that persons who are more mentally and physically active succumb to Alzheimer's disease at a slower rate. This means that
   a. You should insist that your residents be as accurate as possible and always keep a grip on the "truth."
   b. You should frequently point out to the resident exactly what he is forgetting so that he is as aware as possible.
   c. You should provide as many activities as possible at levels that encourage residents to participate.
   d. You should work to keep the resident in the "conversation game" as often and as long as possible.

IN-SERVICE 10 QUIZ:
Handling Difficult Communication Situations

Directions: Circle one correct answer for each question.

1. When a resident has a catastrophic reaction
   a. Communicate calmly with a nonverbal approach: move slowly, keep your arms down and your hands open. Maintain a friendly smile.
   b. Use a loud, high-pitched voice so that the patient can hear you clearly.
   c. Refrain from using eye contact; eye contact is always threatening to a patient with Alzheimer's disease.
   d. Avoid asking for another staff person's help.

2. One of your communication goals for caring for a resident who responds with extreme and inappropriate emotion to a situation is to
   a. Apply physical restraints quickly so that the resident will not harm others.
   b. Prevent the director of nurses from finding out.
   c. Try to understand the meaning behind the person's reaction.
   d. Maneuver the resident to the nursing station immediately so that your colleagues can appreciate how difficult the person is to control.

3. Inappropriate or repetitive behaviors
   a. Must be ignored; they are a product of Alzheimer's disease and there is little that anyone can do except endure them.
   b. Are not manifestations of the disease but are caused by irresponsible use of pet therapy.
   c. Can sometimes be reduced or made less annoying by changing staff responses or environmental arrangements.
   d. Have no meaning as far as the patient's communication is concerned.

4. A resident's hallucinations
   a. Can be useful if you want to demonstrate to the family or the physician how poorly the person is doing.
   b. Should be corrected immediately by using consistent reality orientation techniques.
   c. Can be accepted by you as a moment of conversation if the person is not upsetting others.
   d. Can only be attributed to a toxic drug reaction.

5. When residents constantly repeat questions or phrases
   a. Ask them to write down their questions and you can read them when you have time.
   b. Refer them to the bulletin board where the day's or week's activities are listed.

c. Sit with them at least 10 to 15 minutes twice a day and talk to them.

d. Make a binder or wallet with a few single words or pictures to remind them of the information they wish to remember.

6. Many times when residents resist the caregiver
   a. It is because they feel they are being treated like children.
   b. They do so with the deliberate intention of upsetting the caregiver.
   c. They have resisted authority all their lives and do not know how to react differently.
   d. They are having an adverse reaction to drugs.

7. A resident's resistant behavior might be avoided if the caregiver
   a. Stands above the person's eye level, uses firm body language, such as hands on hips or arms crossed, and adopts a serious face and a clear voice of authority.
   b. Adopts a cheerful tone of voice, a little louder than usual, and coaxes the persons with terms such as "sweetie" and "lamb chop."
   c. Rephrases rather than repeats the request exactly as one way of helping an Alzheimer's disease patient understand.
   d. Avoids all body language and says the key words only one time so that the person does not become confused by too many messages.

8. Residents who wander the facility and pilfer through other people's belongings
   a. Are looking for where they belong or for their own possessions.
   b. Were probably kleptomaniacs before they entered the nursing home.
   c. Are exercising their deep-seated need to clean house.
   d. Seldom get past this agitated phase of their illness.

9. The nature of institutional environments and routines serves to intensify an Alzheimer's patient's wandering and pilfering. Therefore staff should consider
   a. Demanding higher standards of behavior from the residents.
   b. Adding unique symbols to help residents identify their own doorways, name plates, seating spaces, and bed coverings more easily.
   c. Changing the residents' rooms and roommates frequently, to help them exercise their memories and afford them fresh new beginnings.
   d. Removing their own name tags. A name tag is only another sign of "institutionalization" and the residents cannot read anyway.

10. The paranoia over possessions that manifests itself in residents who have Alzhiemer's disease
    a. Is without basis in an institutional setting. No one would dream of taking the possessions of a person who has Alzheimer's disease.
    b. Suggests that they were greedy and possessive before they became ill.
    c. Is difficult for other residents and challenges professional caregivers to use their communication skills as mediators.
    d. Is not the concern of direct care staff. Security regulations should cover these situations adequately.

IN-SERVICE 11 QUIZ:
Direct Intervention Programs: Increasing Communication Opportunities for Residents with Alzheimer's Disease in the Nursing Home

Directions: Circle one correct answer for each question.

1. When residents with Alzheimer's disease are placed into a direct communication intervention program
   a. They have a good chance to be cured of their communication disorders.
   b. Their expressive communication may be worse for a while as their comprehension improves.
   c. Their communication may improve if the program also focuses on improving the responses of caregivers and on improving the arrangement of the environment.
   d. You will not have to work so hard on your own communication skills.

2. Which of the following situations would provide the best opportunity for engaging a patient in conversation?
   a. You meet the patient moving quickly toward the bathroom.
   b. You are wheeling the patient to her next activity; she has a moderate to severe hearing loss.
   c. You are bringing the patient his or her morning snack.
   d. You peek your head into the patient's room and notice that he or she has visitors.

3. The least desirable goal for a communication intervention program would be
   a. To release the patient's early memories and encourage his or her ability to speak about them.
   b. To build the skills of individual caregivers, especially in nursing homes that have a large turnover of personnel.
   c. To develop quick and easy communication techniques for caregivers.
   d. To promote learned helplessness in the patient.

4. A memory notebook serves many purposes. However, it does not
   a. Help to maintain present orientation and early life memories.
   b. Take advantage of the patient's ability to read single words.
   c. Provide a conversation piece to which other patients and caregivers can respond.
   d. Offer the patient a chance to learn about current events.

5. The communication partners program works best if
   a. The volunteer has 10 months of rigorous training in communication skills first.
   b. It is operated as an "English only" program.
   c. The volunteer is able to visit the patient frequently and perhaps even see the patient through the final stages of Alzheimer's disease.
   d. The activities are planned solely around the volunteer's interests and abilities.

6. In programs such as FOCUSED, caregivers
   a. Are given instruction and role-playing practice to improve their communication skills.
   b. Earn a certificate in gerontology.
   c. Learn new skills primarily by viewing videotapes.
   d. Are assured that they have no responsibility in the decline of the communication skills of Alzheimer's disease patients.

7. Which of the following would be the least desirable procedure for an Alzheimer's disease conversation group?
   a. Prevent wandering by placing the table in the corner of the room.
   b. Reward every single effort that every patient makes to communicate.
   c. Serve some food or drink at every session.
   d. Stick to a structured question-and-answer format at all times.

8. Programs such as the Breakfast Club or conversation groups
   a. Rely on the facilitator to do most of the talking and encourage patients to interact with the group facilitator rather than with each other.
   b. Provide a central conversational theme on which the patients can focus and objects they can manipulate, such as food, a Polaroid camera, or plants.
   c. Try to schedule at least 10 patients to a group to stimulate verbalization and increase interactions.
   d. Usually focus on orienting the patient to day, time, and place.

9. The Breakfast Club is a good way to
   a. Teach patients how to cook.
   b. Set up a strict structure for the participants so that they do not have to make any decisions.
   c. Put the patients on a healthier diet.
   d. Stimulate all five senses and allow practice of the procedural skills and social rituals that go with mealtime.

10. A direct intervention program that seeks to help a person with Alzheimer's disease to remember an important piece of information is
   a. Validation therapy.
   b. Spaced retrieval therapy
   c. FOCUSED therapy
   d. Communication partners

IN-SERVICE 12 QUIZ:
Last Things: When a Person with Alzheimer's Disease is Dying

Directions: Circle one correct answer for each question.

1. Palliative care
   a. Is best provided by the resident's favorite caregiver.
   b. Is best handled by the family's faith community or clergy person.
   c. Includes aggressive measures such as daily speech therapy or resuscitation.
   d. Focuses on improved quality of life as a primary goal.

2. One of the goals of complementary and alternative therapies (CAM) is to
   a. Cure the resident of aches and pains
   b. Prolong life
   c. Reduce anxiety and place the resident into a deep state of relaxation
   d. Calm the residents down so that they can say what is really bothering them.

3. If the resident no longer draws or uses information from the environment, caregivers can
   a. Relax about references to the person's medical status while in his presence.
   b. Hold the resident's hand for a few minutes every day to maintain a bond of human warmth.
   c. Turn on the TV so that the resident can enjoy it in a lucid moment.
   d. Encourage the family to take longer breaks between visits.

4. A resident's cries that are inappropriate, repetitive, and inconsolable may be
   a. A sign of undiagnosed pain or illness.
   b. Empty speech.
   c. A sign of impending death.
   d. A deliberate bid for attention.

5. A resident's disruptive vocalizations might decrease if
   a. The staff can no longer hear the cries.
   b. The staff plays audiotapes to the resident of familiar voices, music, or white noise at regular intervals.
   c. A volunteer sits and talks to the patient for several hours every day.
   d. The resident is given a warm bath every day.

6. One way to continue to communicate with a person in the late stages of Alzheimer's disease is to
   a. Talk louder to the resident.
   b. Keep your comments simple and direct: task talk only.
   c. Watch TV while feeding the patient.
   d. Learn how to give one type of complementary therapy treatment.

7. Which statement is not true?
   a. Healing touch does not always involve touch.
   b. Aroma therapists prefer to use scented candles, air sprays, and perfumed powder.
   c. Music therapy is highly individualized and prescriptive. One person's therapeutic music is another's idea of a 5:00 gridlock in downtown Hong Kong.
   d. Massage therapy is a means of reducing the emotional and physical isolation for the dying patient.

8. Which of the following statements is true?
   a. Providing complementary or alternative therapies to residents with Alzheimer's disease is silly because the physician has already said that "nothing more can be done."
   b. Most complementary therapies are expensive, time consuming, inconvenient, and highly risky to learn and administer.
   c. Patients do not have to participate or even be conscious to benefit from most complementary or alternative therapies.
   d. Massage therapists do not need a physician's orders to provide a full body or deep tissue massage.

9. An unobtrusive way of meeting the spiritual needs of dying residents with Alzheimer's disease might be to
   a. Read a treatise on body, mind, and spirit to the staff at your next meeting.
   b. Play a CD of your favorite rock gospel group to residents who are no longer conscious.
   c. Conduct a seance at the residents' bedsides.
   d. Invite a clergy person to your unit to informally meet your colleagues and a few residents.

10. Memorial services for deceased residents achieve spiritual and physical closure by
   a. Allowing staff and familiar visitors to say goodbye to each other.
   b. Honoring the bonds that have developed between professional caregivers and residents within their care.
   c. Giving surviving residents an opportunity to process and grieve the loss of one of their community.
   d. All of the above.

KEYS TO QUIZZES

INTRODUCTION	IN-SERVICE 1	IN-SERVICE 2	IN-SERVICE 3
1. a, b, c	1. c	1. b	1. a, b, c, d
2. a, c	2. b	2. a	2. a, c
3. b, d	3. a	3. c	3. b, c
4. a, b, c, d	4. d	4. d	4. b, c
5. a, b, c,	5. b	5. b	5. a, b, c
6. b, c	6. c	6. b	6. b
7. b, c, d	7. c	7. d	7. a, d
8. a, c, d	8. d	8. a	8. a, d
9. d	9. d	9. d	9. b, c, d
10. b, c	10. d	10. b	10. b, c

IN-SERVICE 4	IN-SERVICE 5	IN-SERVICE 6	IN-SERVICE 7
1. c, d	1. c	1. a	1. d
2. a, b, c	2. a	2. d	2. d
3. b, c, d	3. d	3. b	3. b
4. c	4. d	4. b	4. a
5. d	5. a	5. d	5. a
6. a, b, c, d	6. b	6. a	6. c
7. b, c, d	7. b	7. c	7. d
8. a, c	8. a	8. c	8. a
9. a, b	9. c	9. d	9. c
10. d	10. d	10. c	10. b

IN-SERVICE 8	IN-SERVICE 9	IN-SERVICE 10	IN-SERVICE 11
1. b	1. b, c	1. a	1. c
2. b	2. b, c, d	2. c	2. c
3. c	3. a, c, d	3. c	3. d
4. a	4. a, b, c, d	4. c	4. d
5. d	5. c	5. d	5. c
6. c	6. a, c	6. a	6. a
7. a	7. c, d	7. c	7. d
8. d	8. a, c	8. a	8. b
9. b	9. d	9. b	9. d
10. c	10. c, d	10. c	10. b.

IN-SERVICE 12			
1. d	4. a	7. b	10. d
2. c	5. b	8. c	
3. b	6. d	9. d	

APPENDIX **II**

Overheads

INTRODUCTION OVERHEADS

COMMUNICATION: *Communication* occurs when we send or receive messages or when we assign meaning to another person's signals.

Related words:

- Environment
  - Physical aspects
  - Psychosocial aspects

- Source and receiver

- Spoken words

- Expression

- Body language

Effective communication: Effective communication occurs when the message we intend is accurately understood by another person, who then replies appropriately.

Communication competence: The more ways we have of expressing ourselves, the greater the likelihood that we will be able to communicate effectively in any situation.

Verbal communication: Verbal communication consists of the actual words that we speak.

Nonverbal communication: More than 90% of our communication lies in the nonverbal realm:

- Expression

- Touch

- Body position

- Facial expression and eye contact

- Body orientation

- Personal appearance

- Gesture

- Personal environment

From Santo Pietro MJ, Ostuni E: Successful communication with persons with Alzheimer's disease: an in-service manual, St. Louis, Copyright © 2003, Mosby.

- We communicate most of our information nonverbally.

- Nonverbal communication can augment, repeat, substitute for, or even contradict verbal information.

- Our style of nonverbal communication is determined by our cultures, families, and individual personalities.

- Some people use nonverbal communication more effectively than do others.

- The ability to use and interpret nonverbal information helps us work effectively with Alzheimer's disease patients.

We communicate:

- To exchange information.

- To meet our physical needs.

- To meet our social and emotional needs.

- To engage in self-disclosure.

- To control, exert power, manipulate.

- To meet the needs of others.

- To have a therapeutic effect on others.

From Santo Pietro MJ, Ostuni E: Successful communication with persons with Alzheimer's disease: an in-service manual, St. Louis, Copyright © 2003, Mosby.

Effective communication:

- Saves time.

- Prevents mistakes; saves work later on.

- Calms patients; calms caregivers.

- Defuses power struggles; prevents catastrophic behaviors;
reduces the potential for abuse.

- Prevents learned helplessness in patients.

- Reduces isolation and depersonalization of patients and
caregivers.

- Promotes personal bonding between patients and
caregivers.

- Promotes self-esteem in patients and caregivers.

- Reduces worker stress; reduces high rate of caregiver
burnout.

- Saves facility money.

OVERHEAD 6 REQUIREMENTS FOR EFFECTIVE COMMUNICATION

- A place

- A shared language

- A common frame of reference

- A certain set of mental abilities: perception, attention, intellectual understanding, and memory

- Openness

- Expectation of response

- Respect and trust

From Santo Pietro MJ, Ostuni E: Successful communication with persons with Alzheimer's disease: an in-service manual, St. Louis, Copyright © 2003, Mosby.

IN-SERVICE 1 OVERHEADS:
Communication Problems and Strengths of Persons with Alzheimer's Disease and Related Disorders

Communication disorder: A communication disorder is a condition that interferes with a person's ability to be understood or to understand the communication of others.

Learned helplessness: "Learned helplessness arises when persons learn through repeated experiences that their actions have little effect on the outcome of the situation—especially in the 'restricted' environment of the nursing home." (Foy S, Mitchell M, *Phys Occup Ther Geriatr* 9:1, 1990)

Communication breakdown: Communication breakdown occurs when the listener does not understand the words or the intent, or both, of the speaker's message; it is *not* necessarily the result of a communication disorder.

OVERHEAD 1-2 EARLY-STAGE COMMUNICATION LOSSES DUE TO ALZHEIMER'S DISEASE

Memory

Patients lose
- Time orientation
- Some long-term and short-term memory (not always apparent in conversation)
- Recently acquired information
- Ability to retain five-item lists and telephone numbers

Understanding

Patients lose
- Ability to understand the following:
  - Rapid speech
  - Speech in noisy or distracting environments
  - Complex or abstract conversation
  - Sarcastic humor or innuendo
- Ability to process language rapidly

Speech and language skills

Patients lose
- Ideas of what to talk about
- Ability to process language rapidly (slow processing apparent in pauses and hesitancies)
- Rapid naming ability—use related words, such as "salt" for "sugar" (ability to self-correct is retained)

Social skills

Patients lose
- Ability to stay on topic
- Control over anger; become argumentative
- Conversational bridges; speech seems blunt and rude
- Ability to pay attention to speaker for more than a few minutes

From Santo Pietro MJ, Ostuni E: Successful communication with persons with Alzheimer's disease: an in-service manual, St. Louis, Copyright © 2003, Mosby.

OVERHEAD 1-3 MIDDLE-STAGE COMMUNICATION LOSSES DUE TO ALZHEIMER'S DISEASE

Memory	Understanding	Speech and language skills	Social skills
Patients lose	Patients lose	Patients lose	Patients
• Time and place orientation (not person)	• Ability to understand ordinary or prolonged conversation	• Naming abilities, especially abstract or specific words	• Lose ability to see things from another's point of view, become more egocentric
• Additional long-term and short-term memory (apparent in conversation)	• Ability to focus and maintain attention in presence of distraction or noise	• Fluency; there are more pauses, revisions, and sentence fragments	• Ask fewer questions
• Abstract vocabulary and concepts	• Ability to understand what is read, although reading mechanics are preserved	• Ability to self-correct	• Start fewer conversations
• Ability to remember names of less familiar people	• Some ability to read facial clues, although perception of emotional meaning is retained	• Loudness of voice and vocal expression in conversation	• Make less eye contact
• Ability to remember three-item lists or three-step commands		• Creative "propositional" use of language	• Seldom comment or self-correct
• Ability to retain information soon after presented			• Lose "niceness" in conversation

From Santo Pietro MJ, Ostuni E: Successful communication with persons with Alzheimer's disease: an in-service manual, St. Louis, Copyright © 2003, Mosby.

OVERHEAD 1-4 LATE-STAGE COMMUNICATION LOSSES DUE TO ALZHEIMER'S DISEASE

Memory	Understanding	Speech and language skills	Social skills
Patients lose	Patients lose	Patients lose	Patients lose
• Orientation to time, place and person • Ability to form new memories • Ability to recognize family members	• Ability to understand most word meanings • Overall awareness (do not seem to know when being spoken to)	• Ability to finish sentences • Grammar and diction; speak in jargon • May lose speech altogether; may become mute	• Awareness of social interaction or expectations • Apparent desire to communicate

OVERHEAD 1-5 CHARACTERISTIC CHANGES IN COMMUNICATION OF ALZHEIMER'S DISEASE PATIENTS

- Stereotypic language

- Empty speech

- Paraphasias

- Violations of conversational rules

- Windows of lucidity

From Santo Pietro MJ, Ostuni E: Successful communication with persons with Alzheimer's disease: an in-service manual, St. Louis, Copyright © 2003, Mosby.

- Loss of physical and financial independence

- Loss of livelihood and social role

- Loss of physical attractiveness and grooming skills

- Loss of energy

- Loss of family and friends

- Loss of familiar environments

- Loss of communication partners who speak the same first language

COMMUNICATION ABILITIES PRESERVED IN THE MIDDLE STAGE OF ALZHEIMER'S DISEASE

- The use of procedural memories

- The ability to access early life memories

- The ability to sing, recite, and read aloud with good pronunciation and grammar

- The ability to engage in social ritual

- The desire for interpersonal communication

- The desire for interpersonal respect

IN-SERVICE 2 OVERHEADS:
Additional Communication Disorders in Older Residents with Alzheimer's Disease

Speech: Speech is the way words sound when we talk.

Language: Language is composed of vocabulary, grammar, and intention to communicate—that is, putting words together into sentences to express ideas and feelings.

Voice: Voice is the sound produced by the vibrations of the vocal cords within the larynx, or "voice box," in the throat.

Hearing: Hearing is the sensory process by which sound is transmitted physically and neurologically from the environment to the brain, where it is interpreted as a message. The ear has three parts:
- Outer ear and ear canal
- Middle ear
- Inner ear

From Santo Pietro MJ, Ostuni E: Successful communication with persons with Alzheimer's disease: an in-service manual, St. Louis, Copyright © 2003, Mosby.

OVERHEAD 2-2 COMMUNICATION DISORDERS RESULTING FROM SENSORY IMPAIRMENTS

Hearing loss:

- Conductive loss
- Sensorineural loss
- Recruitment
- Tinnitus

Vision disorders:

- Cataracts
- Glaucoma
- Macular degeneration
- Loss of acuity

Definition: *Aphasia* is a problem understanding and expressing language that generally results from a stroke or other injury to the left side of the brain.

Types of aphasia:

- Fluent aphasia

- Nonfluent aphasia

- Global aphasia

Problems associated with aphasia:

- Hemianopsia

- Transient ischemic attack (TIA)

- Multi-infart dementia (MID)

Definition: *Dysarthria* is a speech problem caused by muscle weakness resulting from nerve damage.

Types of dysarthria:

- Flaccid dysarthria

- Spastic dysarthria

- Ataxic dysarthria

- Hypokinetic dysarthria

- Hyperkinetic dysarthria

- Mixed dysarthria

Definition: *Dysphagia* is difficulty swallowing due to neuromuscular weakness.

Swallowing takes place in four stages:

• Anticipatory phase

• Oral phase

• Pharyneal phase

• Esophageal phase

Definition: If a resident's voice is so quiet or hoarse that he cannot be heard by other residents or staff, he has a *voice disorder*.

Definition: Persons with tracheostomies breathe through stomas in the neck and cannot produce voice unless the stoma is completely covered.

To support residents with voice problems or tracheostomy:

- Support resident upright.

- Eliminate background noise and interruptions.

- Cue patient to "speak up" or "cover stoma."

- Provide amplification if necessary.

- Keep magic slate nearby for communication.

OVERHEAD 2-7 MEDICAL PROBLEMS NOT RELATED TO ALZHEIMER'S DISEASE THAT CREATE COMMUNICATION BREAKDOWNS

- Chronic illnesses

- Drug and medication problems

- Problems with oral hygiene and nutrition

- Clinical depression

- Balance and movement problems

IN-SERVICE 3 OVERHEADS:
Making Changes in the Physical Environment That Support Communication

Communication-impaired environment: "A communication-impaired environment is one in which there are few opportunities for successful, meaningful communication." (Lubinski R, *Dementia and communication*, Philadelphia, 1991, BC Decker.)

Physical environment: The physical environment includes the nursing home buildings and grounds and all the objects contained within. The physical environment also is the manner in which space is used and decorated and the sights, sounds, smells, tastes, and textures of each unique place.

- Poorly arranged or inadequate lighting, glaring or unfiltered light, shiny surfaces

- Lack of visual accessibility

- Missing or inadequate signs and information display (e.g., print that is too small, illegible; too much print matter)

- Too little visual stimulation

- Too much visual stimulation or clutter

- Too much ambient noise

- Lack of proper amplification where sound and voice must be heard

- Not enough pleasurable or soothing auditory stimulation, lack of familiar sounds and voices

FACTORS INTERFERING WITH THE ENJOYMENT OF AROMAS AND TASTE

Aromas:

- Lack of pleasant aromas

- Poor control of unpleasant odors

Tastes:

- Lack of positive taste experiences

- Staff inattention to residents' tastes and food preferences

- Unpleasant dining experiences

Holistic facility design:

- The Heritage Woods program

- The Eden alternative

- Gardening therapy

- The Snoezelen multisensory room

A sudden change in the patient's customary way of communicating can signal a serious medical problem or emotional crisis. Be alert to the following:

Sudden changes in speech:
- Speech becomes slurred, indistinct, or "mumbly."
- Patient is unable to speak; has facial droop or drooling.

Sudden changes in language:
- Resident becomes rude, agitated, more repetitive, even combative.
- Resident reverts to first language.
- Resident becomes restless or distraught in activities that were formerly enjoyed.
- Resident begins cursing, swearing, or using abusive language.

Sudden changes in voice:
- Resident's voice becomes very weak or "wobbly."
- Resident's voice becomes hoarse or "raspy" for prolonged periods.
- Resident's voice sounds wet or "gurgly," especially after eating or drinking.

IN-SERVICE 4 OVERHEADS:
Making Changes That Support Communication in the Psychosocial Environment

Premise: "Although it is unrealistic to assume that lifelong social roles can be completely retained, it is possible to cultivate a social environment that encourages self-sufficiency, independence, contribution, and self-expression to the degree possible for the individual." (Lubinski R, *Dementia and communication*, Philadelphia, 1991, BC Decker.)

Communication impaired environment: "A communication impaired environment is one where there are few opportunities for successful, meaningful communication." (Lubinski R, 1991).

Psychosocial barriers: Psychosocial barriers exist when:

- The environment and staff do not support the preserved abilities of the patient.

- The residents are not treated with regard or respect by the staff or other residents.

- The resident's privacy and personal space have low priority in a nursing home's daily operation.

PSYCHOSOCIAL BARRIERS TO COMMUNICATION—
COGNITIVE FUNCTIONS

Factors affecting preservation of cognitive functions:

- Too few activities appropriate for the Alzheimer's disease resident's level; insufficient transportation provided to and from activities

- Staff unawareness of a resident's personal history; disregard of cultural preferences and practices

- High staff turnover and absenteeism, precluding development of relationships between caregiver and resident

PSYCHOSOCIAL BARRIERS TO COMMUNICATION—
SOCIAL INTERACTION

Factors interfering with social interaction:

- Poor arrangement of rooms and furniture; drab and boring decor

- Unnecessarily restrictive institutional "rules" or unspoken policies

- Staff members who use primarily impersonal, task-related communication with residents; orders the residents; seldom take time for social conversation or companionship

- Lack of attention by staff to residents' personal hygiene and appearance

PSYCHOSOCIAL BARRIERS TO COMMUNICATION—
PRIVACY AND PERSONAL SPACE

Factors interfering with residents' rights and needs for privacy and personal space:

- Lack of sufficient space for private conversations or solitude

- Staff members and visitors who fail to respect residents' rights to privacy and personal space

- Inadequate procedures for protecting residents' personal possessions; claims of loss or theft not taken seriously

IN-SERVICE 5 OVERHEADS:
Communication Strengths and Problems of Professionals Who Care for Persons with Alzheimer's Disease

Communication style: *Communication style* is the set of verbal and nonverbal behaviors that a person typically uses to send or receive messages. Your personal communication style varies depending on the people involved, the circumstances, and your communication goals for the moment.

OVERHEAD 5-2 COMMUNICATION ADVICE FOR PROFESSIONAL CAREGIVERS

- Acknowledge your own communication strengths and weaknesses.
- Be willing to improve your personal communication style.
- Understand communication losses and retained abilities of Alzheimer's disease patients.
- Believe that good communication skills increase the patient's cooperation and decrease troublesome behaviors.
- Take responsibility for communicating with Alzheimer's disease patients.
- Know and use the personal histories of Alzheimer's disease patients as a resource for successful communication.
- Recognize and respond quickly to a patient's efforts to communicate.
- Adapt your personal communication style to meet each patient's communication needs.
- Be sensitive to changes in the patient's communication or other behaviors as a crisis prevention skill.
- Maintain a calm communication style, especially during crises.
- Be willing to ask for help in tough communication situations.
- Use stress management techniques to relieve personal tension.

From Santo Pietro MJ, Ostuni E: Successful communication with persons with Alzheimer's disease: an in-service manual, St. Louis, Copyright © 2003, Mosby.

OVERHEAD 5-3 POTENTIAL COMMUNICATION PROBLEMS OF PROFESSIONAL CAREGIVERS

- Speech, language, voice, and hearing problems

- Gender, status, and age biases

- Cultural and linguistic differences

- Personality factors

- Education and experience

- Situational influences

- Responses to burdens of professional caregiving

OVERHEAD 5-4 FINAL NOTE ON THE COMMUNICATION PROBLEMS OF PROFESSIONAL CAREGIVERS

Communication success or failure does not rest entirely on the skill level of the Alzheimer's disease patient. Success or failure rests heavily on *your* communication skills as well.

From Santo Pietro MJ, Ostuni E: Successful communication with persons with Alzheimer's disease: an in-service manual, St. Louis, Copyright © 2003, Mosby.

IN-SERVICE 6 OVERHEADS:
Multicultural Issues in Nursing Homes

Culture: Culture consists of the customary beliefs, social forms, and material traits of a racial, religious, or social group.

Ethnicity: "Ethnicity" pertains to a large group of people classed according to a common racial, national, tribal, religious, linguistic, or cultural origin or background. "Ethnic," a more precise term than "culture," refers to genetic markers and blood relationships as well as traditional behaviors and beliefs.

Company culture: A company culture determines the unspoken "rules" of a particular company that govern the employees' behavior, jokes, and manner of speaking and dress. The culture is rooted firmly in a company's:

- Product or service

- Mission statements and goals

- Hiring practices

- Requisite professional vocabulary

- Effective communication is at risk when people of diverse cultures work and live together in a closed community.

- Often, 30% to 40% or more of direct care staff members are from different countries, races, and cultural backgrounds from residents.

- Certified nursing assistants comprise the highest number of culturally diverse employees. They also provide 80% to 90% of the care for residents with dementia.

- Ninety percent of residents in most nursing homes are white, American- or European-born persons who speak English as a first language.

- Finding compatible methods of communication is critical to the smoothly functioning environment needed by patients with Alzheimer's disease.

From Santo Pietro MJ, Ostuni E: Successful communication with persons with Alzheimer's disease: an in-service manual, St. Louis, Copyright © 2003, Mosby.

FOSTERING GOOD COMMUNICATION IN A MULTICULTURAL SETTING: FOR SPEAKERS OF ENGLISH AS A FIRST LANGUAGE

- Learn to correctly pronounce the names of coworkers from foreign countries.
- Tolerate differences in communication styles if they are effective, even if they are culturally different from your own.
- If an individual's manner of speaking puzzles you, tactfully express your interest in learning about differences.
- Trust that others intend to say the right thing.
- Consider carefully who should counsel a coworker whose communication style is offensive to residents.
- Notice and support your colleagues' efforts to develop more effective ways of communicating.
- Develop a communication ethic of multicultural acceptance, and actively discourage toxic talk that involves racial slurs and embarrassing questions.
- Support your facility's diversity training programs.
- Develop mentoring programs between American-born staff and persons from another nationality, or between experienced staff and new immigrant recruits.

From Santo Pietro MJ, Ostuni E: Successful communication with persons with Alzheimer's disease: an in-service manual, St. Louis, Copyright © 2003, Mosby.

FOSTERING GOOD COMMUNICATION IN MULTICULTURAL SETTINGS: FOR EMPLOYEES WHO SPEAK ENGLISH AS A SECOND LANGUAGE

- Do not assume that communication breakdowns are always the fault of the non-native speaker of English.

- Keep a cool attitude when dealing with ethnically inspired insults from residents who have dementia.

- Never argue with the resident who has spoken offensively. When a resident's remarks hurt or frustrate you:
  - Speak with your supervisor.
  - Assess what happened just before the insult occurred; learn to look for other or additional triggers.
  - Evaluate your own style of communication and behavior.

From Santo Pietro MJ, Ostuni E: Successful communication with persons with Alzheimer's disease: an in-service manual, St. Louis, Copyright © 2003, Mosby.

IN-SERVICE 7 OVERHEADS:
The Toxic Effects of Verbal Abuse and Communication Neglect

Verbal abuse: Verbal abuse is one of several types of psychological mistreatment. One person speaks to another with the intention of causing emotional pain or controlling another's behavior through violent words.

Communication neglect: Communication neglect is a second type of psychological mistreatment. A person deliberately avoids looking at, talking to, or touching others as a means of withholding emotional warmth and nurturing.

In many states, verbal abuse and communication neglect are criminal acts and punishable by law.

- Inadequate governmental oversight and protection of residents' and caregivers' rights

- Administration failure to create and enforce policies that support caregivers and residents, or that enhance the facility's working conditions

- Personnel inexperienced in crisis prevention and intervention

- Inadequate staff training in how to prevent verbal abuse and communication neglect

- Staff members under extreme work-related stress, approaching "burn-out"

- Employee history of solving problems with violence

- Negative staff attitudes toward the residents (e.g., the residents "are like children and need to be disciplined," "can't tell anyone what I'm doing," or "will never know the difference")

- Repeated provocation by verbally aggressive residents upon staff members

OVERHEAD 7-3 THE SERIOUS RISKS OF NOT REPORTING AN INCIDENT OF ABUSE OR NEGLECT

- The resident could be seriously injured.

- The resident could become ill or die.

- The situation between the resident and the employee could become worse.

- The employee could abuse other residents.

- You could be contributing to the escalation by not saying anything.

- The situation could be discovered by the newspapers.

- You (the co-worker) could become legally involved if you knew and did not report and the situation were to be uncovered later.

- You would have it on your conscience.

- You would be compromising your professional integrity.

From Santo Pietro MJ, Ostuni E: Successful communication with persons with Alzheimer's disease: an in-service manual, St. Louis, Copyright © 2003, Mosby.

TEN WAYS TO PREVENT VERBAL ABUSE AND COMMUNICATION NEGLECT IN YOUR WORK SETTING

1. Guard against toxic talk inside and outside the workplace.
2. Understand the disease process: a resident's aggressive behavior usually is an expression of a severely compromised brain, but a caregiver's insensitive treatment can easily ignite the behavior.
3. Know your limitations; recognize your feelings and how they affect your work.
4. Trust your experience. Seasoned caregivers learn to stay calm in the face of a volatile situation.
5. Establish an informal "buddy system" for coping with aggressive residents.
6. Observe and learn from more experienced coworkers.
7. Read and know the resident's bill of rights.
8. Be familiar with your state's legal definitions of abuse and neglect.
9. Know your state's legal requirements and rights for reporting suspected abuse or neglect.
10. Speak to a trusted supervisor or a person in the administration hierarchy. Keep the discussion confidential.

From Santo Pietro MJ, Ostuni E: Successful communication with persons with Alzheimer's disease: an in-service manual, St. Louis, Copyright © 2003, Mosby.

IN-SERVICE 8 OVERHEADS:
Communicating with Families:
Same Goals, Different Goals

Family caregiver: The family caregiver is the person in the patient's family who takes primary responsibility for the patient's affairs. One third of primary family caregivers are elderly themselves. Nearly three fourths are women.

Caregiver burden: Caregiver burden results from the many physical, psychological, and financial stresses that Alzheimer's disease places on family members.

OVERHEAD 8-2 PROBLEMS THAT FAMILY CAREGIVERS BRING TO THE NURSING HOME

- Negative perception of the nursing home as a "last resort"

- Personal communication problems of the family caregiver

- Long-standing communication problems with the Alzheimer's disease patient
  - Loss of reciprocity
  - Asynchronies—loss of mealtime and bedtime relationships
  - Deterioration of caregiver's social life
  - Emotional scars from previous domestic violence

- Confusion over the transition in role from primary caregiver to visitor

- Spiritual and emotional neediness
  - Need to deal with feelings of guilt and sadness
  - Need to remain "connected" to the patient
  - Need to find meaning in the disease
  - Need to grieve over the slow loss of a loved one
  - Need to grieve over personal losses—time, energy, and affection

From Santo Pietro MJ, Ostuni E: Successful communication with persons with Alzheimer's disease: an in-service manual, St. Louis, Copyright © 2003, Mosby.

- Failing to ask family members to help with the care of the patient

- Appearing too busy to provide adequate care

- Not being well enough acquainted with patients to transport them to appropriate activities

- Working for the institution and not for the family

- Giving the impression that too many patient care duties have been "dumped" on the family

- Avoiding family caregivers or disregarding their importance to the patient

From Santo Pietro MJ, Ostuni E: Successful communication with persons with
Alzheimer's disease: an in-service manual, St. Louis, Copyright © 2003, Mosby.

IN-SERVICE 9 OVERHEADS:
Creating Successful Conversations

Conversation: Conversation is one avenue of communication when two or more people talk with one another on a subject of mutual interest.

Social conversation: Social conversation is a style of communicating that establishes mutually trusting relationships and nourishes self-esteem. Underlying agenda: adult-to-adult communication.

Task talk: The type of communication that caregivers use to get patients to do something (e.g., "Turn over." "Here's your lunch. Sit up." "Move your arm.") Underlying agenda: maintain efficient caregiving.

Institutional talk: A style of communicating defined by a partronizing attitude and tone of voice. Underlying agenda: parent-child relationship.

From Santo Pietro MJ, Ostuni E: Successful communication with persons with Alzheimer's disease: an in-service manual, St. Louis, Copyright © 2003, Mosby.

Conversational success: True interaction spoken between peers, lasting for as little as 5 seconds.

You will be more successful in your conversations with an Alzheimer's disease patient if you do the following:

- Watch carefully for signs that the patient wishes to communicate.

- Accept responsibility for keeping the conversation alive.

- Introduce topics that the patient enjoys and that are at his or her level of understanding.

- Accept even brief exchanges as being worthwhile.

- Stop worrying about the "correctness" or "logic" of a patient's utterances.

OVERHEAD 9-3 TECHNIQUES FOR SUCCESSFUL CONVERSATIONS WITH ALZHEIMER'S DISEASE PATIENTS

Use:

- **Choice questions:** Questions that contain the word "or" and give the person two choices.

- **Matching comments/associations:** Responses that draw from the caregiver's personal experience or opinion.

- **Closure:** An unfinished sentence that the patient is encouraged to complete.

- **Repair:** A word or statement that corrects the patient's error in a positive way by filling in missing information or replacing a vague term with a concrete one.

From Santo Pietro MJ, Ostuni E: Successful communication with persons with Alzheimer's disease: an in-service manual, St. Louis, Copyright © 2003, Mosby.

- **Direct orders:** Meeting a patient's resistance with a command

- **Affirmations:** Giving brief, agreeable responses that do not give enough information to help the patient think of an answer

- **Insistence on the "truth":** Insisting on reality in conversation, constantly correcting a resident's memory errors, repeatedly asking that the resident accurately report personal information

- **Yes-or-no questions:** Questions that can be answered with a simple "yes" or "no" that allow the person with Alzheimer's disease to respond in the shortest, easiest way possible without making any effort to add information to the conversation

From Santo Pietro MJ, Ostuni E: Successful communication with persons with Alzheimer's disease: an in-service manual, St. Louis, Copyright © 2003, Mosby.

DOS AND DON'TS FOR MAINTAINING SUCCESSFUL COMMUNICATION WITH ALZHEIMER'S DISEASE PATIENTS

1. Use adult language.
2. Maintain eye contact.
3. Use visual cues whenever possible.
4. Use simple words and short sentences.
5. Keep your explanations short.
6. Paraphrase, don't just repeat.
7. Avoid saying, "Don't you remember -?"
8. Use touch.
9. Do not shout.
10. Try not to interrupt.
11. Avoid competition.
12. Use a calm, reassuring tone of voice.
13. Do not talk about the patient in his or her presence.
14. Be realistic in your expectations.
15. Allow extra time for the patient to respond.
16. Pay attention to patients' nonverbal communication.
17. Remember that catastrophic reactions are not necessarily manipulative.
18. Listen carefully to "rambling."
19. Be willing to talk about "old times."
20. Continue to enjoy life.

From Santo Pietro MJ, Ostuni E: Successful communication with persons with Alzheimer's disease: an in-service manual, St. Louis, Copyright © 2003, Mosby.

IN-SERVICE 10 OVERHEADS:
Handling Difficult
Communication Situations

Inappropriate and repetitive behaviors: Inappropriate and repetitive behaviors are patterns of behavior that fail to match the social, emotional, cognitive, or linguistic context of the moment. These egocentric and difficult-to-handle behaviors are charged with emotional intensity, have a high rate of recurrence, and are characteristic of persons who suffer from the pervasive deterioration of the brain caused by Alzheimer's disease and related dementias.

Catastrophic reactions: Catastrophic reactions are emotional outbursts, sometimes accompanied by physical acting-out behavior, that appear to onlookers to be inappropriate or out of proportion to the situation. Catastrophic reactions may be triggered by present events or by something from the distant past.

From Santo Pietro MJ, Ostuni E: Successful communication with persons with Alzheimer's disease: an in-service manual, St. Louis, Copyright © 2003, Mosby.

- Catastrophic reactions

- Hallucinations

- Repetitive requests or statements

- Resistance, refusal

- Wandering, pilfering

- Paranoia

OVERHEAD 10-3 GOALS FOR COMMUNICATING EFFECTIVELY WHEN COPING WITH CATASTROPHIC REACTIONS

- Ensure the safety of the resident, yourself, and nearby persons

- Keep the situation from escalating

- Restore the resident to calm and routine behavior

- Understand the meaning of the resident's behavior

From Santo Pietro MJ, Ostuni E: Successful communication with persons with Alzheimer's disease: an in-service manual, St. Louis, Copyright © 2003, Mosby.

GOALS FOR COMMUNICATING EFFECTIVELY WHEN COPING WITH INAPPROPRIATE AND REPETITIVE BEHAVIORS

- Reduce staff and resident frustrations.

- Understand the resident's underlying message.

- Reshape the resident's repetitive behaviors into useful communication.

- Reshape caregiver responses or environment to match the resident's behavior.

IN-SERVICE 11 OVERHEADS:
Direct Intervention Programs: Increasing Communication Opportunities for Residents with Alzheimer's Disease

Communication opportunity: A communication opportunity is any encounter between two persons that offers the possibility for "good communication."

Direct communication intervention programs: Direct communication intervention programs are specifically defined approaches to providing and encouraging communication opportunities for persons with Alzheimer's disease.

From Santo Pietro MJ, Ostuni E: Successful communication with persons with Alzheimer's disease: an in-service manual, St. Louis, Copyright © 2003, Mosby.

- Maintain as many of the Alzheimer's disease patient's residual functional communication strengths as possible.

- Prevent overreaction to disability or "learned helplessness."

- Relieve the burden of caregiving; maintain the health and integrity of the caregiver.

- Improve the quality of life and maintain the human dignity of both patient and caregiver.

- Establish harmonious functioning within the nursing home setting.

From Santo Pietro MJ, Ostuni E: Successful communication with persons with
Alzheimer's disease: an in-service manual, St. Louis, Copyright © 2003, Mosby.

ADVICE FOR CHOOSING A COMMUNICATION INTERVENTION THAT TARGETS PATIENT BEHAVIORS

- Choose activities that allow the patient to practice everyday communication skills, ones that recur in the resident's daily life and that the environment will support.

- Choose activities that match the everyday routines of the nursing home (e.g., do not center activities on a single care provider if there is a high turnover of personnel; do not work on singing if patients are required to keep quiet).

- Choose activities that capitalize on the patient's remaining abilities.

OVERHEAD 11-4 ADVICE FOR CHOOSING A COMMUNICATION INTERVENTION THAT TARGETS CAREGIVER BEHAVIORS

- Target communication behaviors that are likely to occur in the everyday repertoire of the caregiver and the patient.

- Target communication behaviors that are achievable and have tangible results.

- Match the goals of the program to the level of the patient with whom the caregiver is communicating.

DIRECT INTERVENTION PROGRAMS FOR COMMUNICATING MORE EFFECTIVELY WITH ALZHEIMER'S DISEASE PATIENTS

Programs that target the patient's communication skills:

- **Spaced Retrieval:** A one-on-one method for helping persons with Alzheimer's disease remember specific pieces of important information

- **Memory notebooks or wallets:** Albums of pertinent information about the patient that use simple sentences and pictures and serve as conversation or memory devices between patient and caregiver

- **Conversation groups:** Group interaction encouraged by means of reminiscence, current events, games, and conversation

- **The Breakfast Club:** A small group of Alzheimer's disease patients directed in a structured way to prepare, serve, and eat breakfast and to clean up afterward

DIRECT INTERVENTION PROGRAMS FOR
COMMUNICATING MORE EFFECTIVELY WITH
ALZHEIMER'S DISEASE PATIENTS

Programs that target caregiver communication skills:

- **Communication partners:** Volunteers, sought first from among the patient's friends, who are trained to communicate more successfully with the communication-impaired patient

- **The FOCUSED program:** A program for family and professional caregivers who are taught to incorporate seven general principles of good communication when they are with their Alzheimer's disease patients

From Santo Pietro MJ, Ostuni E: Successful communication with persons with Alzheimer's disease: an in-service manual, St. Louis, Copyright © 2003, Mosby.

IN-SERVICE 12 OVERHEADS:
Last Things: When a Person with Alzheimer's Disease Is Dying

Alternative therapy, complementary, or integrative therapy: Alternative therapies are interventions used instead of traditional Western medical practices. In the United States, a patient who chooses an herbal remedy rather than a prescribed drug to relieve pain has selected an alternative intervention. Complementary or integrative therapies are used by patients simultaneously with, or as a complement to, traditional therapies, as when a person elects to try both acupuncture and physical therapy to loosen muscle spasms.

Disruptive vocalizations: Disruptive vocalizations are the inappropriate, repetitive, inconsolable, and very loud noises or words shouted by some residents who are in the late stages of Alzheimer's disease.

Palliative care: Palliative care is active total care of patients who are dying, whose disease is deemed by medical prognosis to be incurable, and for whom life-prolonging procedures are no longer feasible. The principles of palliative care include improved quality of life and intensive pain management, a team approach to care, and treatment of the patient and family as a single unit.

Ruling out physical causes:

1. Have causes of a painful medical nature been ruled out?
2. Are physical needs being tended to sooner rather than later?

Determining a pattern:

3. Is there a predictable pattern to the crying behavior?
4. Could staff or volunteers establish a pattern of visits to the resident?
5. Are there staff members or volunteers who are more successful in quieting the resident?

Making environmental and logistical adaptation:

6. Could an area for the crying patient be fitted with special sound proofing?
7. Could sound buffers be devised to protect others in the vicinity from the noise?
8. Could crying residents be placed closer to the hub of activity for greater stimulation; or further away, to avoid over-stimulation?

Providing direct intervention:

9. Would techniques of behavior modification—that is, giving the resident more attention during quiet periods—be effective?
10. Have a variety of sensory stimuli been consistently tried?

OVERHEAD 12-3 THE DEEPEST COMMUNICATION NEEDS OF THE DYING

- Forgive me

- I forgive you

- Thank you

- I love you

- Good-bye

Complementary treatments

- Allow caregivers to stay in touch when words no longer work.

- Benefit patients after traditional interventions have ceased to be effective.

- Reduce the patient's anxiety and induce a peaceful relaxed state.

- Produce positive results independently of the patient's knowledge or participation.

- Are noninvasive.

- Are low risk of physical or emotional damage or abuse.

- Are provided at the resident's bedside and thus are accessible and private.

- Can be as comforting to the giver as to the receiver.

- Are less expensive than chemical restraints, more humane than physical restraints.

- Can be learned and practiced by family and volunteers as well as health care providers.

The essential issues that bond caregiver to care receiver:

- The importance of social communication and relationships for persons with Alzheimer's disease

- The respect for the dignity of the person with Alzheimer's disease no matter what stage or what condition he or she is in

- The professional caregiver's acknowledgment of human values that include body, mind, and spirit

- The professional caregiver's commitment to quality of service and care

- The right of both direct care staff and residents to environments, procedures, and policies that encourage and support their best efforts

May these "last things" become the cornerstone "first things" of your particular journey in professional caregiving.

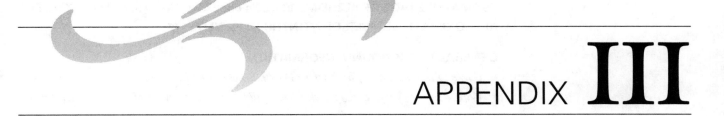

Model Case Study of a Communication-Impaired Resident

INITIALS OF RESIDENT: *T.R.*   **AGE:** *79*   **SEX:** *M*

FIRST LANGUAGE: *Italian*   **LEVEL OF EDUCATION:** *Ph.D.*

PREVIOUS OCCUPATION: *Research scientist, University of Maryland*

ESTIMATED STAGE OF ALZHEIMERS (circle one): Mid (Mid-Late) Late Terminal

APPROXIMATE NUMBER OF MONTHS IN FACILITY: *14*

GENERAL BACKGROUND INFORMATION:

- *Came to U.S. at age 25, just before WWII. Smoker until age 60.*
- *Wife died 1¹/₂ years ago. Two children: Oldest son now a missionary in South Africa. Daughter who lives 60 miles away visits once or twice a month.*
- *Enjoys Italian food. Used to play guitar in a small combo. No religious preference.*

I. COMMUNICATION PROBLEMS CAUSED BY SENSORY IMPAIRMENTS

Hearing impairment or tinnitus: *Mild hearing loss, unaided (never been formally evaluated)*

Vision disorders: *Cataracts, glaucoma*

II. COMMUNICATION PROBLEMS CAUSED BY SPEECH OR LANGUAGE DISABILITIES

Aphasia (at risk for stroke, diabetes):

Dysarthria or dysphagia:

Voice disorders: *Mild but persistent hoarseness (ex-smoker, 40 years)*

Tracheostomy:

Other:

III. COMMUNICATION BREAKDOWNS CAUSED BY MEDICAL PROBLEMS

Chronic illnesses: *Diabetes controlled by diet, mild arthritis*

Drugs and medication problems:

- *Aricept (should stave off some struggle with memory and cognitive challenges)*
- *Halcion*
- *Ibuprofen as needed for arthritic pain*

Problems with oral hygiene and nutrition: *Low-sugar, low-fat diet required*

Clinical depression: *Mild*

Balance and movement problems: *Some stiffness getting out of bed, walking in the mornings.*

IV. COMMUNICATION PROBLEMS CAUSED BY THE AGING PROCESS

Loss of independence: *Yes, but self-sufficient within confines and routine of nursing home*

Loss of livelihood and social role: *Yes. Never receives visits from university colleagues. University is 30 miles away.*

Loss of physical attractiveness: *No*

Loss of energy: *Not severe*

Loss of family and friends: *Wife deceased, one son in Africa, daughter 60 miles away*

Loss of familiar environments: *Yes*

Loss of first-language partners: *Yes*

V. COMMUNICATION BREAKDOWNS CAUSED BY ALZHEIMER'S DISEASE

Memory problems: *Moderate short-term memory loss*

Comprehension problems: *Yes, increasing*

Expressive language problems: *Reverts to Italian with increasing frequency*

Social skills: *Social inappropriateness. Has recently made sexual advances at young CNA*

Empty speech? Stereotypical/repetitive speech? *Severe empty speech*

Mutism? Continual crying out: *A lot of unintelligible speech in Italian*

VI. REDUCING COMMUNICATION PROBLEMS FOR THE RESIDENT

Sensory impairments?

- *Eye exam: Is not wearing glasses that he brought into nursing home.*
- *Label pathways, doors, staff ID badges, and personal possessions in large bold letters.*
- *Direct care staff should be sensitive to how visual and auditory impairments and motor stiffness will decrease attention to conversational speech. They should use appropriate compensations in their speech style (slow rate of speech, low-pitched voice, speaking face to face, light on speaker's face, hold conversation until T.R. can give attention to speaker).*
- *Remove patient to quiet environment when conveying important information.*

Speech, language disabilities?

- *Encourage drinking lots of water or sipping on ice chips to reduce risk of raw throat, inaudible voice due to hoarseness.*

Medical problems?

- *Explore option of antidepressant.*
- *Direct care staff should watch for nonverbal signs that level and frequency of arthritic pain are increasing. T. R. may not be able to adequately express discomfort in words.*

Aging process?

- *Find a communication partner (see In-Service 11) who speaks Italian or who plays the guitar.*
- *Make a memory book to bring distant family members and colleagues closer.*

Alzheimer's disease?

- *Try a memory book.*
- *Remove patient to quiet environment when conveying important information.*
- *Train direct care staff in how to respond to empty speech.*

COMMENTS: *Treatment plan should include methods of spiritual support as T. R. enters final stage of Alzheimer's disease. Desire for early religious symbolism or liturgy may need to be reexplored. Discuss with daughter possibility of complementary therapies such as massage therapy to decrease sexual inappropriateness (perhaps these moments are times when he feels physically and emotionally isolated) or music therapy to help calm patient after times of sexual agitation.*

APPENDIX **IV**

Sample Scripts

DIRECTIONS

The following pages contain excerpts from actual conversations that occurred between several Alzheimer's disease patients and their conversational partners.

SCRIPT 1   In the first example, Joe, the resident, is in the later stages of the disease. Look for and label the four effective conversational techniques: Choice, Closure, Matching Comment, and Repair.

Joe's partner misses a good opportunity to make another repair when Joe says, "They're all gone." How could she have replied?
Your suggestion for repair: _____

_____

[The resident's responses are in italics.]

Resident: *[Sneezes.]*
Conversational partner: God bless you!
God bless you!.
It sounds like you have a cold today.
I do.
This cold weather makes colds come. But today is lovely. Look at that beautiful blue sky. Is it clear or cloudy?
What?
Joe, is it clear or cloudy outside?
It's nice. It's clear.
[Looking at Joe's name tag]: Let me see your name tag. Your name is ____?
Joseph.
Some people are named after their relatives. What about you?
[Nods head] I was named for my grandfather.
[Pause] Our children are gone.
Your children—?
They're all gone.
They're all gone. Oh that happens.
Yeah. Tomorrow or the next day they're coming away.
Your children are coming to see you?
Next day or two.

(End Script 1)

SCRIPT 2   The following script is a good example of how the communication partner avoids getting into a power struggle to keep Joe in the room. She uses choice questions, describes and affirms his impulsive behavior, and redirects him gently with her conversation. Look for and label each choice question and description of the patient's behavior.

Compose your own repair to Joe's last comment: "Yeah, they try to fix it up." Would you choose a clearer verb than *fix* when talking about treating a cold? Also, what words would you suggest to replace *they* and *it*?

_____

_____

[The resident's responses are in italics.]

Conversational partner: Do you want to sit or stand up again?
Resident: *[Stands up.]*

OK, it feels better when you stand up.

Yeah.

Should I stand up next to you or sit down?

I don't care. I want to go back.

We can stay right here. That's not a problem.

No?

No. Let's listen for some music. I hear some big band music out there.

My head's warm.

Yes, it's a little bit warm. I don't think you have a fever. Do you need to go to the doctor?

I don't like doctors. No.

No, you'd rather stay home and take care of it yourself.

Yeah, they try to fix it up.

(End Script 2)

SCRIPT 3   The next conversation demonstrates how even our best efforts are not always successful. Although Kaye seems to recognize the topic, she is probably being asked to process more information than most Alzheimer's disease patients can handle.

If her communication partner had described Kaye's behavior and empathized with her restlessness, Kaye's attention might have returned. Then again, it might not have! If each communication moment is an opportunity for the resident, it is also a challenge for the staff member.

Write a different response to Kaye's remark, "I can't finish this." Use words that describe or affirm her behavior.

_____

_____

[The resident's responses are in italics.]

Conversational partner: I watched a TV show last night about a large ship that sunk in the ocean a long time ago, called the *Titanic*.

Resident: *Oh I remember that.*

You do?

Yeah.

Lots of people were on the Titanic.

[Indicating cake.] I can't finish this.

Oh just put it there and you can have more later. You said you remembered the *Titanic*?

Um-hum.

You remembered it being a big ship?

A big ship. Yes. I can't finish this.

That's OK, you can put it right down there. The *Titanic* was hit by a big iceberg.

I can't finish the tea either.

You can just sit with it. The *Titanic* was hit by a big hunk of ice. The boat rocked back and forth.

And it sunk.

It sunk. I don't think many people survived.

Right. I'm gonna go back.

(End Script 3)

SCRIPT 4   In this example, the conversational partner repeats many nouns to help a resident, Beth, develop the topic. Beth is very soft-spoken and never initiates conversation on her own. But if her partner takes her to a quiet corner with no distractions, Beth still shows an amazing ability to converse.

In the next to the last conversational turn, Beth cannot think of the word for spring. Once her partner uses the label, however, Beth recognizes it and uses it in her next response. This is a good example of how a repair (supplying the noun for the vague term) effectively supports further replies from the resident.

- Circle every noun (names of things) that the communication partner uses. How many are there?
- Read this successful conversation aloud with one of your colleagues. How long did the entire exchange take you to read? Seconds? Minutes?

[The resident's responses are in italics.]

Conversational partner: Seeing that shirt you have on makes me . . .
Resident: *[Interrupting.] Isn't it? It's too much though. I think it's too gaudy.*
I think the colors and the flowers are lovely.
I had it hanging in the closet and thought I'd better wear it.
I see one flower there that really makes me think of spring.
This one, the lilac.
I thought I saw a daffodil right there, see.
A daffodil. Oh yes, that's right.
Daffodils are one of the first flowers of spring. Right after the crocuses.
Right. I've noticed one thing out, the crocuses. They're popping up right now, aren't they, the crocuses?
Yes, the crocuses are popping up now.
I thought so because it's almost time for it.
Um, it's almost time for spring.
Spring, right.

(End Script 4)

INDEX

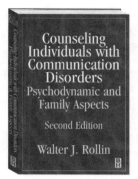
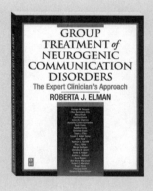
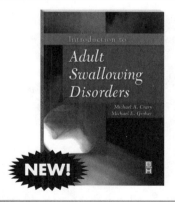
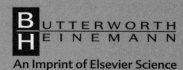

Green
fingers

IDEAS AND ADVICE
FROM TV'S LEADING
GARDENING EXPERTS

Edited by **Adam Pasco**

This book is published to accompany The Greenfingers Appeal.

Published by BBC Worldwide Ltd
Woodlands, 80 Wood Lane, London W12 0TT

First published 1999
Reprinted 1999 (twice)

ISBN 0 563 55114 3

One pound from the sale of this book will be donated to The
Greenfingers Appeal. In 1999 the Greenfingers Appeal is
benefitting Learning through Landscapes (registered charity
number 2485660), The Prince's Trust (registered charity number
803234) and Thrive (registered charity number 277570). In future
years other charitable projects will benefit.

Edited and designed by Cooling Brown
Cooling Brown team: Arthur Brown, Helen Ridge, Rachel Hagan,
        Peter Cooling, Tish Mills
BBC team: Vivien Bowler, Rebecca Hughes, Khadija Manjlai,
        Ellen Wheeler, Vicki Vrint

Set in Trade Gothic and Berkeley Italic, cover set in Officina
Printed and bound by Butler & Tanner Ltd, Frome and London
Colour separations by Radstock Reproductions Ltd,
        Midsomer Norton
Cover printed by Belmont Press Ltd, Northampton

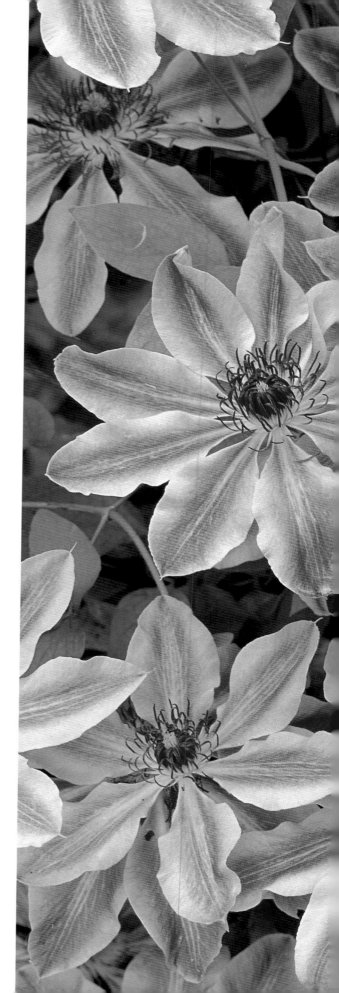

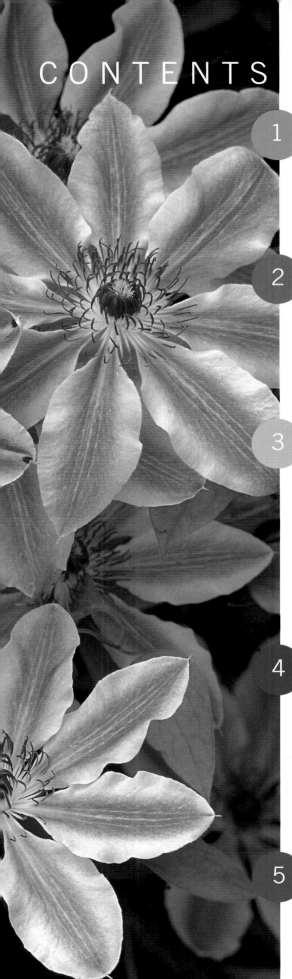

CONTENTS

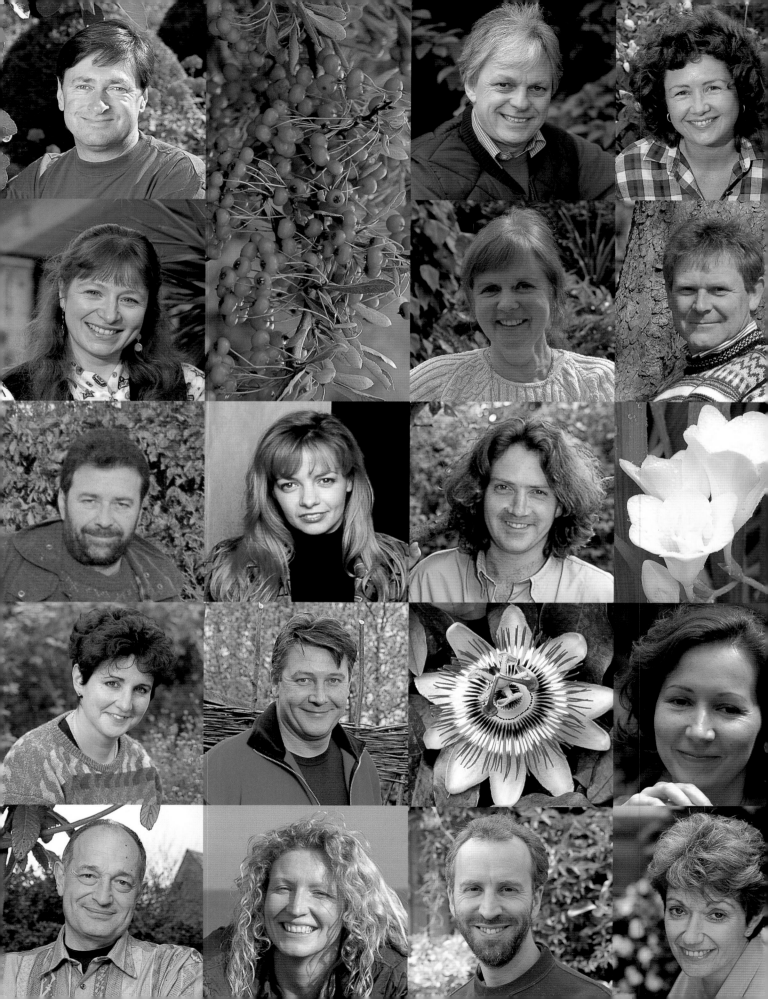

Green fingers

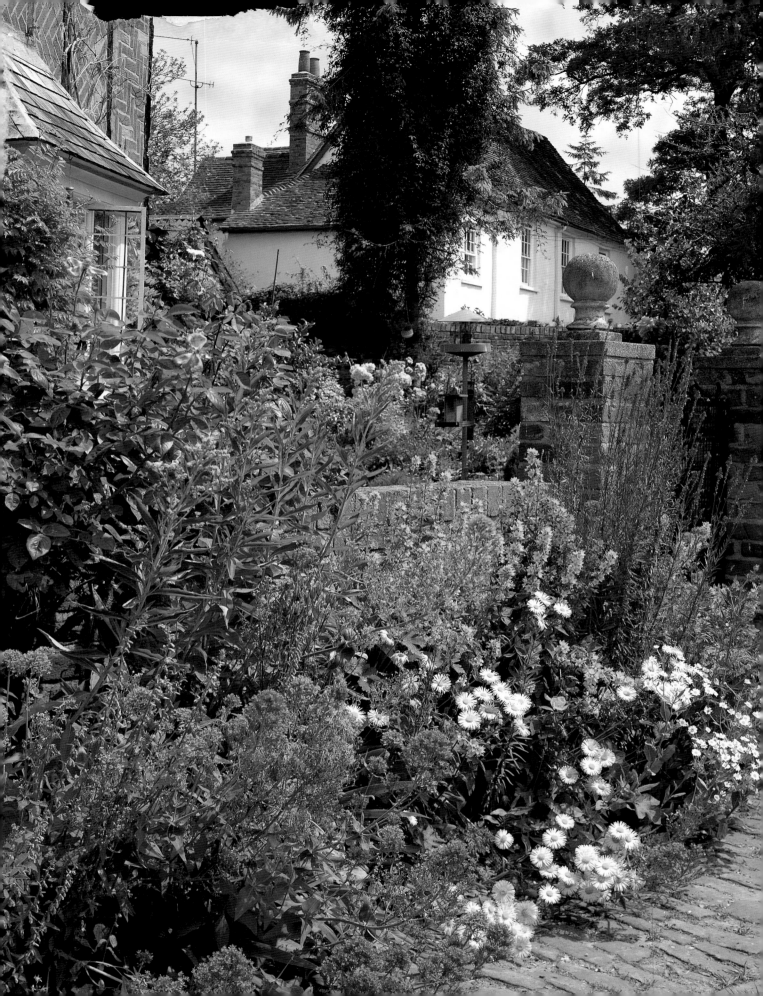

Foreword

Richard Jackson

What, another charity appeal? Well, yes, but this one's a bit blooming different. Gardeners up and down the country are raising money for the Greenfingers Appeal. We're digging deep to help those in need.

Everyone's doing their bit to help, from celebrity television and radio gardeners to students at horticultural colleges, garden centres to growers, and seedsmen and women to landscapers. This book is just one of the many money-raising schemes, and we're extremely grateful to all the writers, photographers and illustrators who have contributed their work free of charge. Without their generosity and enthusiasm, this book would never have appeared.

This book is just the tip of the iceberg. We've planned something to appeal to everyone during the Greenfingers 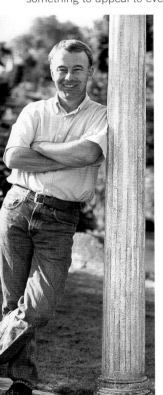 Appeal, for gardeners and non-gardeners alike. One of the wackiest is the Most Unusual Planted Container Competition. Truly extraordinary things are being planted up, from rusty cars to old bras! For children, there's the opportunity to take part in a nationwide Garden in a Seed Tray competition, while the more athletic among us will be attempting the National Wheelbarrow Challenge, in which enthusiastic gardeners will do everything (legal!) that's possible with a wheelbarrow. Plans are also afoot for other exciting activities, from marathons to formation barrow pushes. Hot favourites for this event include a team called the Red Barrows!

Later in the year, on the weekend of September 11 and 12, some of the top commercial growers will be opening their garden gates to the public. It's a unique opportunity to see how thousands of plants are grown from scratch. Pick up a few tips, enter competitions and get some of your gardening questions answered at the same time.

That's just a few of the events. There will be even more happening at flower shows, garden centres and nurseries, so check gardening magazines and your local press for details.

The Greenfingers Appeal is applying to become a registered charity so that its work can continue into the millennium. During 1999, the appeal will be supporting three national charities and using locally raised funds to support other charities, too. The aim is to cover all administration costs through donations from the gardening industry so that net proceeds from the sales of this book can go to the following three charities: Learning through Landscapes, The Prince's Trust and Thrive.

Learning through Landscapes is dedicated to helping schools improve their grounds for the benefit of pupils and the local community as a whole. Any money received from the Greenfingers Appeal will be used by the charity to support thousands of school grounds improvement projects in the UK.

The Prince's Trust aims to help young people succeed by providing opportunities that they would otherwise not have. In particular, they help those who, through disadvantage or lack of opportunity, are failing to reach their full potential. Any money raised through the appeal will be used to support the Prince's Trust Volunteer programmes, which are run from some 200 locations throughout the UK.

Thrive (previously called Horticultural Therapy) works on behalf of more than six million people in the UK who live with sensory or physical impairment, learning difficulties or mental ill-health. Thrive believes that gardening can enable these people to build the skills and confidence needed to change their lives. Money raised by the Greenfingers Appeal will help the charity support a national network of community projects that use gardening for training, rehabilitation or leisure.

By buying this book, you will be directly helping some very worthy causes. Thank you for supporting the Greenfingers Appeal, and happy gardening!

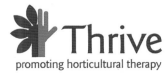

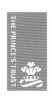

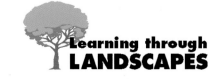

Alan Titchmarsh
It's a **Gardener's World**

When I started gardening for a living, I had to call it 'horticulture', to give it a bit of street cred in the eyes of my mates. Gardening? That was something their grandads did on the allotment at the weekend. Lads of my age didn't do it as a hobby, let alone take it up as a career. My dad was surprised to discover that you could actually train for it. His own father and grandfather had been jobbing gardeners who simply turned up, dug and weeded and then went home.

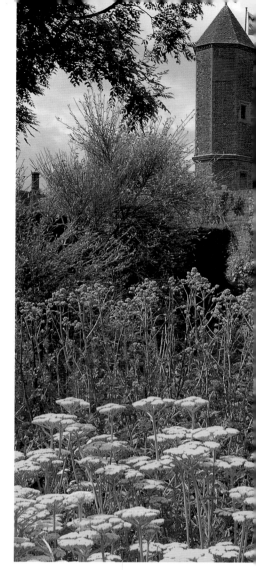

Funny how life changes. These days they call gardening 'the new sex', the new rock 'n' roll. I bet those lads who went into banks and insurance firms, local industry and farming wish they'd spent more of their youth in the garden, instead of spending it all indoors doing maths and accounting.

Why has it happened? Well, like all things, I think gardening has found its time. In the early part of the century, right up to the sixties in fact, gardening was a necessity. You grew vegetables to supplement the family income and you kept the front garden 'tidy' to keep up with the Jones's, a legacy that persists today but which is, thank goodness, gradually being eroded.

Over the last thirty years or so, the horticulture industry has worked hard to show people that a garden can be a place in which to relax, an area that can be transformed, without too much hard labour, into another room of the house where you will want to spend as much of your free time as possible.

Instant Gardening

The advent of the garden centre in the sixties gave us container-grown trees, shrubs and perennials that could be planted at any time of year, even when they were in flower. Until then, the planting season had been restricted to the period between November and March, which are not the most pleasant months for gardening. Now it really was possible to have an instant garden.

Gardening books appeared in increasing numbers, even rivalling cookery in terms of quantity. As more households acquired colour televisions, gardening programmes took off, with *Gardeners' World* appearing on BBC2.

Viewers could now see plants and flowers in all their glory, and Percy Thrower became a household name.

During the seventies and into the eighties, the garden became trendy and landscape designers started to experiment with more contemporary layouts. At the same time, however, there was a huge retro-move to formal gardens that harked back to the seventeenth century. Potagers popped up everywhere and Vita Sackville-West's garden at Sissinghurst in Kent became a horticultural Mecca. The Chelsea Flower Show became so popular that the Royal Horticultural Society had to restrict the numbers of tickets sold because of complaints of overcrowding.

From the eighties onwards, more and more flower shows were launched, from Hampton Court to Malvern. The National Gardens Scheme 'Yellow Book' offered 3,500 gardens to visit, almost all

The Borogrove Folly *This eye-catching combination of elegant topiary and bold colours made a strong impression at the Hampton Court Flower Show in 1995.*

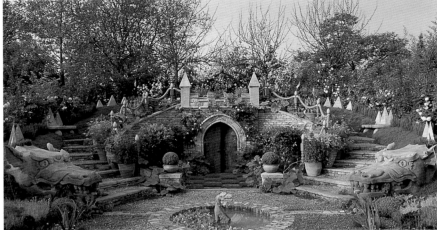

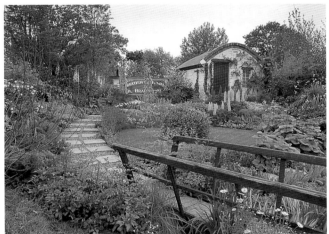

Fun and fantasy *Two impressive displays from the Chelsea Flower Show. The Herbalist Garden, above, designed by Bunny Guinness in 1998, is a magical and symmetrical arrangement of containerised herbs and dragon statuary. The* Sunday Express Garden, *left, evoking impressions of a peaceful rural idyll, was designed by Peter Hogan in 1995.*

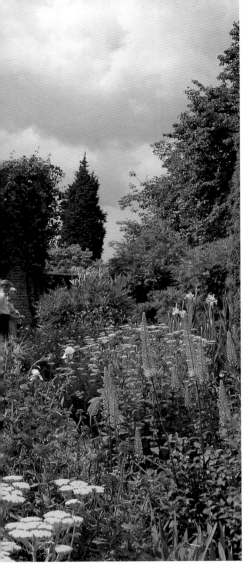

Fairytale castle *The world-famous garden of Sissinghurst, created by Vita Sackville-West and Harold Nicolson, has at its heart a wildly romantic Elizabethan mansion.*

of them belonging to keen amateurs. *BBC Gardeners' World Magazine* appeared, quickly reaching a circulation figure of over 375,000 (more than double the number of copies sold by its nearest rival). Television, too, became aware of a new breed of gardener and people under the age of forty began to present gardening programmes.

In the nineties, the garden make-over programme arrived. *Ground Force* on BBC1 showed what could be done by three people in two days. Most importantly, the schemes tackled by the team could be achieved by any householder with a bit of common sense and application, and they didn't cost a fortune. In addition, Charlie Dimmock introduced a touch of glamour. Audience

figures soared and the programme now attracts more than 11 million viewers.

The secret, I think, lies in showing that gardening is no longer the mystique-filled province of sage old men in baggy trousers. Yes, gardening is a skill, but one that can be learnt by anyone with an aptitude for it. I have spent thirty-five years gardening for a living. I learn more about it every day, and I enjoy it hugely. If that pleasure can be communicated to others, perhaps they will find the Latin names and the hard graft less daunting.

Programmes like *Ground Force* have shown people that there is a patch of ground alongside their house just waiting for them to express themselves. With surfaces like pebbles and decking, such areas need not be muddy and out of bounds for half the year. Instead, they can be transformed into places of year-round pleasure, which can look modern and trendy or old and cottagey.

Flowers and plants are things of great beauty. Most of them grow with little need of further pampering, if they are planted properly and in the right place. By showing how to do this in a no-nonsense and enthusiastic way, gardening programmes have opened up the whole subject to a wider audience.

We have never had a greater range of plants than we do today. Nurseries and garden centres are brimful of new things, and the gardening market is now worth a staggering £3 billion a year. I can think of no other area where the customer gets such value for money.

Britain has, in my opinion, always produced the best gardeners, and they have, in turn, created the best gardens. I have no doubt that gardening will become even more popular in the next millennium. The more I think about it, in fact, the more I am convinced that Adam must have been a Brit.

Gardening on the box

In the lead-up to a new century, we take an affectionate look back at some of the BBC television gardening series and characters of the last 63 years.

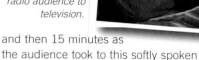

Gardening shows were already an essential part of the output on radio when the first television programmes were broadcast from the station at Alexandra Palace in 1936. The BBC was quick to realise the potential of a gardening programme and so it turned to radio for the presenter of the first television gardening programme, *In Your Garden*. Cecil Middleton brought a loyal audience from his radio broadcasts and his regular column in the *Radio Times*. Round spectacles and impeccable dress belied his wry sense of humour and easy style of presentation, and his popularity swiftly grew.

In Your Garden always had a practical content, with Mr Middleton, as he was known, advising the viewers on topics such as building a rock garden and pruning roses and shrubs. At first, gardening techniques were illustrated on a blackboard until, in May 1937, the first outside broadcast was made in the newly designed television garden at Alexandra Palace, with the huge transmitter towering in the background.

The television service closed down at the beginning of the Second World War and, when it resumed in 1946,

In Your Garden was presented by another man who was to become a gardening legend. Fred Streeter began work aged 12, leading the pony that pulled the mowing machine, for 3s 6d a week. Several years later, he was in charge of 26 gardeners at Petworth House, Sussex.

His style was very much that of a head gardener. Advice was given in a rich Sussex accent and, although always dressed in a suit, this practical man abandoned his jacket in favour of rolled-up sleeves. In Fred, the viewers had a real sense of a man who loved plants.

In the 1950s, Fred was joined on the programme *About the Home* by television's first woman gardener, Frances Perry. Frances was much more than an attractive female sidekick. In an area that is so dominated by men, she worked extremely hard to be recognised as an equal to her male counterparts.

The 1950s saw the emergence of another great character. Percy Thrower began his television career as the gardening expert on *Country Calendar*. The live seven-minute slot gradually stretched to ten

1937
CH Middleton brought a keen radio audience to television.

and then 15 minutes as the audience took to this softly spoken and patient man.

Percy then moved on to *Gardening Club*, one of several 'club' programmes, such as *Inventors' Club*, *Smokers' Club* and *Asiatic Club*. These fell by the wayside, but *Gardening Club* continued its weekly broadcasts until the next great revolution in television history: colour.

Switching on to colour

The change to colour was gradual but gardening programmes were some of the first to benefit from it. So began *Gardeners' World* in January 1968. Percy and co-presenter Arthur Billitt broadcast from several different locations, including their own respective home gardens: The Magnolias and Clack's Farm. The men were firm friends from before the war and their obvious rapport was one of the reasons why the series was so widely enjoyed.

Percy left *Gardeners' World* in 1976, but remained a familiar face on the BBC as the *Blue Peter* gardener. He introduced thousands of young

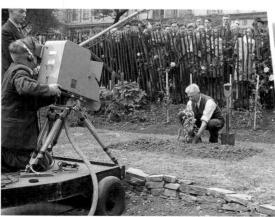

1946 *Fred Streeter's broadcasts from the Alexandra Palace garden attracted crowds of spectators.*

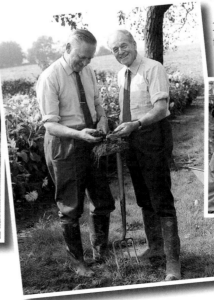

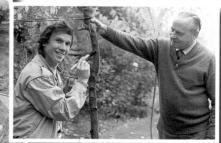

1968 Gardeners' World *presenters Percy Thrower and Arthur Billitt (left). Percy, seen with Peter Duncan, became the* Blue Peter *gardener (above).*

viewers to gardening through the tiny plot that he designed behind Television Centre at White City in London.

Just as the 1950s and 1960s had been Percy's heyday, so Geoffrey Smith reigned supreme in the 1970s. Geoffrey was superintendent at Harlow Carr, the Northern Horticultural Society's garden, when he met the producer of *Gardening Club*. Soon afterwards, this indomitable Yorkshireman found himself in front of the cameras, talking alone and live for 18 minutes on Michaelmas daisies. Countless other programmes followed this initial triumph, including eight Mr Smith's series, his *World of Flowers* series, and the live phone-in programme from Leeds, *Gardeners' Direct Line*.

Familiar faces

Gardening programmes and series reached a peak of popularity during the late 1970s and 1980s. More enduring favourites emerged during this time: Peter Seabrook got his first television break in the *Dig This* slot on *Pebble Mill at One*, while a very young Alan Titchmarsh graced the screen on *Nationwide*. Harry Dodson introduced a new audience to the joys of traditional gardening during the 1980s in *The Victorian Kitchen Garden*, illustrating how the craft of gardening still helps maintain the great gardens we enjoy visiting today. And of course, Geoff Hamilton made his first appearance on *Gardeners' World*, the show he was to make so much his own in the years that followed.

Geoff developed many new and innovative gardening series, including *First Time Garden*, with Gay Search, *The Ornamental Kitchen Garden*, *Old Garden New Gardener* and *Cottage Gardens*. His last series, *Paradise Gardens*, was completed just before his untimely death in 1996. Since then, Alan Titchmarsh has taken over the helm on *Gardeners' World*, with regulars Pippa Greenwood, Stephen Lacey and Gay Search.

The latest gardening phenomenon has been *Ground Force*, where Alan is joined by Charlie Dimmock and Tommy Walsh to carry out amazing garden transformations in just two days on a limited budget. Its creative makeover format has captured the imagination of millions and introduced the joys of gardening to a new audience.

With an ever-increasing range of channels to choose from, viewers will be able to enjoy old favourites as well as many new television series in the future. One of the most exciting is the *BBC Gardener of the Year Competition*, which will be broadcast in autumn 1999, searching for the best gardener in the country. Could it be you?

The history of gardening on television has been rich in characters who have fired the public imagination with their diverse personalities and approaches to gardening. Let's hope the next century is just as fertile.

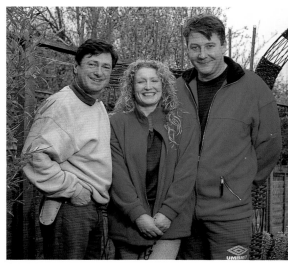

1999 Ground Force *has become a firm favourite with viewers.*

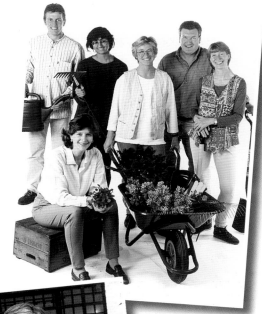

1996
The innovative format of Gardening from Scratch *set a new presenting style.*

1994
Female gardeners take the lead, with Gay Search presenting Front Gardens.

1975 *Viewers first saw Peter Seabrook on BBC1's* Pebble Mill at One.

1979 *Geoff Hamilton was the new face on* Gardeners' World *in this vintage year.*

A weekend makeover?
May the GROUND FORCE be with you

Television's favourite gardening troubleshooters, Charlie Dimmock, Alan Titchmarsh and Tommy Walsh, regularly transform the most unpromising spaces into beautifully designed oases with the minimum of fuss, money and effort. Here, BBC2's *Ground Force* team demonstrates how, with a little organisation and forward planning, you can give your garden a true *Ground Force* makeover.

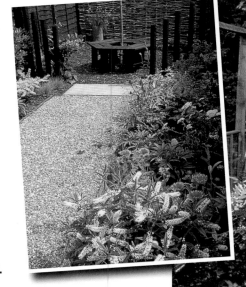

The first step is to decide which sort of effect you would like to create in your garden. This can be easier said than done, so if you do not know where to start, draw inspiration from visits to gardens, magazine pictures and books. Gather together your own photographs, images from catalogues, postcards and paintings that appeal to you. Use these to create what designers call a storyboard, summing up the style you are after. But do not feel you have to stick to just one style. It can be highly effective to divide the garden into different sections, with differing moods.

Check the orientation of the garden and work out which parts are in sun and which are in shade for most of the day. You may find that making little sketches of the shade patterns at regular intervals will help. This information is invaluable if you want to make a shady seating area, a sunny patio and, most important of all, when deciding which plants will be suited to a particular site.

Draw up a rough plan of the garden with a soft pencil and then start to sketch in the features you would like. Drawing on squared graph paper makes it easy to keep your plan to scale. As you work, make sure you have an eraser to hand and don't be afraid to use it.

Be ruthless. Decide which existing trees and shrubs are staying and which are for the chop. Before removing any trees or undertaking any major structural work, contact your local council's Planning Department to find out if you live in a conservation area or if any trees in your area are protected by a preservation order. They may also be able to recommend a qualified tree surgeon to do any work. Try to leave at least a few established shrubs to act as a skeleton framework. Also take a cool look at any existing paths and paved areas and, if they are not exactly what you want, consider getting rid of them.

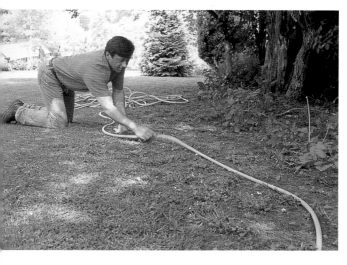

Laying out a hosepipe to plan the shape and size of a border is a good way of getting the right proportions. The hose can be adjusted until the border is in scale with its surroundings.

Clear the ground of perennial weeds, unwanted turf and plants before you start to mark out the features on the soil. If you have a convenient corner, stack cut turfs to rot down into rich compost but, if you are not completely sure of your composting skills, it is probably best to dispose of weeds rather than risk recycling them via a compost heap.

Mark out the shape of paths using trails of sand and use tall canes to represent other major features, then eye them up from all angles before you commit yourself to your design. Try to set up interesting views from key windows in the house, remembering you look out from upstairs as well as down.

Concentrate on one area at a time and complete the work there before you move on. Having a completed section will give you the encouragement to proceed still further.

When you are trying to get a lot done in a little time, forward planning is the key to success. Decide which order to approach the work in, and be realistic about how long you think it will take. To speed things up, gather together all the plants and hard landscaping materials you need before you get started. If you can persuade some friends to come in for a day and have a real blitz, the slog will feel more like a party.

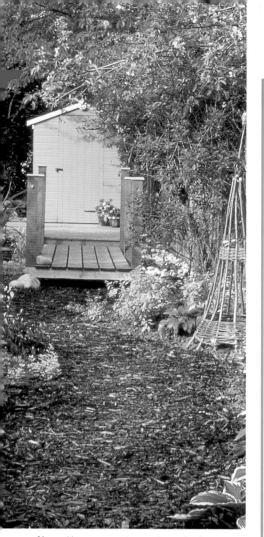

Above *You can create an atmospheric woodland setting by making a winding path of bark mulch through a selection of shade-tolerant plants under the trees.*

Inset, above *Plants with a low, spreading habit are perfect for softening the straight lines and hard edges of paths.*

It is important to use materials that have a strong texture, such as timber, pebbles, bricks and bark. These will give a distinct identity to your garden and, provided you choose them carefully, they will really enhance the overall effect of the planting scheme.

Use bold foliage plants for creating impact and as focal points. Although such plants can be rather expensive, if you choose well they will be a great investment. And don't think that it's necessary to have a big garden to have big plants. One or two carefully chosen specimen plants can transform a small space completely and, strangely enough, really make it feel much larger.

Weekend warriors

If you only have a weekend to transform your unsightly, overgrown plot, then help is at hand. Armed with these personal tips from the *Ground Force* team, the perfect garden can quickly and simply be yours.

ALAN TITCHMARSH designs the *Ground Force* **gardens, shaping the owners' aspirations into achievable plans before helping to turn them into reality, while keeping a close eye on the clock.**

'If you are worried about the success of transplanting a shrub, cut around it with a spade in autumn to sever sideways-spreading roots, but leave the plant in situ. Move it in spring. This way the shock of the move is less traumatic.'

'When making a large area of deck, build several separate sections of decking and fit them together. If any valuable items, such as jewellery or money, should fall through a gap, one section can be easily lifted to retrieve the item without damaging the deck.'

CHARLIE DIMMOCK is the plantswoman on the *Ground Force* **team, and her knowledge and experience of water features are second to none.**

'Always wash stones or pebbles thoroughly before using them in a pool. This gets rid of any surface lime, which may harm fish or raise the pH of the water. Buy a pH testing kit from your local garden centre and test the water at least once a year.'

'Place upturned pots over plants before applying a mulch. This way, you will avoid getting grit or bark on the leaves. Plants that have hairy leaves, or alpines with delicate blooms, may be harmed by wet conditions in the winter, and may therefore need to be covered by a sheet of glass to keep off the rain.'

'To make large container-grown plants easy to move around the garden, mount them on castors or small wheels. For wooden tubs, you can screw the wheels directly on to the bottom. Use wheels big enough to support the weight.'

TOMMY '2-days' WALSH, as he is now known, specialises in hard landscaping, the part of gardening that doesn't involve planting.

'With patios, decks and foundations it is vital that the rectangular or square base is made up of right angles. Make a builder's set square to achieve the perfect right angle. It's costly to remedy mistakes at a later stage if you don't get it right.'

'To mark out accurately where a fence post should go, cut a 2m (6½ft) cane to a length of 1.9m (6ft 4in), which equals the width of a panel plus the thickness of the post. Lay the cane along the string line and knock a peg in at the end of it. This will be the centre of each post.'

It's all in the name

Stephen Anderton

Clematus 'The President'

Why are so many plants named after celebrities? Stephen Anderton takes a wry look at the underlying significance and humour that can be derived from growing big names in your garden.

Are you a gardener? You know, one of those people who likes growing things? Can you remember soil? Well, if so, keep quiet about it. You are seriously out of fashion. Gardening is all about Wacky Personalities these days. Gardens are a measure of one's wackiness. Gardeners who fail in the wackiness stakes, whose jeans are blue and not orange, and who cannot even speak with a strong regional accent, are advised quietly to go indoors and subscribe to *Philately Week*. But fear not, ye men and women of minimal wack. There is a plan, a means by which real gardeners can rise again. So close that copy of Susan Hampshire's *Ultimate I-Want-It-Now Patio Companion*, switch off *Ready, Steady, Garden!*, and read on. Revenge will be as sweet as a pea.

Let's start at the beginning. It's hard to think, isn't it, that a mere two years ago, gardening was heralded as 'the new sex'? Not any more. Time has moved on and it's 'Gardens R Us' now. To be fashionable, a gardener requires a towering, exhibitionist ego, half Geoff Hamilton and half Ruby Wax. Hyperventilate like a television presenter on speed and the media masters will feature you and your garden, and probably your cat, in a glossy magazine. Remember to stock up on pebbles before the photographer comes; they are the sun-dried tomatoes of horticulture. Buy a cream linen jacket, wet it and screw it up in a ball for a week before you put it on, and they may even give you a television series.

But does having a cripplingly extravagant, D-cup personality actually make these people any good at gardening? Can they grow things? Is their idea of a wide range of plants to have both grasses and bamboos? Do they think an auricula is a new kind of miniature mobile phone? Worst of all, do they make you feel less than adequate as a gardener simply because you ain't wacky?

Well, if that's the case, here's what you do. You take all those plants named after egomaniac celebrities, those poor, sweet, unsuspecting plants lumbered with other people's names, and you plant them; and then you play with them. In the imagination, you can be as wicked as you like. Ignominy begins at the bottom of the garden.

Show-biz celebrities

So, who's for the bog garden then? Well, surprise, surprise, there's not a celebrity in sight. No one who's anybody wants to be a bog plant, apparently. No one wants to share with bog myrtle. There are bog plants named after ordinary gardeners and breeders, salt-of-the-earth types like *Iris* 'Aunt Martha' and Primula 'Wendy', but the big names of show-biz don't want to know.

What the celebs want is a bit of glitter, something with finesse, something with perfume. Not a potato or a tomato, but a rose. Like 'Angela Rippon', for instance: been around a bit, orange face, but not as leggy as you'd think. Or 'Anna Ford': a master of presentation with a yellow eye. When it comes to roses, you could plant enough celebrities to make a film by Kenneth Brannagh.

Of course, big names have been attaching themselves to roses ever since Napoleon's Empress Josephine made her world-famous garden at Malmaison and began selling 'Souvenir de la Malmaison' in the shop. There are endless old roses named for 'Madame This' and 'Sir Something That'.

As for clerics, roses have always had an association with the clergy. In the British collective unconscious, country parsons in half-moon glasses and rather crumpled linen jackets potter perpetually about the garden, smiling at 'The Nun' and bending low to breathe deep of the 'Great Maiden's Blush'. Gardeners have long recognised how impossible it is to restrain a 'Rambling Rector', torn between the delights of a 'Smooth Lady' and a 'Smooth Angel'.

Somewhere in this hot-bed of clerics there would have to be room to plant *Dahlia* 'Bishop of Llandaff'. The bishop is, of course, notorious for finding favour in traditional English gardens, despite being black and red. It really is just too, too daring! Curious, also, how at home the bishop seems to be in the company of the scarlet *Crocosmia* 'Lucifer'.

It might be possible to plant an unperfumed garden using nothing but roses named after the great couturiers. For all their proud reputations, they have all been more than happy to give their names to roses with not a hint of perfume. Pack them in: 'Christian Dior', 'Givenchy', 'Lagerfeld', 'Lancôme', 'Lanvin', the lot.

top left: *Rosa* 'Angela Rippon'
top right: *Rosa* 'Anna Ford'
bottom left: *Rosa* 'Blairii Number Two'
bottom right: *Rosa* 'Christian Dior'

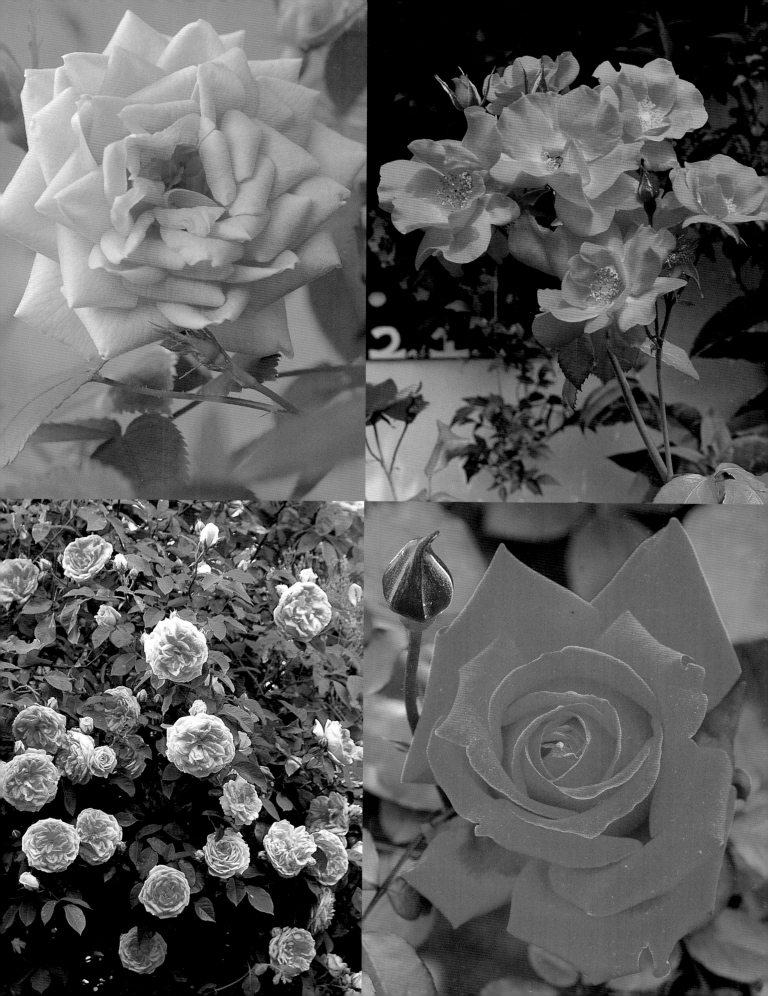

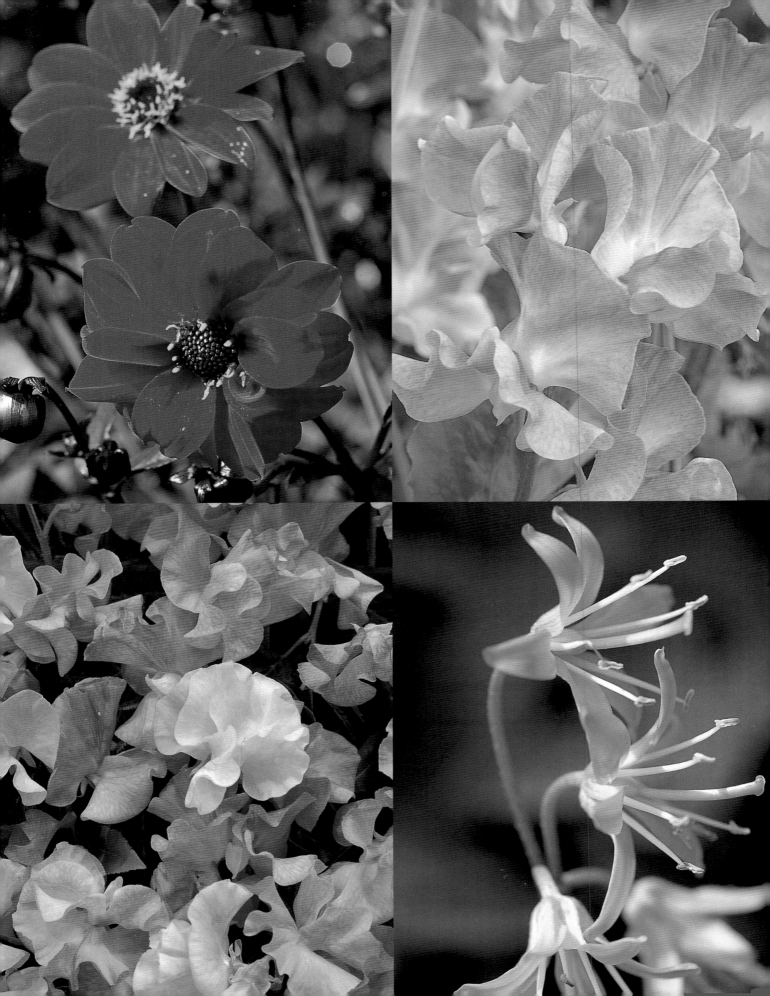

British celebrities and, in particular, gardening celebrities have been much keener to be immortalised by perfumed plants. Sweet peas, it seems, are the focus of the Britpack celebrities. Where else can you find 'Percy Thrower', 'Alan Titchmarsh' and 'Rosemary Verey' all clinging to the Netlon?

Royal blooms

The royals, too, have had their fling with sweet peas. You could, in fact, plant the entire History of the House of Windsor in sweet peas. I envisage an early bed of 'Frolic' and 'Queen Mother', followed by a mid-season display of 'Sandringham', 'Windsor', 'Balmoral', and 'Majesty'. Then, in a more eye-catching position, a Jekyllean colour sequence of 'Purple Prince', 'Royal Wedding', 'Honeymoon', and the various Spencer hybrids, the whole delicately underplanted with 'Kiri Te Kanawa' and yet more 'Rosemary Verey'. The garden ends in a medley of 'Mixed Ripples', 'Supersnoop' and 'Royal Flush', with a closing flourish from 'Early Spencer'. Alternatively, it might end with 'Charlie's Angel', although I doubt this would associate well with 'Her Majesty'.

For gardeners who are less interested in perfume, our Windsor Garden might be planted entirely with clematis, although there would have to be certain substitutions, such as 'Duchess of Edinburgh' for 'Her Majesty', and 'The First Lady' for Mrs Verey. 'Kiri Te Kanawa', such a reliable old war-horse, naturally remains the same, and crops up in almost every popular family.

But with the approach of the Millennium and the House of Lords for the chop, the lords and ladies celebrated in the plant kingdom will become much more a thing of the past. We should be planting now with a new sense of republican duty, free from all these feudal hang-ups. A garden for New Labour perhaps? Roses, as ever, would lead the way. I envisage a 1930s-retro

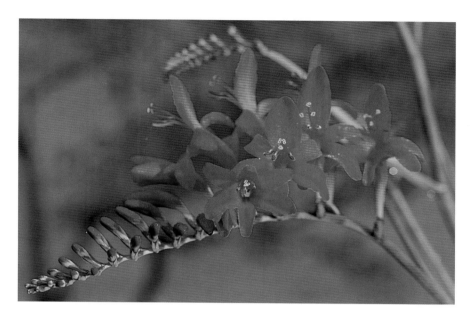

Crocosmia '**Lucifer**'

massed planting of 'Blairii Number One' to express Labour's popular roots. Opposite this will be a mass of 'Blairii Number Two', representing New Labour. It's an old rose, I know, and has been around for years under various different names, but this is a chance to make a real splash with it. If it is a bit lax, it can always be trained. For height, in this otherwise very level bed, I envisage a repeating focus of 'Fascination' in groups of three. 'Fascination', 'Fascination', and 'Fascination'. It's the old gardener's rule of using things in groups of threes, fives and sevens.

Heads of state

Surrounding this joyful scene would, of course, be the horticultural doldrums, where worn-out personalities are left to end their days. *Rosa* 'Margaret Thatcher' is distinctly lacking in vigour these days, but neverthless might be relied upon to survive in the rough, planted around a rustic sundial perhaps, inscribed with the traditional motto *ridicula terra antiqua est*, or, as they say in Finchley, 'It's a funny old world'. Bulbs of *Narcissus* 'President Carter' could be naturalised nearby, but whether *Rosa* 'Desert Peace' would survive the associated planting here is uncertain.

Heads of state have always figured largely in plant names. Sir Winston

Churchill has almost as many plants named after him as Kiri Te Kanawa. (Perhaps his voice wasn't so strong?) Someone even felt moved to call a rose 'Helmut Schmidt'. And there are presidents by the dozen, in roses, clematis, fuchsias, daffodils, rhododendrons, and probably many more. The luckiest presidents get a whole genus of plants named after them, like *Clintonia*.

So, for our Presidential Garden, I propose a raised bed, in a shady position, which should suit clintonias perfectly. The great advantage of a raised bed, of course, is that there is no need to bend down to it.

Fuchsia '**Winston Churchill**'

top left: *Dahlia* 'Bishop of Llandaff'
top right: *Lathyrus* 'Kiri Te Kanawa'
bottom left: *Lathyrus* 'Queen Mother'
bottom right: *Clintonia borealis*

Stephen Anderton is the gardening correspondent of *The Times*. **He has written** *Rejuvenating a Garden* **(Kyle Cathie).**

Gardening tips from the celebrities

NIGEL COLBORN

Never allow your soil to become compacted. The less you walk on your borders, the better the soil structure will be. Passing feet will press soil particles together, driving out air, restricting free drainage and ruining the soil's structure. Therefore, design your growing areas so that they can be serviced from pathways, stepping stones or paving, and use wide planks to walk on when you are digging over. Also, consider growing vegetables in raised beds, and never work with soil when it is too wet.

▽ **If you want your planting to work, imitate nature. Before you decide to replant part of your garden, conjure up some natural scenery in your mind or, better still, go and study it for real! When you have become familiar with the mood set by scenes such as a** stretch of springtime woodland, flowery May meadows, summer roadside verges, luxuriant river banks or even a heatherclad moorland, you will find it much easier to make your borders look natural. This technique is not slavish imitation, but rather the selection of key features of those wild landscapes, scaled down to a domestic level.

PETER SEABROOK

Always cultivate heavy clay soils in drying conditions. If the top layer dries a little after being disturbed, it will not then turn to mud after rain and dry bullet-hard.

▷ **Rotovators should not be used on heavy clay soils from late October to early March. Pulverising wet land at this time destroys the structure of the soil and makes it difficult to cultivate in spring and summer.**

DAPHNE LEDWARD

When planting new bare-root roses, prune back the roots by about a half. This will encourage the young bushes to make many new fibrous roots and will help get them off to a good start in the first twelve months.

Most vegetables grown closer than generally recommended will make smaller individual plants, although the total yield will actually be higher. This is handy if you enjoy lots of freshly harvested mini-vegetables.

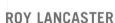

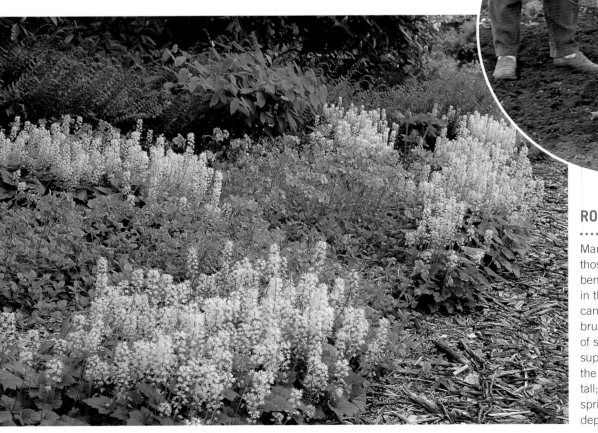

ROY LANCASTER

Many tall perennials or those with slender stems benefit from some support, in the form of linked wires, canes and twine or brushwood. The secret of success, though, is to support them early, before the shoots have grown too tall; this usually means spring or early summer, depending on the perennial.

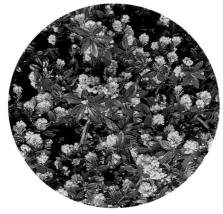

△ Nothing annoys and deters trespassers and burglars more than having to negotiate a viciously spiny bush or hedge. There are many candidates, but few can compete with *Berberis* 'Goldilocks', a dense, strong-growing shrub, which will reach about 2.5m (8ft) and is covered with an armour of thorny stems. Its glossy dark green foliage and clusters of deep yellow flowers in April are a bonus. It can be pruned, if necessary, and will grow in most soils.

ADAM PASCO

Use flowers in your battle against greenfly this summer. Many colourful annuals, like the poached egg plant or cheerful tagetes, encourage adult hoverflies to feed on their nectar. The larvae of these insects have quite an appetite for greenfly and aphids, so by encouraging hoverflies into your garden to feed and lay their eggs you are helping to control pests in a natural way. Remember to plant flowers all around the garden, including in the vegetable plot and around any fruit trees and bushes.

▷ **Plants love a regular meal, especially during the summer months, and feeding encourages strong, healthy growth, flowers and fruits. To avoid forgetting the fortnightly feed, mix slow-release fertiliser granules into the compost when planting up your containers, baskets and growing bags. Or fit a fertiliser dilutor into your hosepipes so that a small dose of feed is included every time you water your plants.**

GAY SEARCH

When planting a climber like ivy, train the stems horizontally along the ground in each direction at the base of the fence or wall you want it to cover. The stems will soon root at each pair of leaves and produce new vertical shoots, covering a much wider area more quickly.

▷ **If you have only half an hour to make the garden look tidy, trim the edges of the lawn rather than mow it.**

A folded disposable dishcloth, laid along the bottom of a window-box before planting, will let water out through the drainage holes but keep the compost in, preventing brown splashes on the window-sill or down the wall.

ALAN TITCHMARSH

An old spoon can easily be made into the perfect implement for removing mud from your tools. First, saw through the bowl of the spoon half-way along its length, then flatten the remaining part with a hammer. Finally, file the cut edge to reduce its sharpness.

When cultivating the soil, it is all too easy to damage or sever the base of clematis with a hoe or fork. To protect it, plant the young clematis through a small section of plastic drainpipe.

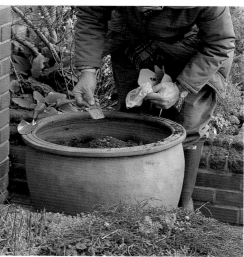

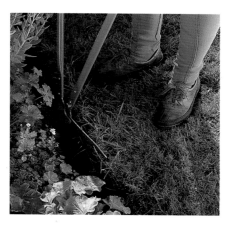

ANNE SWITHINBANK

Repotting prickly cacti is so much easier if you use the old pot as a template. First, knock the cactus out of its old pot. Put a little compost over the base of the new pot, then place the old pot inside it and firm compost all around it. Slide the old pot out to leave a hole, which should match the rootball exactly. Lift the cactus using a newspaper collar and drop its roots gently into the hole.

▽ **Twiggy sticks from pruned shrubs are invaluable for staking herbaceous perennials. They're easy to use, have lots of fork-shaped support and make the best natural-looking props.**

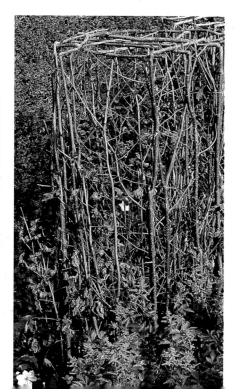

Bringing in the experts

Where do you start when looking for something to grow in your garden? After all, the choice can be bewildering, since there are over 70,000 different varieties of plants currently available at British nurseries. Not all of them are good garden performers, either, and, although fascinating to a plant connoisseur, they may not be suitable if you are looking for a plant that is hardy, reliable and with a long season of colour and interest.

So, instead, why not ask for some expert advice from someone who knows a thing or two about plants and can give personal recommendations? Not only will you be sure of picking the very best varieties, but you will also know that you're in good company when growing them.

On the next few pages, some of the country's best-loved gardeners pick their favourite plants. Each has chosen a 'top ten' theme, and gives a personal selection of those plants you should look out for. Of course, each of them could have made their selection many times over, but by choosing any of these plants you will not be disappointed with their performance or garden display.

Looking at what other people are buying can also be helpful. When Peter Seabrook compiled his list of top ten shrubs, he turned to a major nursery to find out which were the best-selling shrubs in the country. These shrubs are the most popular because, as well as being attractive, they are highly versatile, performing well in a wide range of sites, situations and soils. They also reflect current trends in popularity, so you will be sure of growing the most fashionable new varieties.

Another way to pick the best garden plants is to look for those with an Award of Garden Merit, the AGM. These are rather like plant Oscars, presented by the Royal Horticultural Society to plants that have performed well in

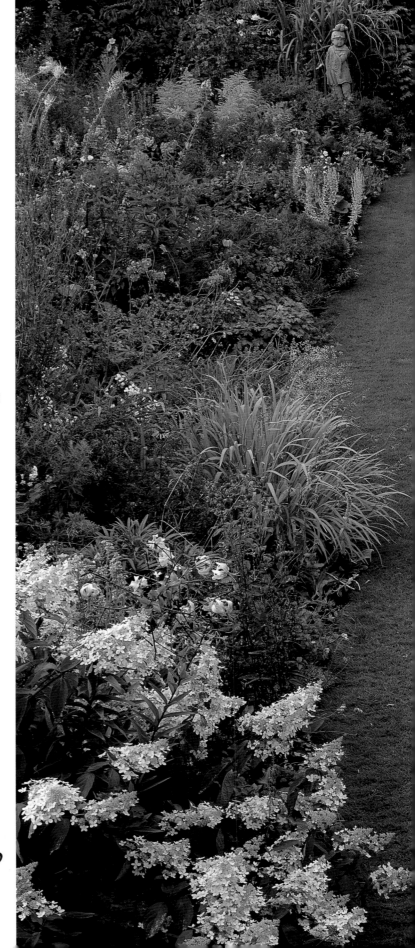

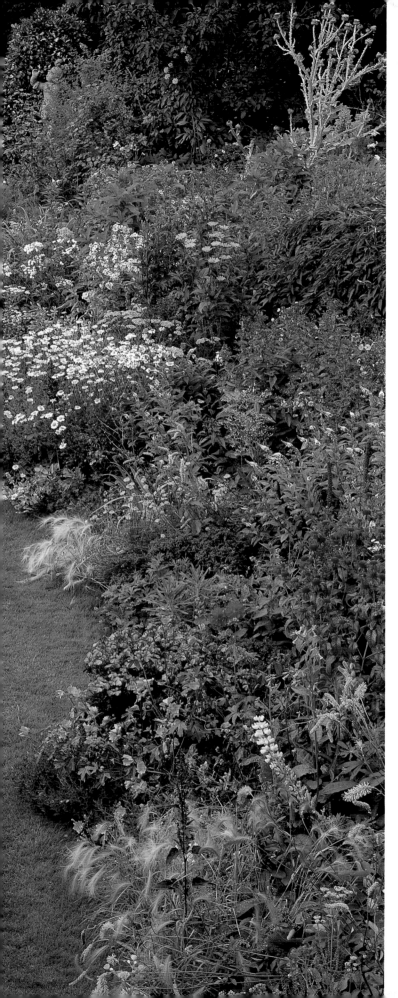

growing trials at the RHS gardens at Wisley in Surrey. Those winning the AGM may be highlighted with a trophy symbol in books, magazines, catalogues or on their plant label. More than 6,000 plants have received an AGM over the years, and a special booklet listing them all has just been published.

When choosing roses, look for those with the accolade 'Roses of Special Merit', given by the Royal National Rose Society. All these varieties have been tried and tested by the RNRS and selected for their health, vigour, flower quality and performance. You should find the 'Roses of Special Merit' rosette on the plant label. Roses are one of the most versatile groups of garden plants and, in addition to highlighting the varieties, this award scheme also shows some of the ways in which they can be grown. Traditionally, roses are grown on their own in beds and borders, and there are plenty of low-, medium- and tall-growing ones to choose from. Very low-growing and spreading varieties are becoming more popular for ground cover, while compact roses are ideal for patio pots and baskets. Walls can be covered with roses, while a garden arch offers the perfect support, especially in partnership with honeysuckle, clematis and other climbers.

Finding your plants

Local garden centres and nurseries are the best places to start looking for plants, but their range can be quite limited. Many nurseries exhibit at the ever-increasing number of flower shows around the country, and at some, like the BBC Gardeners' World Live every June, plants are available to buy. Others advertise through the pages of the hobby gardening magazines, offering plant collections or promoting their mail-order catalogues. While some specialise in seeds or bulbs, others sell trees, shrubs, perennials, young bedding plants, fruit trees and roses. It is certainly worth building up a collection of catalogues to keep for reference.

Once you have become a little more adventurous, or develop an interest in a particular plant, you will certainly want to consider some of the 70,000 other plants available, so pick up a copy of *The RHS Plant Finder*. This useful directory lists mail-order and nursery suppliers for all these plants, including those featured in our experts' choices, and turning its pages will be the start of many new gardening adventures.

To contact the Royal National Rose Society, call 01727 850461. *The RHS Plant Finder* 1998–99 is published by Dorling Kindersley at £12.99. A booklet of Award of Garden Merit plants is now available at £5.95 plus £1.25 p&p from RHS Enterprises (01483 211320).

Pippa Greenwood's Top Ten
FLOWERS

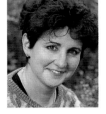

It is an almost impossible task deciding on my ten favourite flowers. When it comes to plants, I must admit that I fall in love easily and, like the wicked woman I am, I don't fall out of love with those I have admired before, but instead accumulate more and more favourites! So, to make this task easier I have 'cheated' and included some broad categories, not just single species or varieties. After all, I have more than ten favourite sweet peas alone. Even as I write I can feel myself changing my mind and thinking of other flowers that I should perhaps include, but I will stand firm and include the first ten I jotted down. So, here goes.

Pippa Greenwood is a regular presenter on BBC2's *Gardeners' World*. An expert on plant pests and diseases, she is the ideal troubleshooter for Radio 4's *Gardeners' Question Time*. Her latest book is *The Flower Garden* (Dorling Kindersley).

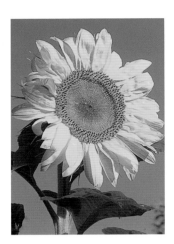

◁ Sunflowers
Wow! What more is there to say? I love them all, from some of the more recent, smaller introductions such as 'Toy Box' to the traditional 'Titan', and the most common of all 'Giant Single'. Last year I grew a row of sunflowers along the back of a small vegetable plot and every time I looked out of the bathroom window they brought a smile to my face.

◁ Tiarella cordifolia
The tiny starry flowers of the foam flower are extremely delicate, and form a sort of haze above the wonderful rounded mound of attractively shaped leaves. The plant grew particularly well in my last garden, which was rather shaded, and really did help to brighten up dull corners.

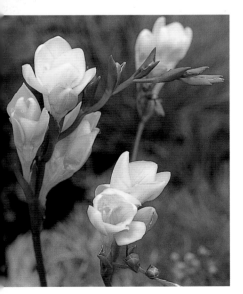

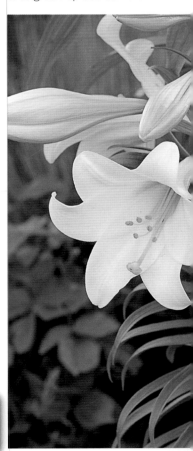

◁ Single freesias
Single freesias possess the perfect scent, so why on earth aren't perfumes like this made for us to buy? I find it positively intoxicating and combined with those smooth, almost velvety flowers in rich colours, what more could you ask for? Every special occasion in my life has been marked by freesias, including most birthdays and the birth of my son, when I was lucky enough to receive many bouquets, most of which included freesias.

▷ Lilium longiflorum
It's that combination of perfume and elegance again, this time on more stately, pure white trumpet flowers, that is the appeal of these lilies. As they can be a little on the tender side, I grow mine in pots so that they can be moved easily to protected areas during the winter, and, without fail, they come back year after year. Sometimes, when I've had a particularly trying day, I treat myself to a bunch. Extravagant, I know, but worth it!

If it's flowers you're after, then there is one regular feed you shouldn't forget: a high potash liquid fertiliser. Give plants either a special flowering plant feed or the same feed that you use for tomatoes.

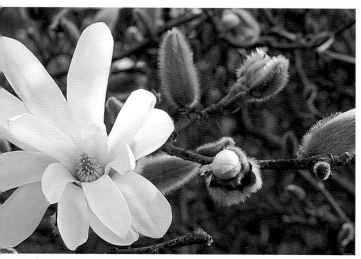

△ **Magnolia stellata**

Although the perfume of this magnolia is very subtle, early in the year on a still day it's very enjoyable. For my 30th birthday, my sister Jennifer gave me £30 to buy 'something you really want'. A friend then gave me a token torn from the local paper that promised '50% off all plants' at the garden centre. The result, a large *Magnolia stellata*, then about 1.2m (4ft) tall. It's now considerably larger and we've managed to move it successfully from our old garden to our new one.

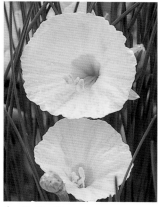

△ **Daffodils**

Cheap and cheerful, and I simply adore them! I've got lots of favourites, ranging from the tiny *Narcissus bulbocodium* to the elegant *N. poeticus*, or Old Pheasant's Eye. The only ones I don't like are those that look like bright yellow crepe paper pompoms – ugh!

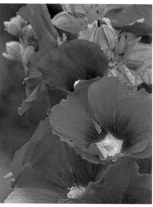

△ **Hollyhocks**

There is something crazy and untamed about these gorgeous giants, and I find it hard to resist their charms. Again, it's singles only for me; the pompom things are definitely not welcome in my garden. The only drawback is fungal rust disease and, yes, mine get it too.

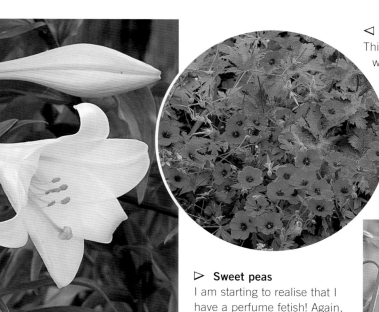

◁ **Geranium psilostemon**

This is another plant that did well in the clay and shade of our previous garden, growing to much greater heights than the books suggest because of the shade. Its bright pink, dark-centred flowers looked stunning when they grew up to meet the nearby 'Maigold' rose.

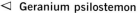

▷ **Sweet peas**

I am starting to realise that I have a perfume fetish! Again, there are none I dislike, but those with a good perfume are something I cannot do without. As a child, I was fascinated by the perennial sweet peas growing at our local underground station at East Putney, and was inspired to grow a few annuals myself.

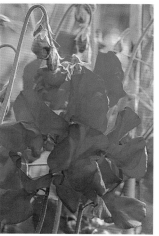

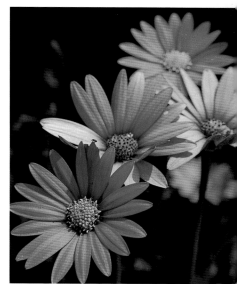

△ **Osteospermum 'Stardust'**

Where I live now it is too cold, and I suspect the soil too heavy, for this somewhat tender perennial to survive the winter without help. But, again, it does do well in a pot and can then easily be given winter protection. What better plant for a sunny doorstep?

Peter Seabrook's Top Ten
SHRUBS

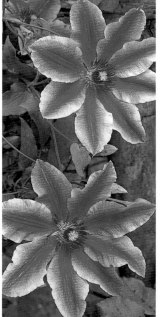

There are so many lovely shrubs available for the garden that choosing my Top Ten proved impossible because I knew my list would certainly change with the seasons and my mood. So, instead, I have listed Britain's top sellers, the same way it's done for the record charts. One of the country's largest nurseries, which grows shrubs for garden centres and DIY stores, kindly gave me their most up-to-date sales information from which I compiled this list. All of these plants are attractive and adaptable, flourishing in all sorts of conditions, as well as being reliable and rewarding. They do, in fact, number among my personal favourites.

Peter Seabrook is a garden consultant, writer and broadcaster. His book *Shrubs for Everyone* (Floraprint) gives lots of helpful advice on selecting and growing shrubs.

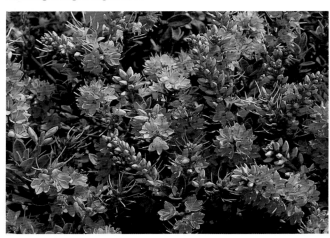

△ **Hebe**
Commonly called veronica, hebes are a very versatile range of compact evergreens. Variegated and silver-leaved kinds are useful for patio pots and window-boxes, especially as winter decoration. Larger-leaved kinds are less hardy and have bigger flower spikes. 'Margret' is the best-loved.

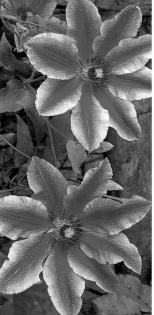

▷ **Vinca**
With their lush green stems, evergreen foliage and bright blue flowers that last for months, periwinkles are hardly shrubs as they will reach only 50cm (20in) in height. The small-leaved, excellent ground-covering *Vinca minor* is the most popular species. It is also widely grown in patio pots for year-round decoration.

◁ **Clematis**
It comes as no surprise that clematis is the number one selling shrub in the country when we remember that there are so many large- and small-flowered kinds, as well as those with attractive winter seed-heads. Many gardens have at least half-a-dozen climbing up walls and fences and scrambling through other plants.

◁ **Euonymus**
The most popular are the variegated types of *Euonymus fortunei*, like 'Emerald Gaiety', 'Emerald 'n' Gold' and 'Silver Queen', which are used for ground cover, in patio containers and even for low hedging and climbing. The silver-leaved euonymus turn pink in cold weather and look particularly good growing up through the deciduous, purple-leaved berberis.

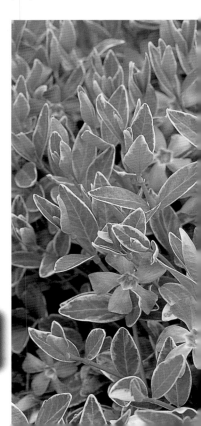

If you are choosing your top ten shrubs, select one that will be in flower for each month from February to November to ensure year-round colour. Most winter-flowering shrubs flower from November to February.

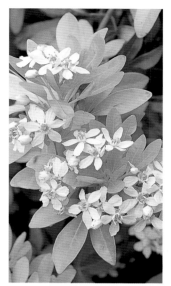

△ **Choisya**
The mock orange has attractive evergreen foliage, which is aromatic when crushed, and fragrant white flowers which appear in late spring and again in autumn after hot, dry summers. The yellow-leaved 'Sundance' accounts for many of the plants grown. All choisya are better in a sheltered position because severe winter frost can kill them.

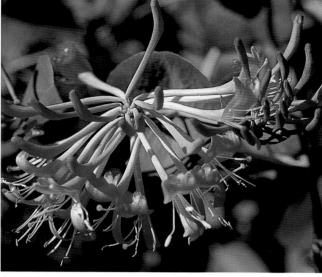

△ **Lonicera**
Honeysuckles are excellent climbers, and are also hugely popular for their scent. Several introductions, including the bright orange-red 'Mandarin', are increasing in popularity. Honeysuckles should be sprayed to control greenfly in early spring if the leaves become sticky.

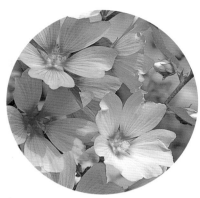

△ **Lavatera**
Growing rapidly to a height of 2m (6½ft), tree mallows flower non-stop through the summer. When they become tall and ungainly, they can be pruned back hard in spring. This delays flowering by two or three weeks, but if it is done every other year, a shapelier plant will result.

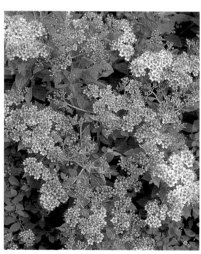

◁ **Spiraea**
These shrubs grow up to 1m (3ft 3in) high, with brightly coloured young shoots in spring. The taller, white-flowered kinds have attractive light green leaves. All of them are very good-natured, doing well in a wide range of soil types. The dwarf ones respond well to hard pruning in winter.

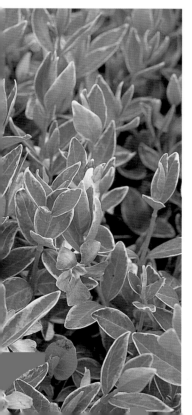

▷ **Potentilla**
These compact shrubs suit modern, smaller gardens and do a good ground-covering job, smothering weeds. But, most important, they flower freely for months. They respond well to regular feeding and new growth bears the best flowers. 'Red Robin' is the most popular cultivar.

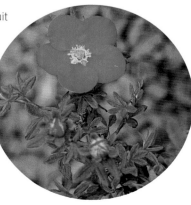

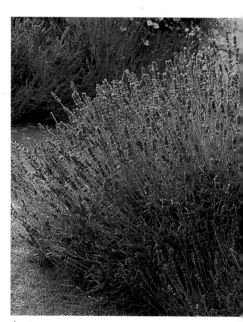

△ **Lavender**
Many gardens are planted with several lavenders, some used in quantity as low hedging. Popular varieties include 'Hidcote' and 'Imperial Gem'. Lavenders are best as young plants with their rich silver-grey leaves. The plants benefit from a light trim after flowering.

Roy Lancaster's Top Ten
PERENNIALS

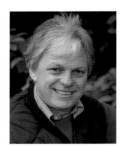

Perennials are commonly used in gardens as accompaniments to the major league plants, like trees and shrubs, but they are quite clearly characters in their own right and can play a huge role in a garden's success. Take my own garden, for instance. When I first moved here, 16 years ago, I planted lots of woody plants and used perennials to fill the gaps. Now, every time I remove an overgrown tree or shrub, I tend to replace it with perennials, as I get more for my money and greater variety. Perennials come in all shapes and sizes and, in addition to flowers, many offer fine foliage effects. Anyone who can count their favourite perennials on the fingers of only two hands is a fibber or else a greenhorn, so let me offer the following selection as ten of the best.

Roy Lancaster is a plant hunter, lecturer, television presenter and author. He has written a number of gardening books, including *What Perennial Where* (Dorling Kindersley). He was awarded the OBE in January 1999.

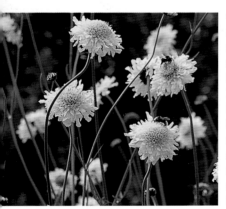

◁ **Cephalaria gigantea**
A big one, this, and appropriately named the giant scabious. Given space, it is impressive, with branching stems that grow to 1.8m (6ft), providing numerous large, primrose-yellow flower-heads in early summer. A great draw for all the bees, butterflies and hoverflies in the garden, it also has pleasing clumps of deeply divided foliage. Easy and hardy in most soils.

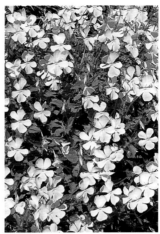

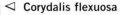

▷ **Geranium macrorrhizum 'Album'**
There are several selections of this wild cranesbill in cultivation and I like most of them for their semi-evergreen, pleasantly aromatic leaves, carpeting habit and easy-to-divide and grow-anywhere characteristics. Most have pink or purple flowers, but in 'Album' they are white with contrasting reddish calyces borne prolifically in late spring. It suits almost any soil, in sun or shade, and provides brilliant ground cover and weed smother.

◁ **Viola cornuta 'Alba'**
Few perennials are as free- and long-flowering as *Viola cornuta* and its selections, of which the white-flowered 'Alba' is my favourite. The low clumps are quite vigorous and lush but they can be cut back, if required, to encourage a more compact habit. An excellent choice for growing beneath roses or as an edging to beds and borders, it can be planted in full sun or half-shade.

◁ **Corydalis flexuosa**
This popular choice for gardens has clumps or patches of ferny foliage through winter and spring, topped by brilliant kingfisher-blue flower clusters in spring. It needs half-shade and an open-textured, moisture-retentive soil. I grow it in large containers filled with compost. Remember, it is summer-dormant, so don't panic when the foliage dies down in summer.

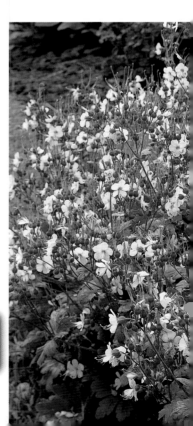

All these perennials are easily increased by division, which is generally best done in early spring or as growth commences. The exception is *Corydalis flexuosa*, whose tiny tubers should be gathered and replanted after growth has died down in summer.

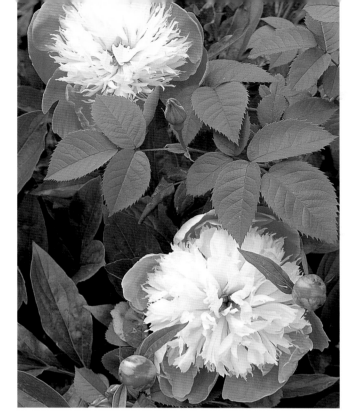

△ **Paeonia lactiflora 'Bowl of Beauty'**
I enjoy herbaceous paeonies from the moment the fat red shoots break through the soil in spring to the often richly tinted dying foliage of autumn. This one is a show-stopper, with vivid pink blooms filled with narrow, creamy white petaloids. Its flowering in June is comparatively brief but utterly memorable. It is happy in most soils, as long as you give it full sun.

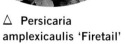

△ **Persicaria amplexicaulis 'Firetail'**
This is the perfect perennial for the back of the border or on its own in an island bed. It also looks good by water or in a bog garden, where the luxurious clumps of bold foliage provide an excellent foil for the branching stems. It grows to a height of 1.2m (4ft) and bears erect slender spikes of bright crimson flowers which last from late June until well into the autumn.

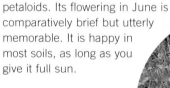

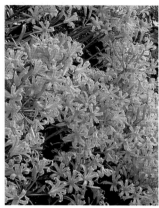

△ **Nerine bowdenii 'Mark Fenwick'**
No hardy bulb attracts more favourable comment in my garden than this. It is so reliable in its autumn display of trumpet-like, rich pink flowers. The strap-shaped leaves appear afterwards, dying away in summer. Give it a warm, sunny, well-drained position, with a wall backing in colder areas, and don't plant the bulbs too deep.

▽ **Acanthus mollis 'Hollard's Gold'**
I admire acanthus, or bear's breeches, because it tolerates both full sun and shade. It also provides a bold ground cover with its huge, deeply cut leaves. The flowers are like mauve-pink foxgloves, in tall, stout spikes that reach 1.5m (5ft) in late summer. I particularly like 'Hollard's Gold' for its yellow-suffused foliage in late winter and spring, which is a real bonus.

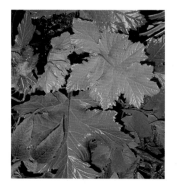

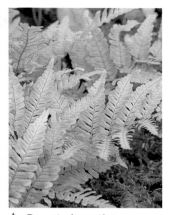

△ **Dryopteris erythrosora**
Generally speaking, hardy ferns are a neglected group of garden plants but I would not be without them. This is one of the most notable, with glossy, evergreen, much-divided fronds growing 60cm (2ft) long, unfurling to a contrasting rose-bronze when young. Thriving in most garden soils, preferably in shade or half-shade, it makes a useful container plant, too.

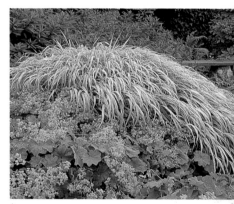

△ **Hakonechloa macra 'Aureola'**
Ornamental grasses, like ferns, are not everyone's first choice for the garden, but they have a lot to offer, and this one more than most. Its tiny flowers are carried in delicate sprays in late summer but the golden-striped leaves last from spring to autumn. Mounds of leafy shoots grow to 30cm (12in) and make superb container plants in shade or sun.

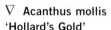

Adam Pasco's Top Ten
CLIMBERS
and WALL PLANTS

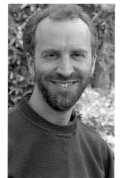

While many plants just fill a gap or spread to cover the ground, climbing plants can clad walls, obscure boring fences or completely envelop a garden arch. Climbers are clever plants, each developing its own way to head for the heavens. The most successful are those that cling onto almost anything they can find, with no assistance from us at all. Others need something to twine around, a support of some sort to get them on their way. A few well-placed hooks or wires can help, or perhaps a piece of ornamental trellis attached to the wall. Popular varieties include clematis, roses and honeysuckle, and, as these have all been recommended by other experts, I have chosen some of my other favourites.

Adam Pasco is the **Editor** of *BBC Gardeners' World Magazine* and one of the UK's most highly respected gardening journalists.

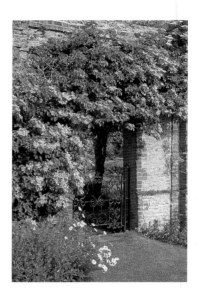

◁ **Climbing hydrangea**
Ask any expert for a climbing plant to suit a north wall, and *Hydrangea petiolaris* will be recommended. Its hardy constitution makes it an excellent choice, while the stems stick to walls without your help. Although it is deciduous, the fresh foliage and lacecap heads of summer blooms make it a favourite. *Schizophragma hydrangeoides*, a relative, is also worth considering.

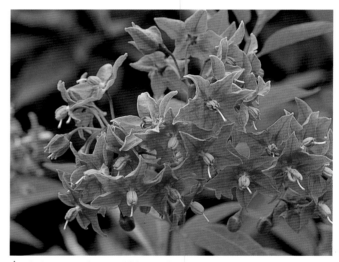

△ **Solanum crispum 'Glasnevin'**
This flowering relative of the potato needs tying up to cover a trellis panel, but it grows rapidly to reach a height of 2m (6½ft) or more in a single season. Flowering from as early as June to the end of summer, it is hardier than many people think and requires regular pruning to keep it in check.

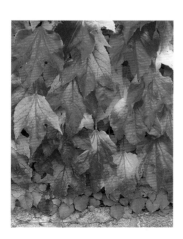

◁ **Boston ivy**
An agile self-clinger, *Parthenocissus tricuspidata* 'Veitchii' is good at clothing a wall, reaching perhaps 15m (50ft) or more. Ivy-like leaves are green all summer, falling in autumn, but putting on a blazing show before they do. At home in sun or shade, this and other varieties of Virginia creeper produce the perfect overcoat for any house.

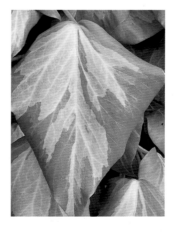

◁ **Hedera colchica 'Sulphur Heart'**
There are many excellent ivy varieties to choose from, including my namesake 'Adam', but this variegated, large-leaved variety is excellent. When first planted, peg all the stems down to soil level along the base of the wall. These will root into the soil, sending up sideshoots over the next few years to cover their support.

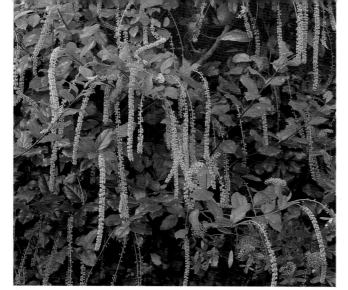

△ **Itea ilicifolia**

At the height of summer, this unusual evergreen wall shrub from China, with holly-like leaves, is a sight to behold, its long, trailing, pale green flower stems transforming it completely. It can be grown as a free-standing plant or trained to wires fixed to a wall. Of no relation, but also with long catkins and creating a similar effect, this time in winter, is *Garrya elliptica* 'James Roof', the perfect shrub for a north wall.

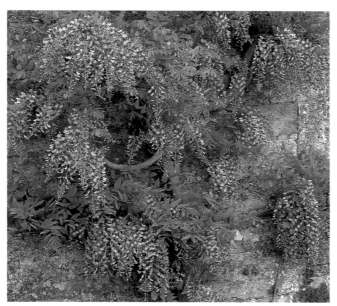

△ **Wisteria**

Despite their short flowering season, nothing matches wisteria for elegance and beauty. Train shoots as they grow to cover their support, and encourage flowering by pruning sideshoots in mid-summer and again in winter. Be sure to buy a named variety, avoiding any shy-flowering seedlings.

Regularly tie in new growth of climbing plants so that it grows in the direction you want it to go and helps cover its support completely. Pinching out the tips of long shoots, or tying them down to a more horizontal position, often encourages sideshoots to form and creates a bushier habit.

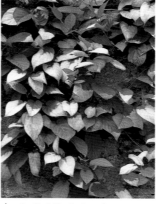

△ **Actinidia kolomikta**

This climbing shrub, related to the kiwi fruit, looks as if some child has been set loose with pots of cream, pink and green paint. Although deciduous, it has wonderful leaves, perfect for training up trellis or along wires on a warm, bright wall. The new leaves and shoots are tender and can be scorched by frost.

▽ **Humulus lupulus 'Aureus'**

Within weeks, the golden hop twines its way up posts and over arches, creating a bright cloak of foliage, followed by hanging hops. It looks stunning alongside purple neighbours, but leave it space to be rampant without crowding out its companions. Shoots die back after the first frost and can be cut down to ground level, but the hardy roots remain, ready to send up new shoots the following year.

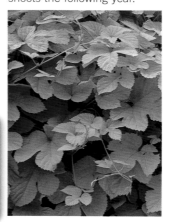

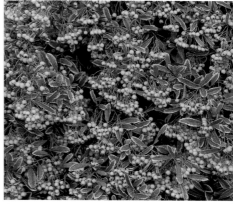

△ **Firethorn**

Popular for all the right reasons, pyracantha is the perfect evergreen shrub for training along walls and fences, especially for extra boundary security! Flowers in early summer are followed by red, orange or yellow berries, often carried well into winter. Pyracantha looks stunning trained as an espalier.

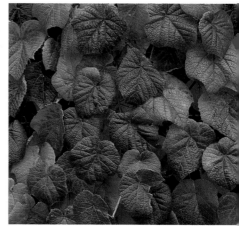

△ **Ornamental vine**

If you've space for a vigorous climber, then look no further than *Vitis coignetiae*, a hardy grapevine from Japan which has enormous, heart-shaped leaves. Deep green for most of the year, they turn fiery red in autumn, before falling. Tie shoots to wires for support, but be prepared for them to grow up to 10m (33ft). Feed and water regularly to get the biggest leaves.

Nigel Colborn's Top Ten
ROSES

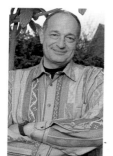

All flowers can be romantic, but nothing beats the rose for poetic inspiration! Blooming throughout those long summer days, sometimes with a luscious fragrance, roses are the basis of almost every good planting scheme. Even out of season, their young foliage, flushed with coppery tones, makes a warm contrast with such bright spring flowers as tulips and daffodils. Every rose grower treasures the first perfect blooms, and by mid-summer the abundance of flowers can be astounding. Some roses even go on to provide a dazzling autumnal display of bright red or orange hips, with leaf colours that burnish to gold just before they fall. Roses need care and attention to give their best and, in certain varieties, diseases can cause problems. For this short list I have selected only varieties that are simple to look after and high on performance.

Nigel Colborn is a regular panellist on BBC Radio 4's *Gardeners' Question Time,* the author of a number of gardening books and a floral judge for the Royal Horticultural Society.

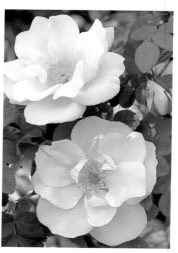

◁ **Nevada**

'Nevada' is a big shrub rose with a loose, open habit that is easy to prune to the desired size. In winter, the stems are a dark purplish colour but, in early summer, they develop garlands of large, creamy white flowers that are faintly blushed with pink at the petal edges. Sporadic blooms follow the main flowering period. Disease-resistant as well as easy to establish.

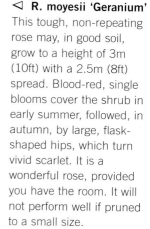

◁ **R. moyesii 'Geranium'**

This tough, non-repeating rose may, in good soil, grow to a height of 3m (10ft) with a 2.5m (8ft) spread. Blood-red, single blooms cover the shrub in early summer, followed, in autumn, by large, flask-shaped hips, which turn vivid scarlet. It is a wonderful rose, provided you have the room. It will not perform well if pruned to a small size.

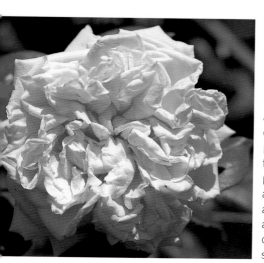

◁ **Gloire de Dijon**

This old climber is still one of the best. The dark purplish stems and lustrous leaves are reddish when young, and large, rounded, very double flowers are produced throughout the summer. The tightly packed petals are a soft apricot-beige, fading to a warm, creamy yellow as they age. A good crop of hips will sometimes follow.

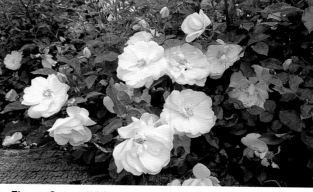

△ **Flower Carpet White**

I have chosen this new, repeat-flowering variety in part for its excellent disease-resistance. The deep green, glossy foliage makes a good foil for the sprays of smallish, creamy white, faintly fragrant flowers. As the name suggests, Flower Carpet White provides ideal ground cover, but it is also excellent as a container plant on the patio. Keep removing the faded flower stems to encourage new buds, and feed during the summer with a high potash fertiliser.

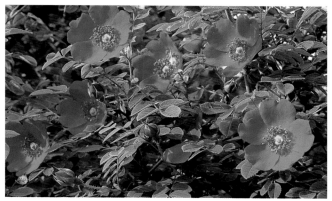

△ **Scarlet Fire**

This vigorous modern climber, or sprawling shrub rose, is an excellent variety, with dark stems, reddish young foliage and huge single, scarlet flowers. Although not a repeating rose, it stays in bloom for a long period in mid-summer, and the subsequent heavy crop of orange hips stays handsome throughout early winter. Sometimes listed as 'Scharlachglut', it looks stunning planted with the purple-leaved vine.

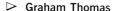
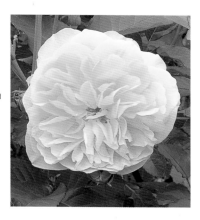

▷ **Graham Thomas**

In my view, this is the best of the modern but old-looking English roses. The tall, lax bushes produce large flowers with incurved petals. When young, these are egg-yolk yellow, fading to a rich primrose just before they fall. A lovely shrub, it needs a big space to develop to its full size.

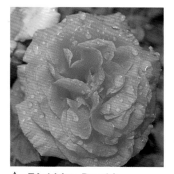

△ **Zéphirine Drouhin**

This thornless rose has rich coppery young leaves and stems. It is equally happy grown as a climber or as a big shrub, and has unique purplish-pink, intensely fragrant flowers, which appear throughout the growing season. This variety is prone to disease but vigorous enough to survive even without spraying and especially if planted on a cool, east wall in rich, moist soil. It will even flower in moderate shade.

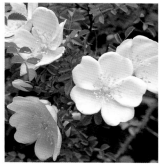

△ **Dunwich Rose**

Sometimes called *R. pimpinellifolia* 'Dunwichensis', this low-growing burnet rose has ferny foliage and bristling stems. The single flowers are pale cream, darkening a little towards their centres, with a gentle fragrance. In autumn, the hips are almost black among foliage that turns bronze as it falls. It flowers early in the season, in May, but is non-repeating. It is disease-free and easy to propagate from suckers.

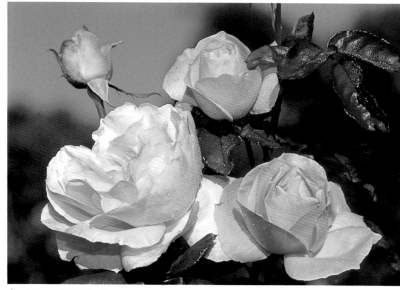

△ **Queen Elizabeth**

This unstoppable floribunda rose thrives in any conditions, producing big sprays of bright pink, non-fragrant flowers from early June until the first frosts. It should be pruned hard each year to prevent the plants from becoming too tall and leggy. Deadhead fiercely after the first main flush, and give the bushes a light all-over pruning to encourage sustained flowering.

◁ **Just Joey**

If you could plant only one hybrid tea rose, this should be it. The neat but vigorous bushes are adorned all summer with large, fragrant blooms in warm, salmon tones, the petals often frilled at their edges. Just Joey is moderately disease-resistant and easy to establish. Regular deadheading of the faded blooms will encourage constant flowering.

> **You should prune your roses in late winter to remove the old shoots and encourage new growth. Feed the plants in spring and mulch with compost to produce the best display.**

HOME FRONT
in the garden

BBC2's *Home Front in the Garden* **team have faced many garden challenges. They have never been fazed. They have created fun, functional and stylish gardens from the most improbable beginnings. Here is what interior designer Anne McKevitt and garden designer Diarmuid Gavin did for one London family in the first series.**

With four lively children under the age of eight, Brian Neeson, a photographer, and his wife, Julie, hadn't had a lot of time to spare for the garden in the two years since they moved into their large terraced house.

The result was scruffy, worn-out lawns, weedy flower-beds and a dull, rectangular layout. The only thing that flourished was a fine crop of wash basins, thanks to Brian's passion for raiding skips. The garden was, frankly, a mess. But the Neesons came up trumps: they called in the *Home Front* team.

Their brief to the team was simple, if a little vague. As well as an exciting play area, Julie wanted 'something colourful without being garish … interesting in a textural way'. For Brian it was 'somewhere we can sit and eat with friends and have a good time'. Their other great concern was that the land behind the garden had been sold for housing, so a design that protected their privacy was vital.

After giving this very sketchy outline, the Neesons blithely decamped for a fortnight's holiday, expressing a touching faith that the team would have completely transformed the garden by the time they had returned.

Undaunted, Diarmuid drew up a rough plan. His first concern was the back of the house. The flight of steps leading straight down from the first-floor level was pretty hazardous for all the children, and especially the new baby. A decking area was what was needed, or even a split-level deck, like an old wooden sailing ship, which would provide room for an al fresco dining area and a safe, stately descent to the garden.

A curving lawn would then lead through to the children's play area at the end of the garden, where Diarmuid was determined to make a bit of a splash! This area also presented the biggest challenge:

Left *The back of the house is bonded to the garden by two-tier decking and lush planting. The new bright yellow surround to the kitchen door and Diarmuid's surreal blue door echo the colours at the other end of the garden.*

Right *The view from the deck: a gentle wash of sea-green lawn, lapped by golden sand and the distant prospect of a seaside funfair. Trees planted behind the wall will eventually form an even denser screen.*

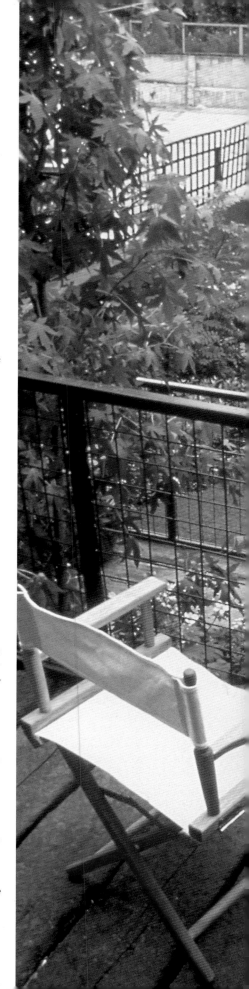

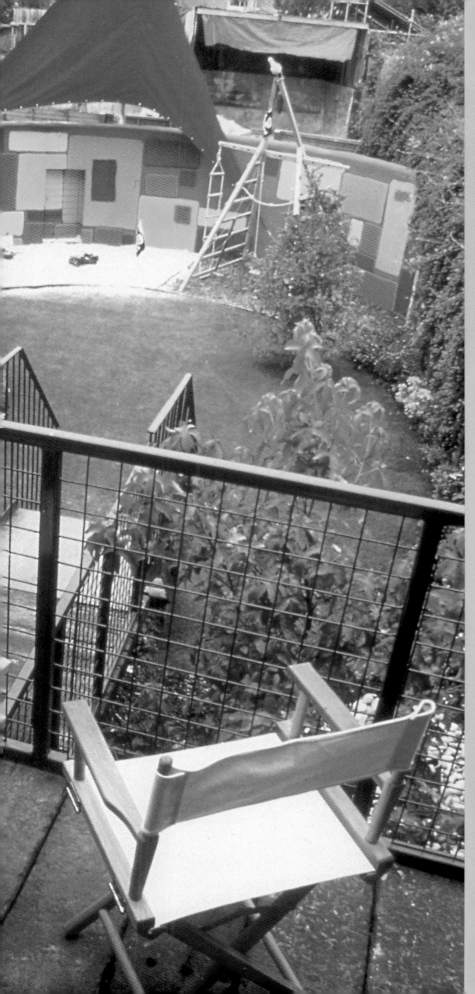

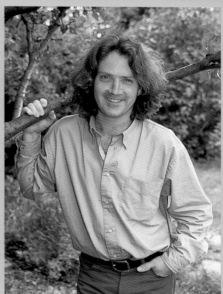

Diarmuid Gavin

the need for privacy. Planning regulations dictated that any permanent structure could not exceed 1.8m (6ft), which was not nearly enough.

Continuing the nautical idea of the deck, Diarmuid suggested a temporary structure, a great sail that would soar and billow over the end of the garden, providing fun for the kids, a wonderful focal point and, of course, privacy.

For the overall colour scheme, he took his cue from the Neesons' kitchen. 'They've painted it a really funky orange colour,' he enthused, 'which gives me great ideas for the rest of the garden.'

Anne, meanwhile, had her eye on the border below the decking – the perfect spot, she felt, for a stunning water feature that could be enjoyed both at garden level and by anyone gazing out over the decking rail. A burbling pebble pool would be the ideal solution, providing the mesmeric sight and sound of water while being child-friendly and very affordable.

With the main plan decided upon, construction could begin, starting with the split-level deck that would provide such a stylish transition from house to garden. Salvaged RSJs provided the support, while massive railway sleepers were used for the two platforms. Made of hardwood, they last for ever, and were a real bargain at only £10 each. More savings were made with the stairs, by simply cutting the

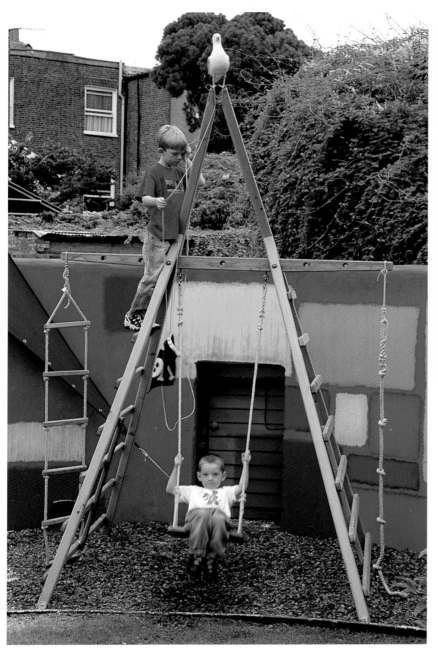

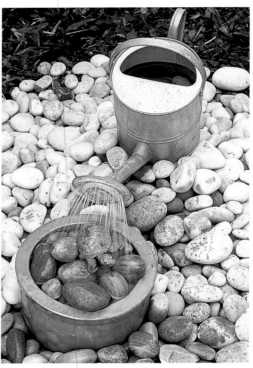

Gentle rain *Anne's calming water feature is simple to make. Dig a hole to form a reservoir, line it with heavy-duty polythene, fill with water and install a pump. Place rigid netting over the reservoir and finer netting on top of that to form a base for the pebbles. A tube from the pump is fed through the base of the watering can.*

A special place for the kids
Seagull ahoy, and hoist the Jolly Roger. Dexter and Jacob Neeson can't believe their luck.

original single flight in two. The mesh railings were chosen with child safety in mind and included a stair-gate on the top deck, so that baby Curtis could have his own secure play area close to the house. The space below the decking was a bonus, creating a useful storage area for toys, tools and for Brian's salvaged wash basins and other skip treasures.

As the decking rose, Anne got down to some serious pickaxe and shovel work to excavate a reservoir for her pebble pool. But once completed, she wasn't happy with the original idea of a simple bubble fountain and pebble surround. It wasn't in keeping with the

garden, she felt, and needed more impact. The problem was solved when she purloined the Neesons' handsome galvanised watering can. With tubing threaded through the base, she angled it over a pebble-filled pot so that a constant gentle rain wetted the pebbles and a silky sheen of water ran down the side of the pot. Anne's high standards were met, and the Neesons had a delightful water feature.

Patchwork of colour

At the other end of the garden, the sail was erected and the team moved on to tackle Diarmuid's curved rear wall. The team originally painted it blue, but everyone agreed that this just wasn't exciting enough. So, Diarmuid suggested trying out swatches of other colours. It was these bright swatches that led to the final design, which created a vibrant patchwork of colour, a bit like a holiday at the seaside. They learned a lesson along the way, too. Introducing a few paler colours just didn't work. For a bold scheme like this, take courage, take advantage of the hundreds of shades of masonry paint, and use only vibrant colours.

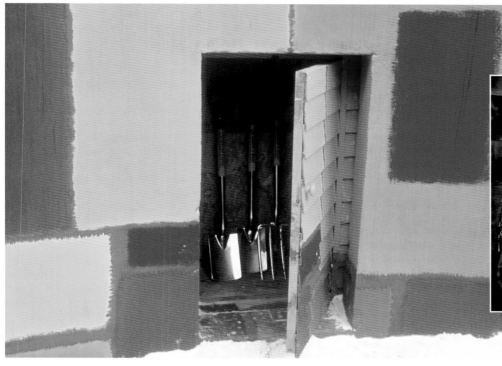

A vibrant hideaway *The rear wall, in all its colourful glory. By trial and error, the team achieved a magnificent result.*

Anne McKevitt

The wall held a few surprises, too. Two little doorways, which were camouflaged by paint, opened to reveal storage cupboards for toys and garden tools. This was achieved simply by placing two small garden sheds behind the wall and butting them against two openings. The team even catered for Fido, the family cat, with his very own catflap painted bright blue at the base of the wall.

With the major features in place, it was time for grass-laying and planting. In the borders, Diarmuid deployed his favourite trick of first laying out all the pots on the ground to assess the finished effect. The decking area was filled with pots and planters, including a splendid steel planter to house a liquidambar, or sweet gum tree, which was echoed by a twin planted at ground level. Chosen to provide instant height, these liquidambars give a fully furnished feel to the back of the house, together with the bonus of spectacular colour during the autumn months.

Last-minute titivations heralded the return of the Neesons from their holiday. A nervous team shepherded them in, but nerves gave way to delight when the Neesons eventually found words to express their amazement. 'It's incredible … it's fantastic!' gasped a dazed Julie. 'I just can't believe it's the same garden. Is that real grass?' The children, meanwhile, were swarming down to their sand and bark-lined seaside play area, scarcely able to believe their luck. Brian wasn't far behind them, and was first on the swing, before spotting Anne's pool which, like the rest of the garden, he absolutely loved.

Up on deck, Diarmuid and Julie surveyed the scene in a moment of mutual euphoria. 'I've got another room out here now,' she sighed appreciatively. Diarmuid pointed half-apologetically to the bright blue door that he had mounted on the side wall and which led nowhere. Julie, happy as a sandboy, smiled and gave her verdict: 'The door is surreal, but it's there, and it looks right. It'll be a constant reminder of you, Diarmuid.' The *Home Front* team had indeed worked its magic.

An industrial planter *Diarmuid is a great believer in looking around you for garden ideas. This impressive planter is made from industrial steel ducting which, at around £30 per cubic metre, is a stylish steal. Simply line it with heavy-duty polythene, make a few holes in the base and top up with drainage material and compost.*

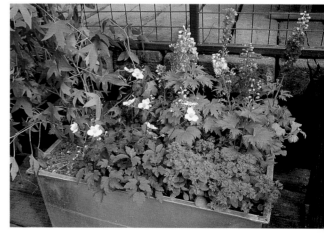

Before planting, lay out your plants on the ground to give an impression of what the final scheme will look like

A Calendar of
COLOUR

We all strive to have colour in the garden for every month of the year, but somehow there always seems to be a time when the border displays start to slump. It wouldn't be realistic to expect your borders to be filled with colour throughout the year, but with careful planning it is perfectly feasible to create focal points of interest from January through to December. It's quite possible that many of your favourite plants are included here, as well as a few that you have not tried before. Added to your garden they should help keep it looking colourful all year round.

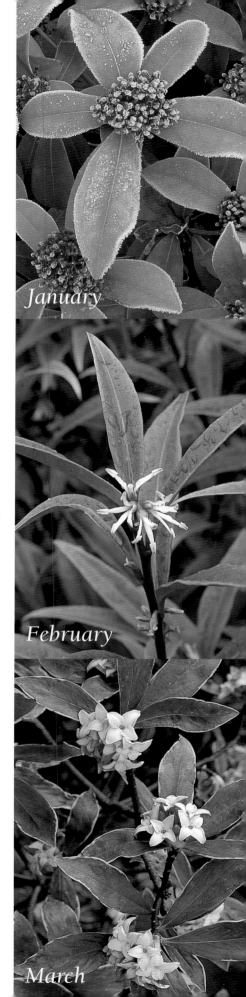

January

February

March

January

Skimmia

Clusters of waxy red berries that persist through the winter and evergreen foliage make skimmias invaluable shrubs. Usually a male and female variety must be grown to ensure fruit, but *Skimmia japonica* ssp. *reevesiana* will set berries on its own. Its habit is more compact than most and is suitable for winter containers. Ensure all skimmias are well fed to prevent the leaves from becoming yellow.

Others to try:
Acer griseum
Chaenomeles
Chimonanthus praecox
Clematis cirrhosa
Cornus stolonifera 'Flaviramea'
Erica carnea
Erica x *darleyensis*
Gaultheria procumbens
Hamamelis mollis
Hedera helix 'Goldheart'
Helleborus niger
Jasminum nudiflorum
Lonicera fragrantissima
Picea pungens 'Globosa'

February

Christmas box

Although small, the flowers of *Sarcococca hookeriana* var. *digyna*, which unfurl along the purple-tinted stems, have a heavy scent that can carry for considerable distances on mild days. It also makes an evergreen contribution throughout the year and increases in size to form a dense slender shrub. All sarcococcas thrive in deep shade, even under large trees, in most fertile soils.

Others to try:
Camellia japonica
Chionodoxa
Cornus mas
Corylus avellana 'Contorta'
Crocus tommasinianus
Cyclamen coum
Daphne mezereum
Eranthis hyemalis
Garrya elliptica 'James Roof'
Hamamelis x *intermedia* 'Jelena'
Helleborus orientalis hybrids
Iris histrioides
Leucojum vernum
Viburnum x *bodnantense* 'Dawn'

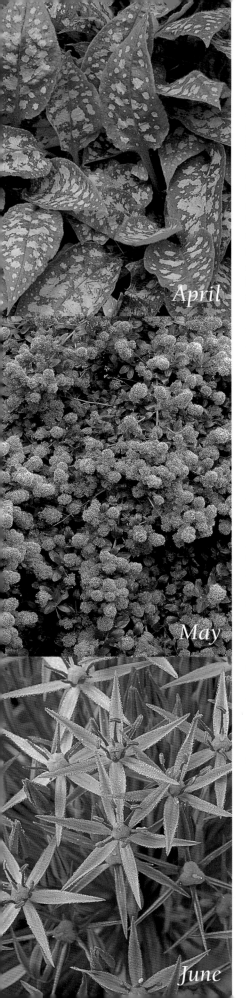

April

May

June

March

Daphne

One of the easiest daphnes to grow is *Daphne odora* 'Aureomarginata', which rewards minimal care with an abundant supply of scented blooms. The evergreen foliage, rimmed in gold, sets off the flower clusters a treat. Young plants are the quickest to establish and benefit from a sheltered position. Feed occasionally through the spring and summer months and prune back any leggy branches.

Others to try:
Anemone blanda
Clematis armandii
Forsythia x *intermedia* 'Lynwood'
Hacquetia epipactis
Hepatica nobilis
Narcissus 'Jetfire'
Osmanthus heterophyllus 'Goshiki'
Primula 'Wanda'
Prunus mume
Salix caprea 'Kilmarnock'
Scilla siberica

April

Lungwort

Many varieties of pulmonarias are available. Mostly evergreen, they are, without exception, true gems, with handsome foliage and spring flowers. *Pulmonaria saccharata* is a spotted-leaved type, although some are plain green or completely silver, and the flowers open pink and gradually turn blue. They make good ground cover in shady places, even self-sowing where happy.

Others to try:
Amelanchier lamarckii
Berberis darwinii
Bergenia cordifolia
Clematis alpina
Convallaria majalis
Corylopsis pauciflora
Doronicum x *excelsum*
Epimedium x *rubrum*
Lysichiton camtschatcensis
Magnolia x *soulangeana*
Ribes sanguineum 'Pulborough Scarlet'

May

Californian lilac

Every garden has places where low colourful cover is required and, if this happens to be a sunny spot, Californian lilac (*Ceanothus thyrsiflorus* var. *repens*) is an ideal plant. Its prostrate stems make evergreen mats of foliage that are hidden underneath the masses of blue flowers in summer. Well-drained soil is essential and plants establish quicker if new compost is added before planting.

Others to try:
Cytisus x *praecox* 'Warminster'
Euphorbia characias ssp. *wulfenii*
Magnolia liliiflora 'Nigra'
Pieris japonica 'Variegata'
Prunus 'Shogetsu'
Rhododendron luteum
Rosa xanthina 'Canary Bird'
Syringa meyeri var. *spontanea* 'Palibin'
Tulipa 'Generaal de Wet'
Veronica gentianoides
Viburnum sargentii 'Onondaga'

June

Ornamental onions

Alliums have become one of the most popular bulbs, bringing their distinctive drumstick shape to borders. They range in size from small and compact to the towering specimens whose bulbs can be planted between perennials or dwarf shrubs. *Allium cristophii* has large spherical purple flower-heads which look good for months and can be dried for indoor arrangements.

Others to try:
Aquilegia vulgaris
Convolvulus cneorum
Cornus kousa var. *chinensis*
Digitalis purpurea
Erysimum 'Bowles' Mauve'
Iris 'Jane Phillips'
Lavandula stoechas ssp. *pedunculata*
Lupinus
Paeonia lactiflora 'Bowl of Beauty'
Rosa 'Graham Thomas'
Wisteria floribunda 'Alba'

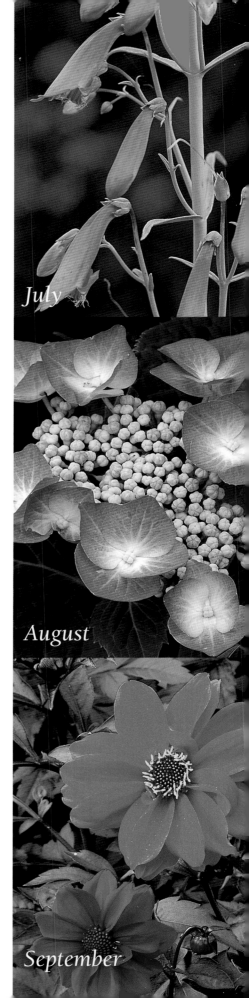

July

August

September

July

Penstemon

The open-faced tubular blooms of this group of tender perennials appear from July through to October. Flower colours include reds, such as 'Flame', whites, pinks, purples, blues and also some bi-colours. *Penstemon barbatus* and *P. ovatus* survive outside as evergreens and other varieties are hardy in most gardens, provided they are given protection. As a rule, the larger the flower and leaf, the more tender the plant.

Others to try:
Astrantia major ssp. *involucrata* 'Shaggy'
Buddleja davidii var. *nanhoensis*
Centaurea
Eryngium
Fuchsia 'Superstar'
Hemerocallis
Hosta 'Francee'
Impatiens
Incarvillea
Lathyrus grandiflorus
Lathyrus odoratus
Lavandula
Leucanthemum
Lilium regale
Lychnis coronaria
Pelargonium
Petunia
Romneya coulteri
Verbascum

August

Hydrangea

These bushy plants are grown for their large flower-heads. The two most common varieties, which are seen flowering in August, are both types of *Hydrangea macrophylla*, which have blue, purple or red flowers, depending on the soil type, and foliage that turns red in autumn. The hortensias have large, domed flower-heads, while lacecaps, like *H. macrophylla* 'Mariesii Perfecta', have flat, open heads.

Others to try:
Achillea
Agapanthus 'Loch Hope'
Argyranthemum
Campanula 'Elizabeth'
Clematis florida 'Flore Pleno'
Crocosmia
Dahlia
Diascia
Hibiscus syriacus
Lavatera 'Barnsley'
Lavatera trimestris
Liatris spicata
Osteospermum
Phlomis russeliana
Rudbeckia var. *sullivantii* 'Goldsturm'
Sidalcea 'Elsie Heugh'
Solanum crispum 'Glasnevin'
Verbena 'Homestead Purple'

September

Dahlia

'Bishop of Llandaff' is a wonderful showy form of dahlia with single, open-centred, dark red flowers up to 13cm (5in) across. The leaves are bronze-green and make an ideal foil for the blooms. Staking may be necessary in windy areas to ensure plants do not topple over. Plants or tubers should be planted in spring once the danger of frost has passed, and lifted and overwintered after the first frosts.

Others to try:
Anemone x *hybrida*
Aster amellus 'King George'
Caryopteris x *clandonensis* 'Heavenly Blue'
Ceratostigma willmottianum
Echinacea
Fuchsia magellanica
Hebe pinguifolia 'Pagei'
Humulus lupulus 'Aureus'
Hydrangea paniculata 'Unique'
Scabiosa
Sedum spectabile
Tradescantia

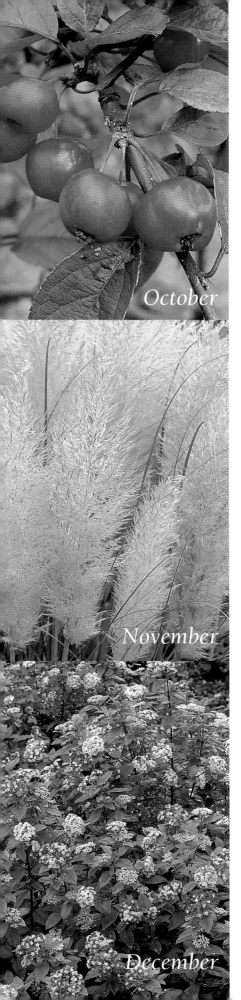

October

November

December

October

Crab apple

These invaluable trees are grown for their masses of cup-shaped spring flowers and brightly coloured autumn foliage and fruits. They will tolerate any soil except one that is waterlogged for long periods. The majority of crab apples have white or pink-white blossom but the fruit vary widely in their colour and size. Look out for *Malus* x *robusta* 'Red Sentinel' for its dazzling red fruits.

Others to try:

Acer japonicum 'Vitifolium'
Aster ericoides
Clematis 'Bill MacKenzie'
Colchicum speciosum
Cotinus 'Grace'
Cyclamen hederifolium
Dendranthema
Euonymus
Fothergilla major

Leucojum autumnale
Leycesteria formosa
Nerine bowdenii
Rosa moyesii
Rudbeckia 'Herbstsonne'
Salvia involucrata 'Bethellii'
Schizostylis coccinea 'Jennifer'
Solidago 'Queenie'
Yucca gloriosa 'Variegata'

November

Pampas grass

Ideal as a fine specimen plant for borders or as the centrepiece to a lawn, *Cortaderia selloana* 'Pumila' is an evergreen grass that is renowned for its silky, silvery flowering plumes in early autumn. Position near a dark background for best effect. Remove the old plumes to their base in spring, but remember to wear gloves at all times as protection from the sharp, roughened leaf edges.

Others to try:

Acer palmatum
Arbutus unedo
Berberis wilsoniae
Cornus kousa
Cotinus coggygria
Cotoneaster
Cyclamen hederifolium
Elaeagnus varieties
Gaultheria mucronata
Geranium wlassovianum
Liriope muscari
Lonicera x *purpusii* 'Winter Beauty'
Prunus x *subhirtella* 'Autumnalis'
Pyracantha
Skimmia japonica 'Nymans'
Sorbus cashmiriana
Viburnum farreri

December

Viburnum

A superb plant for the winter period, *Viburnum tinus* 'Eve Price' produces its clusters of star-shaped flowers until mid-spring. Pink in bud, they open to white above dark green leaves and are then followed by small, oval, blue fruits. Forming a compact shape, this evergreen plant is bushy, slow-growing and hardy. Grow in sun or semi-shade and a deep, fertile soil that does not dry out.

Others to try:

Abies koreana
Acer pensylvanicum 'Erythrocladum'
Aucuba japonica 'Crotonifolia'
Betula utilis var. *jaquemontii*
Callicarpa bodinieri var. *giraldii*
    'Profusion'
Elaeagnus x *ebbingei* 'Gilt Edge'
Erica carnea 'December Red'
Hedera helix varieties
Ilex aquifolium
Iris foetidissima
Mahonia
Phormium tenax
Photinia davidiana
Rubus biflorus
Taxus baccata 'Standishii'
Leucothoe 'Scarletta'

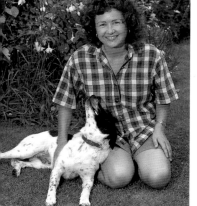

Gardening for children

Clare Bradley

These two unusual projects for young gardeners are enormous fun (for grown-ups as well!). Growing a gourd is so quick and easy, while planting a brick with colourful plants is a really creative way of decorating a garden wall.

Gourd fun in the sun

Gourds like the hot weather, so you will have to wait until early summer before you can start this project. But once you sow the seeds, you won't have to wait long for results as gourds are some of the fastest-growing plants. Close relatives of the pumpkin and marrow, they produce fruit in all shapes, sizes and colours. Many are delicious to eat, but some are grown because they make fascinating autumn decorations when dried out.

Gourds and squashes need to be pampered and grown in a warm, moist soil, which is why they are not sown outside until summer has well and truly arrived. Traditionally, they used to be grown on the top of compost heaps where it is rich and warm, but they will also do well in large pots or in growing bags.

Be careful when you handle the plants as their long stems are rough and covered with small prickles. They climb by gripping with twining tendrils.

Gourds are thirsty plants, and the compost should never be allowed to dry out, and they will probably need watering every day. They will also benefit from a liquid feed from time to time. One that is suitable for flowers and fruit, such as a tomato fertiliser, is ideal.

Flowers and pollination

Gourd plants have yellow male and female flowers. It's easy to spot female flowers because they have a tiny swollen gourd

How to plant your ornamental gourd

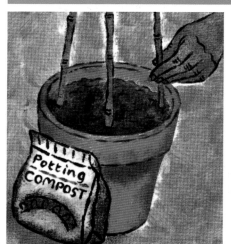

1 Fill a large flower pot, at least 30cm (12in) diameter, with potting compost. Make a wigwam by planting three bamboo canes around the edge and tie them together at the top.

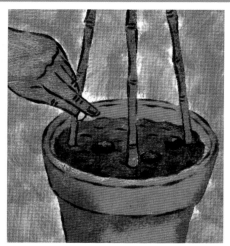

2 Dampen the compost, then sow three seeds in the middle of the pot, about 1–2cm (½–¾in) deep. Plant the seeds on their edge rather than flat as this prevents them from rotting.

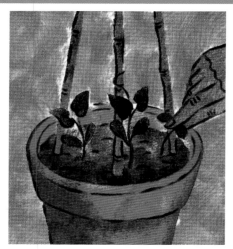

3 There is only room for two plants to grow in this size of pot. It is possible that they won't all grow, but if three seedlings do emerge, all you have to do is pull out the smallest.

behind the petals. Male flowers carry lots of yellow pollen. The female flower needs to be pollinated to make a gourd. This is usually done by bees and insects as they fly from flower to flower collecting pollen, but you can do it by hand. Simply pick off a male flower and dust it against the female flower. The petals quickly fall off as the fruit begins to swell.

On the fruit trail

The trailing stems grow very long, up to 5m (16ft). To keep them within bounds, pinch out the growing tip when it has reached 60cm (2ft). Sideshoots will develop from the stem. Remove their growing points when they are 60cm (2ft) long. Harvest the fruit during autumn, once it is completely ripe.

Clare Bradley is the *Blue Peter* gardener. She has written a number of books, the most recent *The Young Gardener* (Metro).

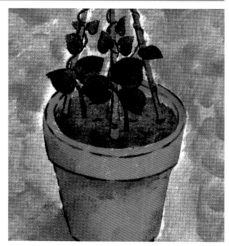

4 As the stems grow, place them so that they branch out and around the canes. Watch out for slugs. Look for them by torch light on warm damp evenings and pick them off.

How to make a wall of colour

Have you noticed how some plants grow in the most amazing places like the cracks of brick walls? With just a few bricks and a selection of plants you can make your own creative wall.

Plants can adapt to survive in impossible situations. Many of the plants you find growing in walls originally grew on mountains where conditions can be just as tough. Known as alpines, lots of these plants are able to grow by clinging to crevices on rock faces, so they make an ideal choice for a dry stone wall or a patio edge. You may not have a wall to plant up, but you could use a few bricks, which cost around 20p each from DIY stores. Make sure you mix grit with the compost as alpine plants need good drainage.

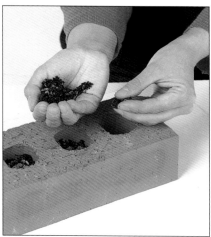

1 Put the brick on a seed tray or outside in the position where you want to display it. Half fill the holes with the mixture of grit and compost.

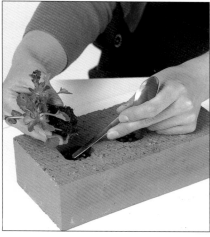

2 I planted a sempervivum, viola and saxifrage. Use a spoon handle to ease the plants into the holes. Add extra compost and grit to fill any gaps.

Aftercare

Plant several bricks for a really stunning display. The plants need to be fed with a liquid fertiliser once a week in spring and summer. They won't last for ever, and your brick will become overgrown, but you can divide plants or take cuttings to use in containers or other wall features.

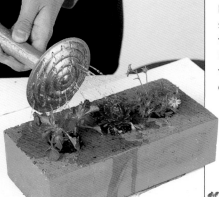

3 Using a watering can or plant sprayer, gently water each plant in, but take care not to wash the soil away. Keep the compost moist but don't overwater.

Gardens and Wildlife:
a natural partnership

Chris Baines

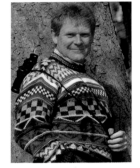

The wildlife that shares our gardens is a great source of pleasure. There's nothing to beat the sound of early morning bird song, the colourful spectacle of butterflies feeding on a buddleia bush, or the thrill of meeting the neighbourhood hedgehog on its early evening slug hunt. Between us we have over a million acres of gardens – a rich mixture of habitats that together adds up to the biggest nature reserve in the country. Think of your own particular patch as a sunny glade, set among the trees of the urban forest, filled with fruits and flowers, and linked into the rich network of hedgerows, railway embankments, town parks, school grounds, cemeteries and other people's gardens. No wonder our gardens are so good for wildlife and, with a little time and effort, they can be made even better.

Nesting boxes *Extra sites for nesting birds and roosting bats can be provided artificially. Put up lots of nesting boxes, choosing well-screened, sheltered sites wherever possible. House walls make much safer nesting sites for garden birds than trees if you are plagued by squirrels.*

Hibernation habitat *It pays to tolerate a little untidiness somewhere in the garden, which is not too challenging a task for most of us. Pile up old rotting logs, bundles of twigs and heaps of fallen leaves in a quiet corner to provide a hibernation habitat for hedgehogs and other secretive wildlife.*

Mini-meadow *A neat lawn is fine, but birds will benefit from a little moss for lining nests and, if you allow some of the grass to grow, there will be scope for planting wildflowers such as cowslips, meadow cranesbill, bugle and snake's head fritillary. You may also have breeding meadow brown butterflies and possibly a hunting kestrel as a bonus.*

Stone wall *Nooks and crannies are at a premium in most gardens, but they make essential hiding places for many of the creatures of the night. Build an open-jointed stone wall, ideally with a bank of soil behind it, and you will have the perfect habitat for overwintering newts and toads, for colonies of bees and for the nests of wrens and bluetits.*

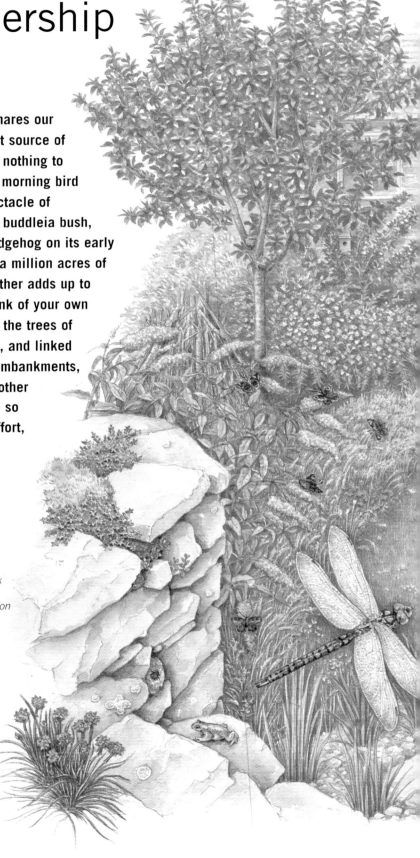

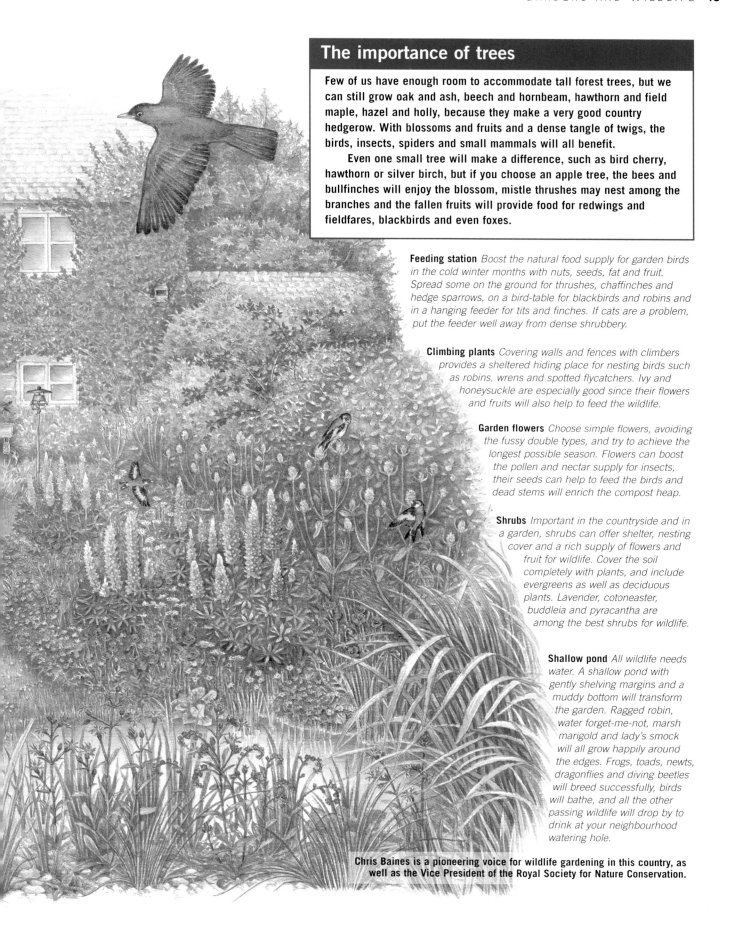

The importance of trees

Few of us have enough room to accommodate tall forest trees, but we can still grow oak and ash, beech and hornbeam, hawthorn and field maple, hazel and holly, because they make a very good country hedgerow. With blossoms and fruits and a dense tangle of twigs, the birds, insects, spiders and small mammals will all benefit.

Even one small tree will make a difference, such as bird cherry, hawthorn or silver birch, but if you choose an apple tree, the bees and bullfinches will enjoy the blossom, mistle thrushes may nest among the branches and the fallen fruits will provide food for redwings and fieldfares, blackbirds and even foxes.

Feeding station *Boost the natural food supply for garden birds in the cold winter months with nuts, seeds, fat and fruit. Spread some on the ground for thrushes, chaffinches and hedge sparrows, on a bird-table for blackbirds and robins and in a hanging feeder for tits and finches. If cats are a problem, put the feeder well away from dense shrubbery.*

Climbing plants *Covering walls and fences with climbers provides a sheltered hiding place for nesting birds such as robins, wrens and spotted flycatchers. Ivy and honeysuckle are especially good since their flowers and fruits will also help to feed the wildlife.*

Garden flowers *Choose simple flowers, avoiding the fussy double types, and try to achieve the longest possible season. Flowers can boost the pollen and nectar supply for insects, their seeds can help to feed the birds and dead stems will enrich the compost heap.*

Shrubs *Important in the countryside and in a garden, shrubs can offer shelter, nesting cover and a rich supply of flowers and fruit for wildlife. Cover the soil completely with plants, and include evergreens as well as deciduous plants. Lavender, cotoneaster, buddleia and pyracantha are among the best shrubs for wildlife.*

Shallow pond *All wildlife needs water. A shallow pond with gently shelving margins and a muddy bottom will transform the garden. Ragged robin, water forget-me-not, marsh marigold and lady's smock will all grow happily around the edges. Frogs, toads, newts, dragonflies and diving beetles will breed successfully, birds will bathe, and all the other passing wildlife will drop by to drink at your neighbourhood watering hole.*

Chris Baines is a pioneering voice for wildlife gardening in this country, as well as the Vice President of the Royal Society for Nature Conservation.

Successful Water GARDENS

Charlie Dimmock

Having a water feature adds an extra dimension, even to a small garden where space is limited. You can grow plants in and around the water, and its presence will help to encourage wildlife into your garden. Water also has a wonderfully calming influence.

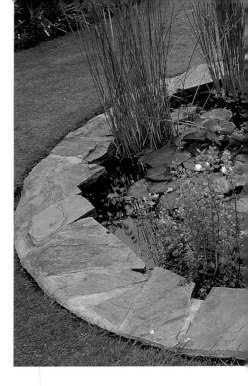

nstalling a pond couldn't be easier. You can buy either pre-cast pond shells, which come in different shapes and sizes, or pond liners for covering the inside of a hole. That's the good news. The bad news is that the holes don't appear by themselves; you've got to dig them.

Liners and pre-cast shells

The simplest way of making a pond is with flexible liners because they are so easy to use. They can be made from a number of materials; generally, the heavier the gauge, the longer they will last. The liners can be moulded into any shaped hole and are easy to repair. They are great if you want a more natural-shaped pond than that provided by a pre-cast shell, and are also easier to put down.

Flexible liners can be punctured quite easily if laid too taut around the hole, but generally a top-grade plastic liner or a thicker rubber, or butyl, one will last around 25 years. They are considerably cheaper than pre-cast shells, and are used on the *Ground Force* programmes because of their many benefits.

Pre-cast shells come in predetermined shapes and sizes, and are made from plastic or fibreglass. Middle-of-the-range pre-cast shells will usually last around 15 years. While they don't puncture as easily as flexible liners, they can crack; the easiest way to repair them is by covering them with a flexible liner. The downside of shells is that the range of shapes and sizes is limited, they can look contrived and tend to deteriorate more quickly than flexible liners.

Pond depth

When planning your pond, decide roughly what size it will be: how long, wide and deep. This is important for establishing the types and numbers of plants and fish that can be introduced. To support a wide range of plants and fish, the depth of a pond at its deepest point should be 60–90cm (2–3ft). This depth will provide adequate protection from predators and harsh winters, while providing an even, constant temperature throughout the summer. Ponds with less than this depth may still be adequate for the fish and plants, but there will be less of a buffer during extreme conditions.

Making a pond with a pre-cast shell

Mark out the shape of the shell with canes and dig out a hole 30cm (12in) bigger than its shape. Put soft sand in the base of the hole to prevent the shell cracking. Place the shell in the hole and check with a spirit level that it is perfectly level. Fill the shell with water and at the same time cram soil in under the shelves and at the sides of the shell to secure it. Hide the visible edges with paving or turf.

Stocking the pond

The size and depth of a pond determine the number of plants and fish that can form a healthy, balanced environment. Choose plants that won't invade your pond and add some oxygenating weed to keep the water clear.

Selecting the right plants

One of the most difficult tasks is finding the right plants to fit the scale of the

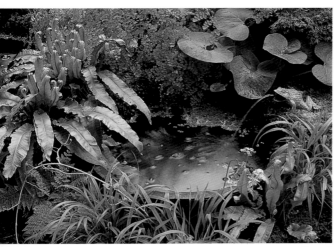

Planting with care *Even the smallest of pools benefits from a thoughtful planting scheme. Here, an interesting range of flower shapes and colours contrasts effectively with textured foliage and varied leaf shapes*

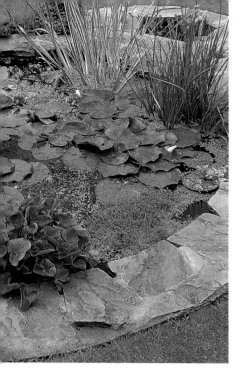

Added value *A pond adds interest to any garden, not least because it increases the range of plants that can be grown. The specialised micro-climate can also play host to lots of wildlife*

pond, and the smaller the pond, the more difficult the problem becomes. Where fish are present, some vegetation is essential. Not only does it provide food and cover from predators, such as herons and kingfishers, it also shades the water, helping to keep it cool.

It is important to have a mixture of plants within the pond because they all perform different functions. Waterlilies and deep-water aquatics, growing in depths of 45–60cm (1½–2ft), provide perfect shelter for the fish; oxygenators are important for the clarity and quality of the pond water; and bog plants and marginals provide shade in the shallow water, where many young fish will congregate.

Floating plants provide cover on the water's surface but they can grow rapidly, blocking out the light and choking all other pond life. Introduce sufficient plants when you stock the pond to colonize only up to one-third of the surface area of the pond. As a rule of thumb, there should be about three plants of whatever kind per sq m (sq yd) of pond surface. Plants to avoid because of their tendency to invade include *Azolla mexicana, Decodon verticillatus, Lemna minor* and *Sparganium erectum.*

How to make a pond with a flexible liner

1 Mark out the shape of the pond; if you want an irregular shape, a garden hose can be laid out until the shape is decided.

2 As you dig the hole to form the contours of the pond, remove the valuable topsoil and store it for later use.

3 As you dig deeper, leave ledges or shelves on which to position planting baskets.

4 Check that the rim is level using a spirit level and plank. Some of the excavated soil can raise any low areas around the rim. Compact the

soil inside the hole. Line the hole with moist sand or old carpets to prevent the liner from being punctured by stones.

5 Unwrap the liner and lay it centrally over the hole. Pour a few litres of water onto it to act as a weight and drag the liner into the bottom of the hole, then it's off with your shoes and socks as you get into the hole and spread out the liner. Fill up the pond with water.

6 Trim any excess liner around the rim, leaving about 15cm (6in). Hide and secure the rim with a layer of turf or a row of paving slabs.

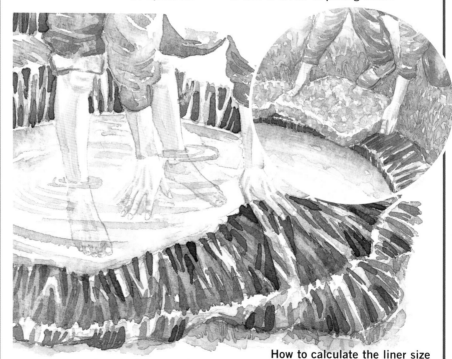

How to calculate the liner size
Length of liner required = length of pond + twice the depth of the pond
Width of liner required = width of the pond + twice the depth of the pond
Always allow a little extra for folds and overlaps

Planting aquatics
Aquatics can be grown in basket-like containers, which are usually made of strong plastic; metal and wood containers can produce toxins which are harmful to fish. These containers make the plants

more accessible for maintenance and propagation.

The plants which are to be submerged or partially submerged are planted in these mesh containers in the spring, using a special soil-based, aquatic plant compost which contains no fertilisers that will foul the water. The upper surface of the compost is covered with a 2.5cm (1in) layer of pea shingle to prevent the compost from floating away and making the water cloudy.

A basket can be lowered into the centre of the pond quite easily: thread a long length of string through its sides and tie the two ends together. You need an assistant to stand on the opposite side of the pond; both take hold of the string and lower the basket into the centre of the water until it settles on the bottom. The string can now be released.

Feeding

Aquatic plants usually need feeding only every year or two. The most common means of feeding involves placing a pellet or sachet of slow-release fertiliser in each basket. This is done by fixing the fertiliser onto the tip of a long cane and inserting it where needed.

Divide and rule

Many aquatic plants are propagated by division in the spring. The containers are lifted out of the water and all the compost is washed away from the plants before they are divided into smaller segments and replanted in new containers. The old central part of the plant should be discarded.

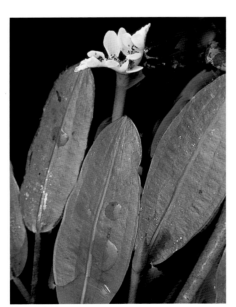

The water hawthorn, *Aponogeton distachyos*

Choice hardy plants

The following plants are suitable for small and medium-sized ponds.

DEEP-WATER AQUATICS
Aponogeton distachyos
The water hawthorn has long, fleshy, light green, floating leaves, with highly scented cream flowers during summer, which turn green as they fade.

Sagittaria sagittifolia 'Flore Pleno'
This beautiful, fancy aquatic has light green, arrow-shaped leaves and white flowers with double rows of petals in mid-summer.

Orontium aquaticum
This strange-looking plant has fine, pencil-like, yellow and white flowers held above the water on slender green stems. The blue-green leaves are lance-shaped and float on the water's surface.

OXYGENATORS
Callitriche species
These plants are very similar to each other in appearance, having light green leaves which form a rosette on the surface. They grow well only when the water chemistry is well balanced, making them perfect indicator plants.

Mentha aquatica
Technically a water purifier, the water mint has oval-shaped, dark green leaves with deeply toothed edges on purple-red stems. The small lilac flowers appear in small round clusters in summer.

Lagarosiphon major
A submerged aquatic with brittle stems, densely clad with small, lance-shaped, deep green leaves that curve downwards. Small tubular flowers, which are green tinged with pink, appear in summer.

FLOATERS
Hydrocharis morsus-ranae
This pretty plant resembles a miniature water lily, with small, mid-green, kidney-shaped leaves. The small summer flowers each have a yellow centre surrounded by three white petals.

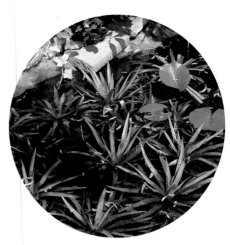

Stratiotes aloides

Stratiotes aloides
The water soldier resembles the top of a pineapple floating on water. The cup-shaped female flowers are creamy white with a papery texture, while the male flowers are carried in tight clusters in a pink, rolled-leaf-like structure; both appear in mid-summer.

Utricularia vulgaris
Bladderwort has showy, bright yellow antirrhinum-like flowers that appear on long stalks above the water in mid-summer. The delicate, bright green foliage has a lace-like appearance, with small flotation bladders mixed among the leaves. Suitable for soft water areas only.

MARGINALS
Eriophorum angustifolium
The cotton grass reaches 45cm (18in) and produces fine grassy foliage topped with fluffy white, cotton-wool-like flowers in early summer. Like all eriophorums, this plant must be grown in a water-logged, acid soil. It's invasive, so regular trimming is needed.

Iris laevigata
The blue-flowered aquatic iris, with sword-shaped, smooth green leaves, grows up to 90cm (3ft) high and forms clumps up to 90cm (3ft) across. There are numerous different-coloured forms.

Mimulus luteus
This musk has green, rounded leaves and green stems up to 30cm (12in) high, which are topped with spikes of bright yellow, snapdragon-like flowers. It flowers all summer and can be propagated by division in the spring.

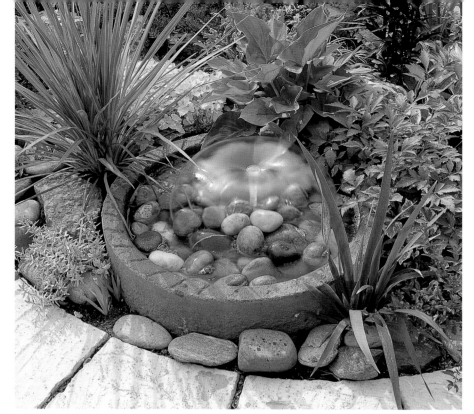

HOW TO MAKE A BUBBLE FOUNTAIN

1 Start by digging a hole at least 25 litres (5½ gallons) in volume to accommodate a reasonable reservoir of water and a submersible pump to circulate it. The easiest way to do this is to buy a small water cistern from a local DIY store. This will have the volume of water indicated on the side.

2 Bed the water cistern on a layer of damp sand and use a spirit level to make sure that the rim is level. Pack loose soil into the gap between the outside of the cistern and the walls of the hole.

3 Put the pump into the cistern, making sure that the sealed electrical connections are not damaged. Set it to an appropriate flow setting before filling the tank with water to a level above the top of the pump. Test the pump to make sure it is working.

4 Cover the tank of water with a sturdy metal grid resting just on the soil surface, with the outlet spout of the pump protruding through it.

5 Cover the grid with a layer of pebbles to hide the top of the pump. Turn on the pump and reposition the pebbles as necessary to make a nice flow.

SUMMER-FLOWERING WATER LILIES
Nymphaea 'Gonnère'
In summer, this plant has pure white flowers with double rounds of petals, which look like snowballs bobbing about in the water. The medium-sized leaves are a fresh pea-green colour.

Nymphaea 'Froebelii'
This popular free-flowering variety has dull purple-green leaves and deep blood-red flowers with vivid orange stamens.

Nymphaea 'Rose Arey'
The large, star-shaped pink flowers have a distinctive aniseed aroma. The leaves are bronze when young, turning deep green with a crimson tinge as they age.

Bubble fountains
What about a water feature without a pond? You can still have noise and movement from even a small amount of water without the extra work that a pond involves. And an easily built bubble fountain is perfectly safe for young children.

Making a bubble fountain
In the aptly named bubble fountain, water bubbles up through a group of pebbles or a large, flat stone, with a hole drilled through it, that is placed in the middle of

Bubble fountains *Pebbles are an attractive way of concealing the water tank hidden below*

a group of pebbles. This type of fountain can occupy an area as small as 30cm x 30cm (12in x 12in), with all the working and equipment totally hidden from view. This gives the illusion that the water is rising up from nowhere, tumbling over the stones and vanishing.

A bubble fountain requires little maintenance. Some water is lost through evaporation, so check the level in the pool regularly, once a week through the summer but less often at other times, and top up when necessary.

Successful pumping
Two types of pond pump are available. One uses a low-voltage electricity supply, and the other runs on the mains supply. Place the pump in the base of the pool and run the cable back to an indoor socket. All cabling must be protected to prevent accidental damage. Fix a circuit breaker into the mains plug: it cuts out the electricity if a fault develops. Always call in a qualified electrician to install an outdoor electricity supply for a water feature or lighting. If any parts are damaged, return the unit to the supplier rather than trying to repair it yourself.

Consider the following when choosing a pump:
1 The kind of feature it will serve, and whether it needs a continuous or intermittent flow.
2 The height, or head, of the fountain or waterfall from the water surface.
3 The outlet, i.e. the type of nozzle.
4 The pond, i.e. the volume of water held in the pond at its normal capacity.
5 The pipes, i.e. their internal diameter, and the distance the water has to be pumped.

The low-maintenance garden Gay Search

If you have a garden that is overgrown and with little worth saving, don't be downhearted but see it as a wonderful opportunity to do something completely different. In this garden, designed by Helen Yemm from BBC2's *Gardening from Scratch***, an awkward, near-derelict site has been quickly transformed into a low-maintenance gravel garden.**

The beauty of a gravel garden is that, once the preparation and planting have been done, the upkeep is minimal – a welcome draw for those who prefer relaxing in the garden to working in it. However, before you can think about relaxing, there is a little work to be done. First of all, getting rid of any visible weeds is essential. This can be done with a glyphosate-based weedkiller. The next step is to lay a membrane to prevent future weed growth and also help to conserve moisture in the soil. If the gravel is to have a cosmetic rather than functional role, a layer of just 2.5cm (1in) is needed to cover the membrane. If any weeds dare to show their faces after this, treat them with glyphosate. Rest assured, they will eventually give up the ghost.

When it comes to choosing plants, an important factor in any gravel garden is the ability to cope with drought. A lack of rain is something all gardeners have to take into account these days, given the trend towards much drier summers and, more significantly, winters. Choosing drought-tolerant plants, therefore, makes a great deal of sense. Fortunately, there are some wonderfully exciting plants that thrive in hot, dry conditions. Plants with silver foliage, such as artemisia and catmint, tend to like dry conditions, as do those with furry leaves, such as lambs' ears and verbascum. Since plants lose moisture through their leaves, drought-lovers never have large, fleshy leaves. Plants with narrow leaves, such as pinks, and spiky ones like sisyrinchium and cordyline, are good choices for the gravel garden. Aromatics, such as rosemary, lavender and *Helichrysum italicum* ssp. *serotinum*, the curry plant, also thrive in dry conditions. A word of warning, though: just smelling a curry plant can cause an allergic reaction.

Hot, vibrant colours and tall, dramatic plants lend themselves perfectly to gravel gardens. *Osteospermum* 'Nairobi Purple', *Phygelius* x *rectus* 'Devil's Tears', *Crocosmia* 'Emberglow', *Verbascum* 'Arctic Summer' and *Dorotheanthus bellidiformis*, or the Livingstone daisy, are particularly good. If you feel like splashing out, try a large cordyline. It really is worth having just one striking mature plant in a newly planted area. Additional focal points in the gravel garden can be created by

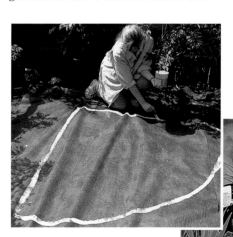

After laying the membrane, mark out the shape of your border with paint (above).

By creating planting areas without membrane, plants can self-seed through the gravel into the soil (right).

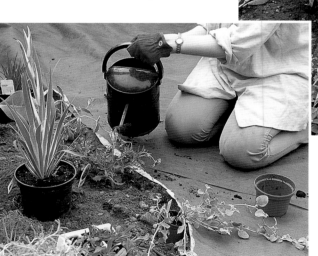

Create a path through the gravel with paving slabs. By using stone slabs that are different shapes and sizes and dotting them around, the path will have an informal feel (above).

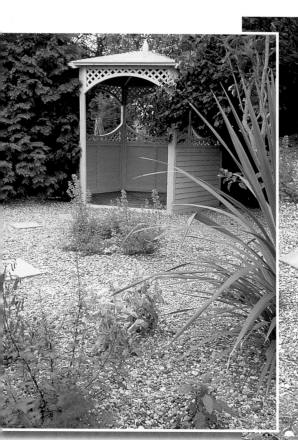

A wooden gazebo, assembled from a kit, provides the perfect place to sit and contemplate the garden. Originally an orangey-brown, the gazebo was painted with a silvery-grey opaque woodstain to complement the planting (above).

One or two strategically placed terracotta pots, containing sun-loving, drought-tolerant plants such as *Lotus berthelotii*, make striking focal points (right).

adding terracotta Ali Baba pots planted with *Lotus berthelotii*, which has foliage like fine silver needles and burnt-orange flowers like miniature parrots' beaks.

It's very easy to plant individual plants through the membrane by cutting generous crosses in it and digging out a planting hole for each one. If you're planting a sweep of plants, you can cut a large area of membrane away. This makes it simpler when putting in a lot of plants fairly close together and allows self-seeders such as bronze fennel to seed themselves around, giving a very soft, natural look. Plants self-seed far better in gravel overlaying soil.

Top tips for gravel gardens

● Even in a small garden, try and have a secret area that is invisible from the house and dramatically different from the rest.
● If you have a really bad weed problem, use a membrane under the gravel. It won't solve the whole problem, since real toughies can work their way through snags and gaps, but it will certainly help.

● Drought-tolerant plants generally don't need rich soil, so don't overfeed them.
● Water new, little plants until they are properly established.
● Don't try to have a neat and tidy gravel garden. The whole idea is that things find their own space and if cats make beds in the nepeta, so what?

Containers for SUMMER COLOUR

Anne Swithinbank

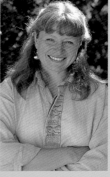

Summer containers are fun to put together because of the exciting plants available and the fast rate of growth during spring and summer. The popularity of container gardening over the past decade has certainly been matched by the range of plants available from garden centres.

Whether the planting becomes a showy, floriferous mass or a demure, shade-tolerant arrangement, whether it consists of native herbs or alpines or is an unusual, drought-tolerant composition, there is one common factor. Even if the plants are small to begin with, they will grow out of all recognition when the magic ingredients of water and food are added to warm summer temperatures and long days.

Most summer containers are planted in spring and cannot be put outside until late spring or early summer when the danger of frost has passed. There is also room for impulse summer planting later in the season, to give extra colour to revive a flagging garden or help celebrate a special occasion.

YOU WILL NEED: 1 pot of *Lilium* 'Reinesse' (3 bulbs); *Lavandula stoechas leucantha*; cream-variegated *Hedera helix*; bedding *Dianthus*; *Impatiens* 'Cherry Blush'; *Antirrhinum pendula* 'Lampion'; glazed terracotta pot, 35cm (14in) diameter, 30cm (12in) high

Anne Swithinbank has written a number of gardening books, including *Container Gardening for All Seasons* (BBC Worldwide), and is a panellist on Radio 4's *Gardeners' Question Time*.

Lily Pot

Lilies rising up from lavender is one of my favourite combinations, and *Lavandula stoechas leucantha* (white French lavender) makes a lovely companion. Distinctive in having white bracts protruding from the top of the flower spike, this has a different perfume from English lavender. A good pot of cream-variegated ivy saved from previous winter containers will balance the white lavender.

Garden centres do still have some bedding plants in mid-summer, but the range tends to be smaller and the plants larger. Inject some strong colour by choosing a bedding dianthus.

It also pays to keep a few spare summer bedding plants, potting them on into 10cm (4in) pots. From my stock, I chose a pale pink, dark-eyed *Impatiens* 'Cherry Blush' (busy Lizzie) and *Antirrhinum pendula* 'Lampion' (trailing snapdragon) to fill in remaining gaps to the front.

When the lily bulbs have finished flowering, remove the dead flowers and let the stems die back naturally. In early autumn the bulbs can be planted out into the garden. At the end of the season you can use the lavender in borders and the ivy in another container.

This display is suitable in sun or light shade.

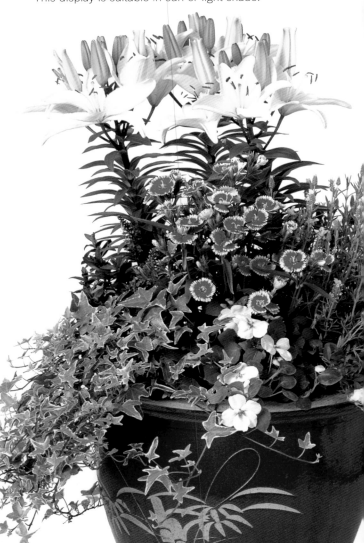

Basketweave Planter

Baskets are a cheaper and more rustic alternative to terracotta, concrete or stone. For a longer life, line them with polythene cut from old compost bags, so that the black side faces outwards. This will also stop compost from falling through the holes. Make slits in the bottom and put in a generous layer of stones or polystyrene so that excess water can escape easily. *Argyranthemum foeniculaceum* produces masses of small, white daisies all summer and is blessed with extra finely cut, ferny, blue-green foliage. Place a good, strong plant to the middle-back of the basket, then position *Fuchsia* 'Annabel' just to the front of it. Lovely pink-tinged, creamy white flowers contrast well against light green foliage. A trailing effect will be provided by a double, lilac-flowered, ivy-leaved pelargonium on one side and a silvery, felt-leaved *Helichrysum petiolare* 'Variegatum' on the other. Place the two pelargoniums so their stems reach towards each other. The helichrysums will then be on the outside. Fill in gaps with three white, large-flowered petunias. For a touch of bright red, three plants of trailing Tyrolean carnations have also been added, but these are optional. At the end of the season, carefully remove and pot the argyranthemum, pelargonium and fuchsia and place them in a cool, bright, frost-free place to overwinter. A good pruning-back in spring will encourage fresh shoots of leaves and flowers.

This display should be planted in late spring and placed in a sunny position.

YOU WILL NEED: *Argyranthemum foeniculaceum*; *Fuchsia* 'Annabel'; double lilac-flowered, ivy-leaved *Pelargonium*; *Helichrysum petiolare* 'Variegatum'; white Grandiflora *Petunia* x 3; wicker basket, 30cm (12in) diameter, 30cm (12in) high

Marigold Pot

Assuming that this arrangement will be seen from the front, first position the five *Salvia farinacea* 'Victoria' in a group, about 8cm (3in) apart, towards the middle-back. This elegant salvia can be bought as small plants or raised from seed. The newer variety *S. f.* 'Strata' is possibly even lovelier, bearing silvery stems and calyces from which the blue flowers emerge. They rise to some 45cm (18in) and will add height.

To each side of the container and at the very back, position three *Plectranthus forsteri* 'Marginatus'. This aromatic plant, with variegated, slightly fleshy leaves, has trailing stems which are quite brittle in comparison with those of ivy. It is a quick-growing plant that roots easily from cuttings.

Find a couple of slots along the front for two more trailing plants of *Lysimachia congestiflora* 'Outback Sunset'. This rather luscious plant bears bright green leaves and clusters of rich gold flowers which appear with regularity and reliability all summer.

Having arranged these tall and trailing plants, fill any gaps with compact *Tagetes* cultivars, or orange and lemon French marigolds, mixing them well. When they are all in place, carefully fill in around the roots with compost.

At the end of the season, lift and repot the plectranthus, which can overwinter as a houseplant. It needs good light and a constantly warm temperature – minimum 13°C (55°F). Take cuttings for next year. *Lysimachia congestiflora* 'Outback Sunset' can be kept in a cool, bright, frost-free place; the other plants should be composted. This display should be planted up in late spring and placed in a sunny position.

YOU WILL NEED: *Salvia farinacea* 'Victoria' x 5; *Plectranthus forsteri* 'Marginatus' x 3; *Lysimachia congestiflora* 'Outback Sunset' x 2; *Tagetes* x 7; terracotta pot, 36cm (14½in) diameter, 30cm (12in) high

Drought-tolerant Basket

To help this hanging basket withstand a dry, windy site, it is packed full of drought-tolerant plants that can endure a little neglect without withering.

Begin by lining the basket and sitting it on a flowerpot for stability while you plant. A small tray of mixed succulent portulaca will yield enough little plants to fit around the sides. These trailing plants are double-flowered varieties of *Portulaca grandiflora*, or sun plant. Their rootballs should be small enough to fit into the mesh from the outside. If they are not, wrap the leaves carefully in a tube of polythene and thread this through from the inside before unwrapping.

Having filled in around the roots with some more compost, place plants in the top of the basket. Plant a bright red zonal pelargonium in the middle of the basket, and surround it with three *Helichrysum italicum* ssp. *microphyllum*. This dwarf curry plant starts off as a compact bush of narrow, silvery, curry-scented leaves. As the planting matures, its stems rise up to produce heads of yellow flowers.

Between the helichrysums add two plants of the succulent *Aptenia cordifolia* 'Variegata' for its cream-variegated leaves and small, starry, bright pink flowers. The third plant is *Nolana* 'Blue Bird'. Tough-looking leaves are joined by rather shy, sky-blue, saucer-shaped flowers.

Although all these plants can survive short drought periods, aim to water them well and apply a liquid feed every week. At the end of the season, pot up the aptenia and possibly the nolana to overwinter in bright, cool, frost-free quarters. The curry plant can be planted in the garden.

This basket should be planted up in late spring and hung in a sunny position.

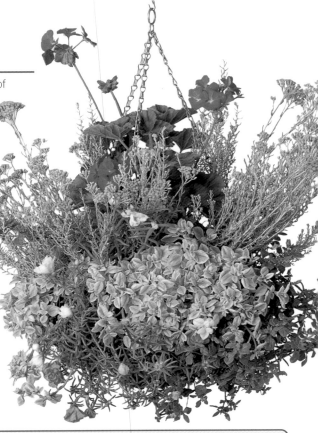

YOU WILL NEED: double, red *Portulaca grandiflora* x 6; red zonal *Pelargonium*; *Helichrysum italicum* ssp. *microphyllum* x 3; *Aptenia cordifolia* 'Variegata' x 2; *Nolana* 'Blue Bird'; plastic-coated wire hanging basket, 30cm (12in) diameter

Shallow Bowl for a Shady Position

Emphasising the all-round effect of this bowl, the *Dryopteris affinis* (golden-scaled male fern) is planted in the middle, snuggled into place with handsome *Hosta fortunei* var. *aureomarginata*. Many gardeners think that foliage plants like hostas should have their flower spikes removed to retain better foliage. I disagree. I enjoy the way a plant changes naturally during the seasons, even if it ruins the symmetry of my planting. To this combination were added the architectural leaves of *Helleborus orientalis* (Lenten rose).

For the rim of the container, take a short-growing *Astilbe* and divide the clump into two. Add to this a potful of *Heuchera* 'Palace Purple' and two of *Ajuga reptans* 'Multicolor' (bugle), arranging them around the edge to complement the foliage of the centre. Fill any gaps between with small plants of pale pink bedding *Impatiens* 'Accent Coral' (busy Lizzie).

It is fine to leave the plants in the container for the winter, although for the most part they will die back and rest. Compost the impatiens. When the other plants burst back into growth the following spring, the gaps can be plugged by more impatiens and the cycle can continue. Alternatively, lift the herbaceous plants and use in the garden if the bowl is to be freed for autumnal plantings.

This bowl, planted up in late spring, is best in shade or semi-shade.

YOU WILL NEED: *Dryopteris affinis*; *Hosta fortunei* var. *aureomarginata*; *Helleborus orientalis*; *Astilbe* cultivar; *Heuchera* 'Palace Purple'; *Ajuga reptans* 'Multicolor' x 2; *Impatiens* 'Accent Coral' x 6; terracotta bowl, 57cm (23in) diameter, 25cm (10in) high

Aromatic Herb Pot

A pot of culinary herbs should look beautiful, smell delicious and deliver plenty of fresh leaves to use in cooking. Herbs are generally far more drought-tolerant than the typical bedding plant, and a successful herb pot should last at least two years. It should contain a good majority of evergreens, like rosemary, sage and thyme, for winter interest and usefulness. A bushy rosemary plant is ideal for the centre of an arrangement. Restricted to a container, in close competition with other herbs and regularly cropped, it should remain within bounds.

To one side of the rosemary place an aromatic sage. For colour *Salvia officinalis* 'Icterina' (tricolor sage), with its sage-green and lime-green leaves, is hard to beat. Take odd leaves for cooking, but also nip out whole shoots if it grows too large. *Thymus* x *citriodorus* 'Aureus' (golden lemon thyme) is great for cooking, too, but select it only if you want its distinctive, lemony flavour. *Helichrysum italicum* is added for its colour and smell. Its silvery-grey leaves smell distinctly of curry. The two herbaceous herbs growing in the back are *Melissa officinalis* 'Aurea' (lemon balm) and *Origanum* 'Gold Splash' (marjoram), both of which die down for the winter, but put up plenty of new spring shoots.

Although continuous cropping will keep these herbs young and fresh, trim the shrubby herbs by about half to two-thirds in spring as they come into growth. Keep them growing together for two seasons, then lift them out in early autumn or spring, and plant in the garden. The lemon balm and marjoram can be lifted and divided.

Plant this container in late spring and stand it in a sunny position.

How to plant a tub or trough

1 Cover the base with crocks to a depth of 2.5cm (1in) or more.

2 Dunk any dry plants in a bucket of water until bubbles stop escaping.

3 Tease out congested roots.

4 In the tub, build up the compost. Add each plant at the correct depth.

5 Fill around all the plants until the compost level is within 2.5cm (1in) or so of the top.

6 Position the container on feet in order to raise it. Water using a watering can fitted with a rose.

How to plant a hanging basket

1 Remove the chain and balance the base on a flowerpot for stability.

2 Fit the liner into place and put soil in the base up to the point where the first plants are to be fed into the sides.

3 Force or cut a hole in the liner. Push through the roots of small plants from the outside.

4 If plants have large rootballs, wrap their shoots in a square of polythene to make a narrow, protective tube. Then feed this through the liner from the inside out.

5 Build up the compost as plants are added, leaving enough space to arrange plants in the top.

6 Fill around all the roots with compost. Reinforce the moss or moss substitute around the rim of the basket.

YOU WILL NEED: *Rosmarinus officinalis*; *Salvia officinalis* 'Icterina'; *Thymus* x *citriodorus* 'Aureus'; *Helichrysum italicum*; *Melissa officinalis* 'Aurea'; *Origanum* 'Gold Splash'; terracotta pot, 34cm (13in) diameter, 26cm (10½in) high

Outdoor Entertaining

Alan Titchmarsh

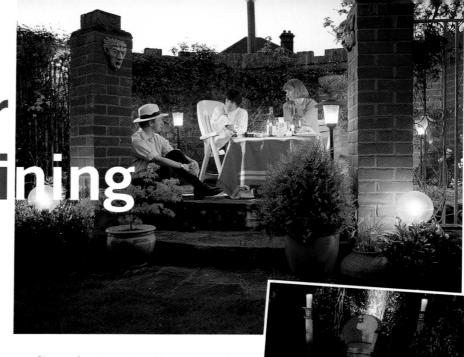

An outdoor room, like any other area of the home, requires furnishing if you want to use it for entertaining. Garden furniture adds both style and comfort. The first consideration is the size of the garden, bearing in mind that even the smallest garden should have somewhere to sit down and relax. If space is really limited, portable seats, such as foldaway chairs, can be stacked against a wall when not in use. Don't forget the decorative merit of garden furniture either – a bench could provide a focal point at the end of a path, or a pretty chair enliven an otherwise dull corner.

Choose furniture that will complement the style of the garden – crisp, white-painted wrought ironwork in a smart town garden, for example, or rustic-style, wooden furniture in a wild cottage garden. Remember that if you do choose wooden furniture, treat it with preservative to prevent it from rotting.

Position tables and chairs near to the kitchen so that there is not far to walk carrying platefuls of food. Garden seats, on the other hand, may be best placed near a scented plant, such as a rose or jasmine. Or, if the garden is quite shaded, you might want to place seating in the spot that gets the most sun.

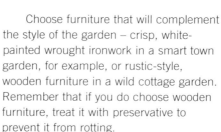

Children's play area

If you have children, making part of the garden an outdoor play area allows them to release energy and have fun. In a large garden there are few limits and you can, for example, make use of a lawn in summer by putting up a net for games of badminton. More permanent features could include a swing or even a tree house. In smaller gardens there will usually be enough space for a sandpit, a paddling pool or Wendy house.

Lighting

Artificial lighting makes it possible to enjoy the garden in the evenings, too. Used skilfully, it can not only show off features, such as pretty statues or striking architectural plants, but create mood. Some lighting is designed to be functional as opposed to decorative, being used to

A sense of the dramatic
Even the simplest of lighting can add mood and atmosphere to an evening's party. Candles can be especially effective providing they are positioned in a sheltered spot.

increase safety rather than create atmosphere. For example, lighting paths, driveways, steps and doorways is a practical measure to increase security. However, bright floodlights cast deep shadows and are therefore counter-productive.

Well-designed garden lighting brings a special beauty to the garden at night, highlighting the best features while drawing attention away from any eyesores. Downlighting illuminates features or areas of the garden from above. It can imitate nature, suggesting filtered sun or moonlight, when the light is directed through a tree or structure, casting soft shadows on the ground below. Uplighting

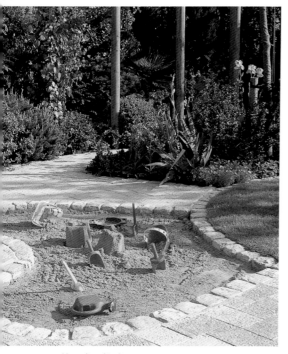

Keeping it clean
A waterproof cover will keep a sandpit clean and allow the children to play in it even after heavy rain.

Flamboyant chef Ainsley Harriott is familiar to many as the larger-than-life host of *Can't Cook Won't Cook* **and** *Ready Steady Cook*. **These delicious barbecue recipes will make a memorable outdoor feast.**

Coco-chicken and Mango Skewers

The smell of these chicken skewers is sensational, and the orange of the mango and green of the mangetout make them into attractive as well as tasty kebabs, flavoured with Thai green curry paste and coconut milk.

Serves 4

450g (1lb) chicken breast fillets
1 large, ripe but firm mango
50g (2oz) mangetout (about 24)

For the marinade:
120ml (4fl oz) canned coconut milk
1 tablespoon Thai green curry paste
1 teaspoon prepared minced lemongrass
    from a jar
1 teaspoon palm or light muscovado sugar
1 tablespoon Thai fish sauce
1 tablespoon groundnut or sunflower oil
finely grated zest of ½ lime
1 teaspoon lime juice
8 x 25cm (10in) bamboo skewers soaked in
    cold water for 30 minutes.

Cut the chicken into 2.5cm (1in) cubes. Mix together all the marinade ingredients, stir in the chicken and leave it to marinate for 2 hours at room temperature or overnight in the fridge.

Peel the mangoes and then slice the flesh away from either side of the thin flat stone and cut it into 1cm (½in) pieces.

Drop the mangetout into a pan of boiling salted water. Bring them back to the boil, drain and refresh under running cold water.

Thread 3 pieces of chicken and 3 mangetout folded around 3 pieces of mango alternatively on to each skewer.

Barbecue the skewers over medium-hot coals for 10 minutes, turning now and then and brushing with the leftover marinade, until the chicken is lightly browned.

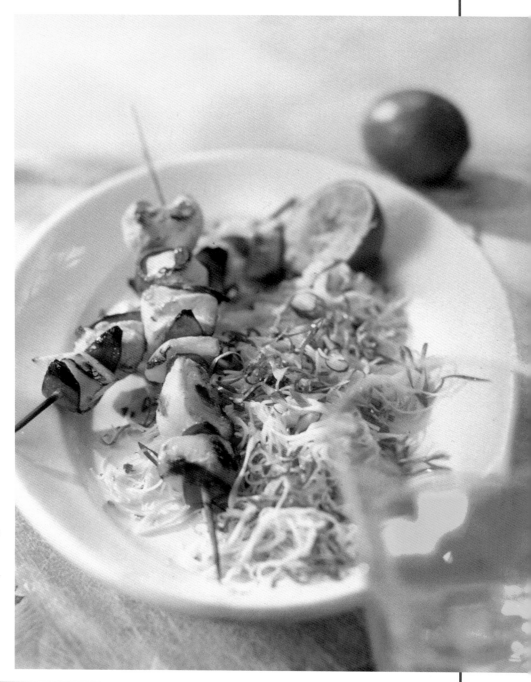

Marinated Halloumi Cheese with Tang! Tang! Dressing

Halloumi is a waxy Cypriot cheese which does not melt during cooking. This makes it perfect for grilling on the barbecue. 750g (11/2lb) of cheese might seem like a lot but it is quite a dense, heavy cheese and it will give everyone 3 thin slices which is just about right for a main course.

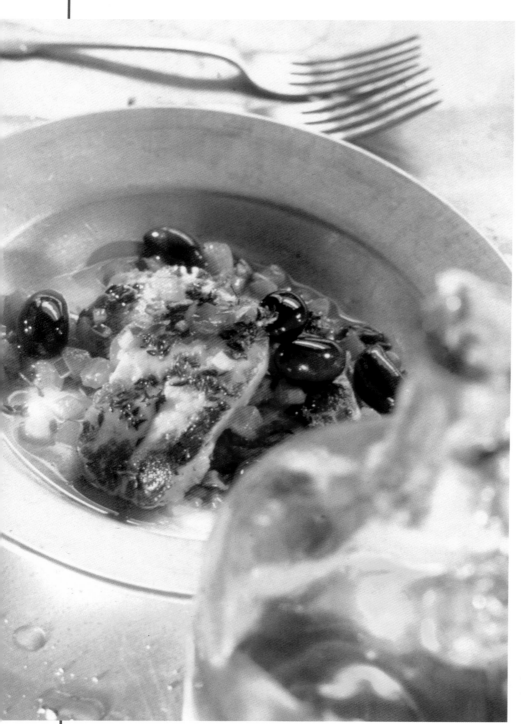

Serves 4 *as a main course or*
8 as a starter

750g (1½lb) halloumi, cut into 12x1cm
(½in) thick slices
2 tablespoons olive oil
1 teaspoon balsamic vinegar
2 tablespoons lemon juice
1 tablespoon chopped fresh thyme
salt and freshly ground black pepper

For the Tang! Tang! dressing:
5 tablespoons extra virgin olive oil
4 plum tomatoes, skinned, seeded
and diced
4 spring onions, trimmed and thinly sliced
½ small red onion, very finely chopped
2 tablespoons chopped fresh flatleaf parsley
1½ tablespoons balsamic vinegar
½ teaspoon crushed black peppercorns
50g (2oz) Calamata or other black olives
to garnish

For the marinade, mix the oil, vinegar, lemon juice, thyme and some salt and pepper together in a large shallow dish. Add the slices of cheese, turn once or twice in the mixture and leave to marinate at room temperature for 1 hour.

Just before you are ready to cook the cheese, mix together all the ingredients for the dressing.

Lift the slices of cheese out of the marinade and barbecue in batches over medium-hot coals for 3 minutes or until they are golden, flipping them over with a fish slice half way through. Stir any leftover marinade into the dressing.

Place 3 slices of cheese on to each plate, spoon over the dressing and garnish with a few black olives. Serve with plenty of crusty fresh bread.

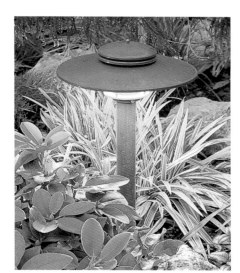

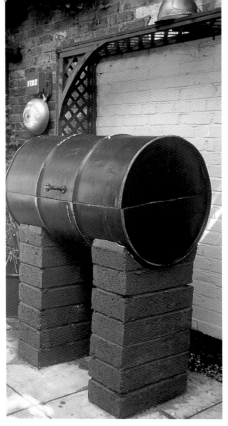

Concealed lighting (left)
Blending into the foliage during the day this lantern downlighter casts a soft, warm glow when required.

Home-made barbecues (right)
Barbecues can easily be made from recycled materials. This oil drum has been cut in half horizontally, painted and placed on brick pillars so that it's at a convenient height for cooking.

directs light up from ground level and can be used to create subtle shadows, throw an outline into sharp relief, silhouette a subject or provide a focal 'glow' in the garden. It can create the most dramatic lighting effects, but is best used sparingly.

Diffused lighting, which scatters the light, should be used in preference to a bright floodlight, which produces glare and ruins an atmosphere of relaxation. Bright light also shortens the garden by creating deep shadows away from the light source, and the areas and features that are lit by floodlighting appear flat and uninteresting.

Garden lighting does not have to be provided by electricity. Oil-fuelled lanterns or lamps, and candles of all sizes look attractive and create soft, atmospheric pools of light. Simply placing candles or nightlights in empty jam-jars or terracotta pots arranged in rows or small groups is economical, and they look very pretty when lit. Metal lanterns holding candles can be hung on wall hooks, but for safety's sake make sure that they are well out of the reach of babies and small children. Scented candles are very pleasant, and some also act as insect repellents – an important consideration on a warm summer's evening.

Barbecues

If you enjoy al fresco eating, a barbecue is essential. Whether you intend to use it only on rare occasions, or on a regular basis, there is a wide range of barbecues

to choose from, from small disposable trays to sophisticated grills set in glamorous trolleys with table attachments and accompanying gadgets.

Think carefully about where you put your barbecue. It needs to be partially sheltered, but positioned to allow easy access to both the kitchen and the eating area. For safety, it is best to situate the barbecue on a level surface and at a height that is comfortable to work at. It is also a good idea to install lighting nearby so that you can see what you are doing when grilling. Do not situate barbecues close to windows, as smoke will billow into the house. Also, keep them away from any wooden structures where they would be a fire hazard.

Many free-standing or mobile barbecues take up little space in the garden and can be conveniently dismantled and packed away when not in use. These are particularly useful for small gardens. On a roof garden or deck, a lightweight mobile barbecue is a better choice than a permanent type, but bear in mind that a barbecue fuelled by bottled gas could be a problem if you have to carry gas bottles up and down stairs.

For regular outdoor meals, a permanent brick or stone barbecue is more practical. Whichever materials you choose, the style of barbecue must be easy and safe to use. For example, in an exposed garden, a partially enclosed, oven-like structure with a chimney will help to disperse the smoke and give better control of the fire.

Always consider the size of the grill and, where possible, choose one larger than necessary for your requirements. The cooking grill for any type of barbecue should be sturdy and well made and, most important, it must be easy to remove for cleaning.

A part of the patio
Static, brick-built barbecues are the ideal solution for those who eat outdoors frequently. This particular one has been designed to complement the paving on the patio. Planting at each side softens the edges of the brick.

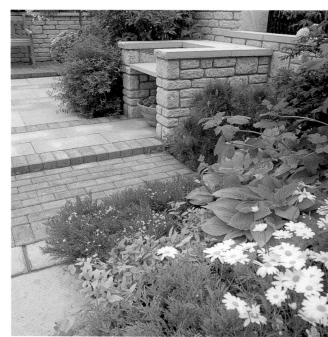

Making a path

Paths are so functional that it's all too easy to take them for granted but, when well laid out, they improve a garden no end. Take a look at your own garden, and you'll probably spot a well-worn trail in the lawn, which is a sure sign that a path is needed. Whether you're planning to make a new path or simply renovate an old one, there's no need to feel apprehensive as the job is surprisingly easy to do. Better still, the time and effort involved will be more than repaid with a path that will last for years.

Gravel has long been a favourite path material, and who can resist the wonderful crunching sound it makes under foot? Be warned, though, if cats frequent your garden, as they are sometimes tempted to use gravel as a litter tray. Even if you are plagued by cats, you can still follow this plan, as the basic techniques used to make a gravel path can be applied to all sorts of different materials, from chipped bark to broken slates. Once you've made your path, its maintenance should be minimal and the plastic membrane laid underneath it will prevent most weeds coming up. Any weeds that do work their way through can easily be tugged out by hand or sprayed with a weedkiller specially formulated for paths.

Edging tiles as an attractive option

Instead of using wooden boards to border a garden path, you could try edging tiles. Their attractive appearance and long life help to compensate for the fact that they are more expensive and will require the extra effort of setting in concrete. Victorian tiles will define your path with a beautifully ornate edge as well as adding a touch of colour.

To keep costs down, look out for second-hand tiles at your local reclamation yard. Alternatively, you could try using concrete ones which are available from DIY stores.

1
Mark out the path with pegs and string, checking that the width is the same along its length. Dig out the base of the path to a depth of 10cm (4in). If it borders a lawn, dig down to 12.5cm (5in) so that the edge is below turf level, making it easier to use a mower.

2
Set the edging boards along the path. These are held in place with pegs put in every 60cm (2ft), alternately placed inside and outside the edging board. If the path is positioned next to a lawn, make sure the edging is about 2.5cm (1in) below the level of the turf.

3
Lay a permeable plastic membrane along the base of the path. If you do need to use more than one sheet, be sure to have a generous overlap to avoid gaps. The plastic membrane will help prevent weeds appearing in the path and should reduce the maintenance needed later on.

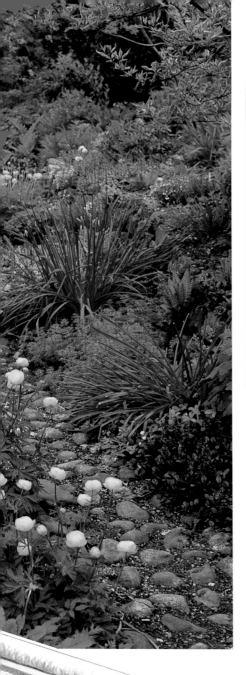

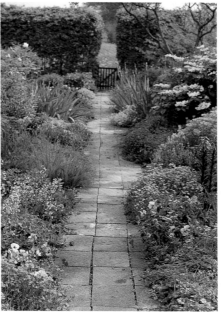

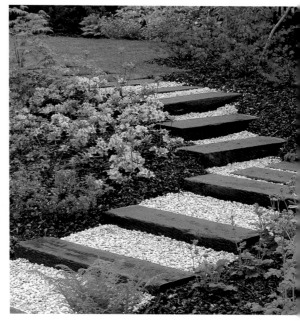

Other ideas for creating a path

If a solid path would look too heavy in your garden, you can set stepping stones into a grass path for access in all weathers. You can use cobbles, bricks, flagstones, even railway sleepers as the risers for steps in a gravel path. And a path doesn't have to be straight. In smaller gardens, a zigzag path can increase planting potential and create the illusion of greater space.

Exploit the creative potential of your paving materials to create patterns in preference to a regimented finish, and soften the hard edges of flagstones with plants that spill over onto the path.

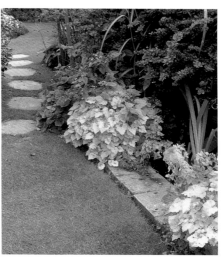

Laying stepping stones

Stepping stones make an interesting alternative to a solid path. You can choose from ordinary paving slabs, log slices or pre-cast stepping stones.

To lay stepping stones, position them at a comfortable stride apart. Cut around the stone and remove the soil underneath to the depth of the stone plus another 4cm (1½in). This avoids damaging any lawnmower blades that pass over them. Wrap log slices with chicken wire before laying them, as they can become slippery in wet weather. Put a layer of sand 2.5cm (1in) deep in the hole and bed the stone in. Firm it in by tapping with a heavy club hammer over a block of wood.

4

Spread the gravel over the membrane to a depth of 7.5cm (3in). For a fine finish use pea gravel at the top. Leave a gap of about 2cm (¾in) between the level of the gravel and the top of the edging board. This prevents the gravel from spilling out and helps to maintain a clean edge.

Laying a patio

Building a patio has to be one of the best ways to enhance a garden. It may seem a major undertaking but the work involved in making a small patio can easily be completed in just one weekend, although you can always do it over several weeks if you want to spread the load.

As your patio will be a lasting feature in the garden, it's worth taking time to get the details right before you start the hands-on work. The site for the patio is perhaps the most important thing to consider. Remember that it doesn't always have to be right next to the house, especially if this doesn't have an ideal aspect. Lay out the rough shape of the patio with some rope, and adjust it until you are happy. As a rough guide, an area about 5m x 3m (16ft x 10ft) will suit the needs of an average family.

When it comes to selecting materials, brick pavers are a great choice to create a good-looking patio that is also easy to build. They are much lighter to work with than traditional paving stones and simpler to lay as no cementing is required on a non-load-bearing patio.

The pattern illustrated here is a basic basketweave but a number of different designs are possible. The more complicated ones will require some cutting of the pavers. With a solid foundation and a sufficient drainage slope, your patio will stand you in good stead for years to come.

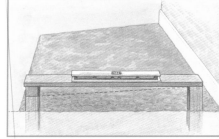

Making a drainage slope
It is important to give the patio a slight slope to allow any rainwater to drain away. A fall of approximately 2.5cm per 2m, or roughly 1in per 6ft, is sufficient. This can be achieved by using marker pegs set 1.8m (6ft) apart, and a spirit level to measure the fall.

1
Mark out the patio area with pegs and string, setting the string at the ultimate level of the patio. This level needs to be at least two bricks below the damp-proof course if the patio borders a house. A builder's set square is useful to ensure all the corners are at right angles.

2
Dig out the patio to a depth of about 15cm (6in) plus the thickness of the pavers. Put in a drainage slope to allow rain to run away from the house. Firm the soil in the patio base by hand or with a plate compactor. Lay edging boards, using a spirit level to check the drainage slope.

3
Put in a layer of hardcore, 10cm (4in) deep, to act as a foundation, then firm it down so that it is level. This layer is very important as it ensures that the paved surface will remain level once it is laid. This type of patio construction will not hold heavy loads such as cars.

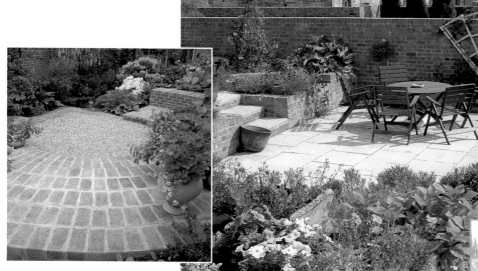

Visual interest *Different paving materials and patterns can be used even in a small area. Here, the bricks radiate out in a fan shape, drawing the eye towards the lush green planting.*

A sunny spot *A well-sited patio, in a sunny corner against a wall, becomes an extra room of the house for al fresco meals.*

Cross-section of a patio
This illustration shows the hardcore base, the sand layer and a paver. After settling the pavers in level with the edging boards, brush the surface over with joint filling sand.

5
Lay the pavers in the desired pattern, butting them up to prevent any gaps. Work from a board placed on the pavers you have already laid so that your weight is spread evenly over the area as you work. Tamp down the finished surface with a plate compactor or a length of board and a mallet.

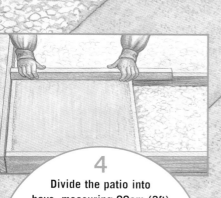

4
Divide the patio into bays, measuring 90cm (3ft) square, with 5cm (2in) sand boards. Add sand and level it to the tops of the boards with a length of wood. This will create a flat surface onto which the pavers can be laid. Remove the sand boards and fill the empty gaps with sand.

Planting a scented border

Whether you prefer the rich perfume of lilies on a warm summer evening or the gentle scent of violets in spring, fragrance is a rewarding element of any garden. While most gardens contain at least one scented plant, why not group a few together to create a melting-pot of fragrances? As well as a mixture of scents, it's possible to have fragrance all through the year from flowers and aromatic foliage.

In this simple design, shrubs, bulbs, perennials and annuals have been used to ensure a fragrant display throughout the summer months and even into the depths of winter. The plants have been selected for a pastel colour scheme but alternatives for a hot and fiery scheme are also given.

Measuring only 3m x 1.2m (l0ft x 4ft), the design uses sweet peas on a tripod and other annuals between the shrubs to enable a range of plants to be grown. Some have been underplanted with bulbs such as lilies and narcissus to make full use of space and add their special fragrances to the design.

1 Regal lily *Lilium regale*
To pack a punch from the back of a border, this fragrant lily won't disappoint. In mid-summer it produces as many as 25 very fragrant flowers. It's also one of the easiest lilies to grow and will do well in large containers. H:1.5m (5ft).

2 Mexican orange blossom *Choisya ternata*
This dependable evergreen has glossy leaves that give off an orange aroma when crushed. Slightly scented white flowers cover the bush in spring. H: 1.8m (6ft) S: 1.8m (6ft).

3 French lavender
Lavandula stoechas ssp. *pedunculata*
This distinguished plant has large purple bracts on each flower-head. The whole plant is aromatic and its flowers make a heavenly scented pot-pourri. H: 60cm (2ft) S: 60cm (2ft).

4 Violet *Viola riviniana* Purpurea Group
Sweet violets, *V. odorata*, are the ones to choose for scent in spring, but this variety, although unperfumed, is still useful for disguising the old leaves of the hyacinths. H: 20cm (8in) S: 30cm (l2in).

5 Mock orange *Philadelphus* 'Sybille'
This hardy shrub will grow in most well-drained soils in a sunny position. It produces white flowers with pale purple centres in early summer, when their strong perfume will waft from the back of the border. H: 1.8m (6ft) S: 1.8m (6ft).

6 Pinks *Dianthus* 'Inchmery'
Many old-fashioned pinks have a strong clove fragrance, which is essential in any scented garden in summer. 'Inchmery' has double, pale lavender-pink flowers. H: up to 45cm (l8in) S: 30cm (l2in).

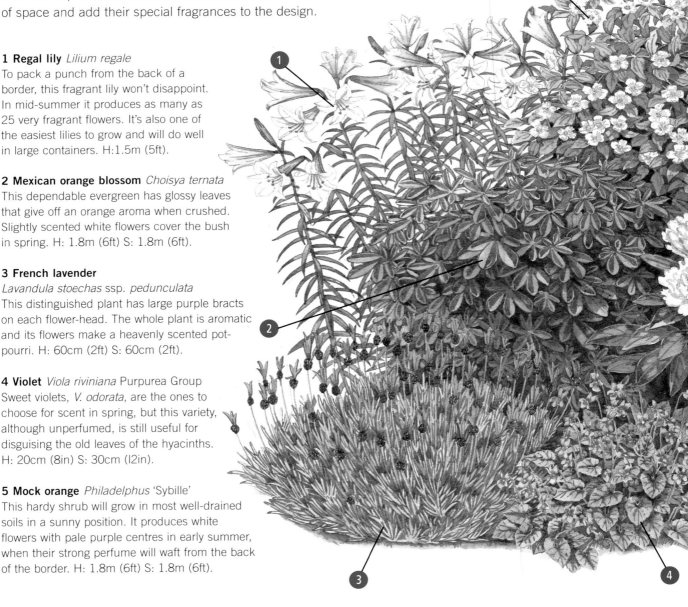

7 Sweet pea *Lathyrus odoratus*
There is nothing equal to the fresh fragrance and intense colours of sweet peas in summer and, best of all, this pretty annual is very easy to grow. Arrange a simple wigwam of sticks in the border for support. H: 2.4m (8ft).

8 Sweet rocket *Hesperis matronalis*
The loosely packed, white or purple flower-heads of this cottage garden favourite appear from late spring to mid-summer. They are most deliciously scented in the evening. It is a hardy but short-lived perennial that normally self-seeds. H: 90cm (3ft) S: 45cm (18in).

9 Christmas box
Sarcococca hookeriana var. *humilis*
This small evergreen shrub is grown for its highly scented, tiny, pink-tinged white flowers which appear in winter, followed by spherical, dark blue-black fruit. It will grow in sun or shade, making a low bush. H: 60cm (2ft) S: 90cm (3ft).

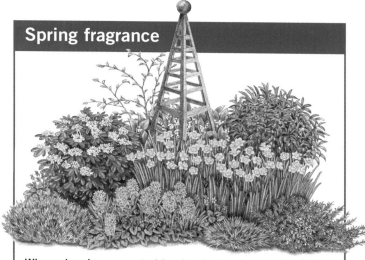

Spring fragrance

When planning a scented border, try to choose plants that will provide fragrance right through the year. Some plants featured in this summer border also provide spring interest, especially when grown through with early fragrant flowers. *Sarcococca hookeriana* var. *humilis* produces richly scented flowers in late winter, while *Choisya ternata* and prostrate rosemary provide blooms in spring. Bulbs such as *Narcissus* 'Cheerfulness' and hyacinths are valuable in small areas when grown through other plants. Spring violets and lily-of-the-valley are perfect for shady corners.

10 Tobacco plant *Nicotiana alata*
These half-hardy annuals produce their best fragrance on warm evenings in late summer. Sow seed indoors in early spring, then plant out once the risk of frost has passed. H: up to 90cm (3ft) S: 40cm (16in).

11 Paeony *Paeonia lactiflora*
'Duchesse de Nemours'
Sniff the fully double flowers of this robust perennial and you'll be rewarded with a blend of sweet and slightly spicy fragrance. Once planted, paeonies shouldn't be disturbed. They are fully hardy, but protect young foliage and flower buds from the damage caused by late spring frosts.
H: 80cm (32in) S: 80cm (32in).

12 Rosemary *Rosmarinus officinalis* Prostratus Group
This low-growing plant is perfect for softening the edge of a path in a warm position. Small blue flowers appear among its narrow evergreen leaves in spring. H: 15cm (6in) S: 1.5m (5ft).

Planting a cottage garden

A traditional cottage garden will look as if nature had a helping hand in creating it. A typical cottage garden border might be around 6m (20ft) long and about 2.5m (8ft) wide, with a path running through the centre, leading from north to south. At the north end, this border is in full light, but at its distant end it runs up to a 1.5m (5ft) wall lying east-west across it, with an old apple tree just inside the wall, overhanging out of the garden. The main aim is to take advantage of the different conditions in the border and to develop a change in mood and style from the hot, dry end to the shaded zone.

Although the general planting can be random and mixed, rather than blocks of colour, it is important that there is a series of central anchor points; these are marked in green on the plan and there are five in all. They will be small evergreen or twiggy outline shrubs.

Shaded area

Under the Bramley tree
Plants to try include *Anemone nemorosa*, *Convallaria majalis*, *Smilacina racemosa*, lots of *Primula vulgaris* and *Primula elatior*, *Epimedium* x *rubrum*, *Cimicifuga simplex* and violas.

On the shady wall
Any variety of ivy will give evergreen interest, while the climbing *Hydrangea anomala* ssp. *petiolaris* is a good one to choose for flowers.

Up into the apple tree
Plant a honeysuckle, *Lonicera periclymenum* 'Serotina', plus *Rosa* 'Wedding Day' or *R.* 'Rambling Rector'.

Plants on the high wall (house wall)
Choose climbing roses, such as *Rosa* 'Albertine' or 'New Dawn'. *Rosa* 'Kathleen Harrop' and *R.* 'Scarlet Fire', planted with *Vitis vinifera* 'Purpurea'. You could also try varieties of clematis: *Clematis* 'Alba Luxurians' and *C.* 'Perle d'Azur' or *C.* 'Madame Julia Correvon'.

Bottom border

Shade end
Cimicifuga, *Primula florindae*, *Smilacina racemosa*, *Hosta sieboldiana*, *Helleborus foetidus* and lunaria all over the place.

Semi-shade
Anemone x *hybrida* 'Honorine Jobert', *Aconitum carmichaelii*.

Sun
Korean chrysanthemums including *Chrysanthemum* 'Mei-kyo' and

'Nantyderry Sunshine'. Pansies, violas, heleniums, solidagos and pinks, especially repeaters such as *Dianthus* 'Diane', 'Doris' and 'Haytor White', plus laced varieties like 'Dad's Favourite' and 'Sops-in-wine'. *Alchemilla conjuncta*, blue lupins, *Papaver orientale*, especially Goliath Group 'Beauty of Livermere' and annual poppies. *Centaurea cyanus* in blue and pink, consolidas, calendula, tropaeolum, iberis, *Malcolmia maritima*, clarkias and nigellas, in fact, an unholy mix.

Top border

Moving back along from sun end to shade end (north to south)
Start with sun-loving plants, such as *Geranium pratense*, or with the hardy cranesbills, such as *G. sanguineum* 'Album', *G. sanguineum* var. *striatum* and the distinctive soft-leaved *G. renardii*.

You could plant more pinks here. This time try different varieties, such as the old-fashioned *Dianthus* 'Camilla', 'London Brocade' or 'Fair Folly'.

This merges to a warm-coloured area with eschscholzias, *Nemesia caerulea* and perhaps *Euphorbia griffithii* 'Dixter'. These hot colours are cooled down with a wild blue *Geranium pratense* and some campanulas. An excellent choice is the plain blue variety, *Campanula carpatica*.

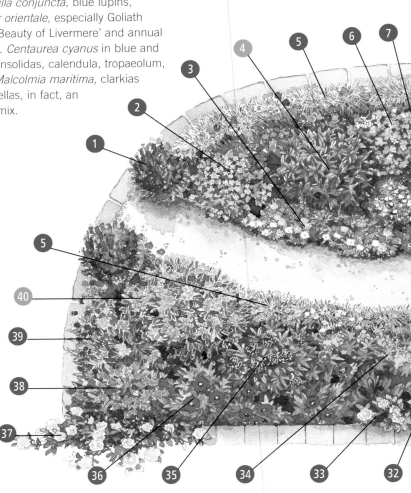

Semi-shade

Aquilegias are the perfect cottage-garden flower. Try cottage varieties of *Aquilegia vulgaris* in shades of blue, pink and white. By the path, try pulmonarias, such as *P.* 'Lewis Palmer' and *P. saccharata*, along with more lunarias. Also, a selection of the plants that grow in the shady area under the Bramley tree. Fill any spaces with *Anemone nemorosa*, violets and primroses.

Containers

Plant your containers with something solid and bold. You could try a big fuchsia, heliotrope, large salvia species, spiky yucca or even a cordyline. It just needs to be something that will make a really solid statement.

Plants to try for a colourful cottage mix

1 Salvia in containers
2 *Geranium endressii*
3 *Papaver rhoeas* Shirley
4 Daphne
5 *Dianthus* 'Fair Folly'
6 *Geranium renardii*
7 *Nemesia caerulea*
8 *Geranium pratense*
9 *Euphorbia griffithii* 'Dixter'
10 *Campanula carpatica*
11 *Mahonia aquifolium*
12 *Lunaria annua* 'Alba Variegata'
13 *Aquilegia vulgaris*
14 *Lunaria annua*
15 *Cimicifuga simplex*
16 Bramley tree, *Rosa* 'Wedding Day'
17 Philadelphus
18 Ivy
19 Violets
20 *Pulmonaria saccharata*
21 *Hydrangea anomala* ssp. *petiolaris*
22 *Smilacina racemosa*
23 *Vitis vinifera* 'Purpurea'
24 *Hosta sieboldiana*
25 Holly
26 *Anemone* x *hybrida*
27 Violas and pansies
28 Chrysanthemums
29 *Clematis* 'Perle d'Azur'
30 Helenium
31 Sarcococca
32 *Nigella damascena*
33 *Rosa* 'Albertine'
34 *Alchemilla conjuncta*
35 Lupins
36 *Papaver orientale*
37 *Rosa* 'New Dawn'
38 Calendula
39 *Centaurea cyanus*
40 *Brachyglottis* 'Sunshine'

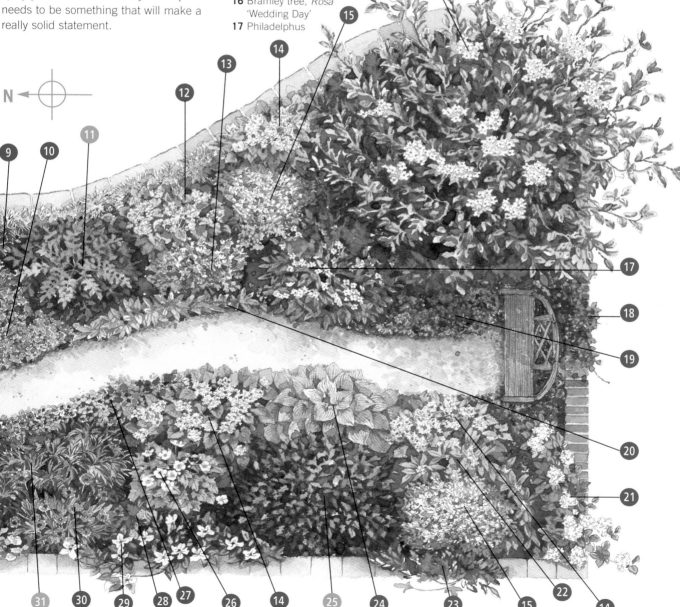

Designing a herb garden

The only herbs anyone seemed to use a few years ago were sage and thyme. Now, with a renewed interest in fresh herbs for cooking, and with an increasing number of international recipes calling for exotic herbs, many more types have become kitchen essentials. To satisfy demand, supermarkets stock packs flown in from all over the world. Yet for the price of just a couple of these packs, you can grow your own supply and pick them fresh just seconds before using them.

It couldn't be easier to grow herbs, even if you've only got space for a window-box. All they need is a bright, sunny spot with free-draining soil. If your soil is on the heavy side, improve its drainage beforehand by adding some grit, or consider planting your herbs in a raised bed which will be naturally free-draining.

Garden centres stock a wide range of herb plants. If you are selecting well-known herbs, look out for those varieties that have more unusually coloured leaves or flowers than the common forms. If there are some herbs that you want to have plenty of, you may prefer to raise them from seed instead to help keep costs down.

Plant your herbs next to a path so that they are easy to reach and also to give you the pleasure of smelling their aroma every time you brush past them. Attractive flower-heads from herbs such as chives are an added bonus. You can simply harvest the herbs as you want, either using them fresh or preserving them for later.

A focal point *Planting herbs according to their potential height and spread can add depth. Here a bed of tall-growing fennel, rosemary and dill makes an attractive backdrop.*

1 Mint *Mentha spicata*
The most often grown mint is perennial spearmint. To help contain its rapid spread, plant into a deep, bottomless bucket that has been sunk into the ground and filled with soil.
H: up to 90cm (3ft) S: indefinite.

2 Coriander *Coriandrum sativum*
Sow this annual herb direct into the ground as it does not like being transplanted. Harvest the leaves when young and fresh, and collect the seeds by placing paper bags over the seed-heads.
H: 50cm (20in) S: 20cm (8in).

3 Golden oregano
Origanum vulgare 'Aureum'
This perennial spreads less than the green-leaved form, but still needs to be lifted and divided occasionally. Give it shade to prevent scorching. If you want to use it in dried form, harvest the leaves before the flowers.
H: 30cm (12in) S: 30cm (12in).

4 Chives *Allium schoenoprasum*
This perennial makes a good edging plant and has attractive purple flowers in summer. The chopped leaves have a mild onion flavour.
H: 30cm (12in) S: 15cm (6in).

5 Dill *Anethum graveolens*
This annual herb should be sown direct into the ground in spring as it doesn't like being transplanted. Pick the feathery leaves before it flowers, then collect the stronger-flavoured seed as it ripens. H: 60cm (24in) S: 30cm (12in).

6 Rosemary *Rosmarinus officinalis* 'Miss Jessopp's Upright'
This vigorous shrub can be used as an informal hedge. Replace plants about every five years. New ones can be raised from summer cuttings.
H: 1.5m (5ft) S: 1.5m (5ft).

7 Fennel *Foeniculum vulgare*
The ferny foliage of this perennial tastes like aniseed. If you don't want the seeds, remove the flower-heads as it self-sows freely. Try *F. vulgare* 'Purpureum' which has purple foliage.
H: 1.8m (6ft) S: 45cm (18in).

8 Bay *Laurus nobilis*
This evergreen tree or shrub is great as a centre-piece to a herb garden. It can be clipped and trained into attractive shapes, or left to form a loose bush. Protect from cold winds which will scorch the foliage.

The aromatic leaves can be used either fresh or dried.
H: up to 12m (40ft) S: up to 10m (30ft).

9 French tarragon
Artemisia dracunculus
A half-hardy perennial. Cut sprigs as you need them or harvest en masse, leaving about two-thirds of the plant to regrow. French tarragon can only be bought as a plant. Tarragon seed found on sale is of the inferior-tasting Russian type. Good with chicken and for flavouring vinegar.
H: 1.2m (4ft) S: 30cm (12in)

10 Purple Sage *Salvia officinalis* Purpurascens Group
Dry the leaves of this perennial before it flowers in summer. As sage can become woody, it needs a trim in spring to keep it bushy and should be replaced every four years or so. H: 80cm (32in) S: 90cm (3ft).

11 Parsley *Petroselinum crispum*
A biennial plant that needs to be fed to perform well. Harvest fresh young leaves, and remove any that are tough and yellow. *P. crispum* var. *neapolitanum* is a flat-leaved type with a stronger taste. H: 80cm (32in) S: 60cm (24in).

12 Sweet basil *Ocimum basilicum*
Sow this annual indoors in late spring. When planted in the garden, it needs to be grown in a warm, sunny spot. The leaves are great in Italian dishes and can be frozen for winter use. There are many different types to try, each with their own distinctive flavours and leaves. H: 30cm (12in) S: 30cm (12in).

13 Thyme *Thymus vulgaris*
Perennial garden thyme is the most commonly grown but there are lots of other types, including variegated *T. vulgaris* 'Silver Posie', *T.* 'Doone Valley' and golden *T.* x *citriodorus* 'Aureus'. Some are upright-growing, while others are mat-forming. All types benefit from trimming over after flowering. H: 15cm (6in) S: 40cm (16in).

Planting a window-box

Growing herbs in a window-box, or any other sort of container, is a great idea when space is at a premium. Use gritty compost, and cover the container's drainage holes with pot crocks or broken polystyrene. Feed, water and trim the herbs regularly. Replant your container every spring.

Productive ideas for small gardens

Fresh produce straight from the garden is something everyone can achieve, no matter how small their garden. Adam Pasco, Editor of *BBC Gardeners' World Magazine*, **shows how, with a little planning, you can grow tomatoes in hanging baskets, courgettes in patio containers, herbs in pots, or fruit trained on walls and fences.**

Food scares are currently making the news on a daily basis, with worries about genetically modified crops and the use of pesticides, so what better way to gain peace of mind than by growing your own produce? If you have plenty of space, such as an allotment or a large kitchen garden, the types and quantities of crops you grow are almost limitless. Where space is restricted, however, you will need to be much more selective when choosing varieties. You will also need to decide on how best to grow them in order to ensure the very highest returns from every crop.

Tubs and baskets can play host to many things, but herbs are perhaps the most successful and popular choice. Placed close to the house, within easy reach of the kitchen, a selection of pots can provide fresh parsley, chives, mint, coriander and basil throughout the summer. Mediterranean favourites, including thyme, rosemary and sage, relish a site in the sun and will flourish on a hot patio. Most herbs can be raised from seed, or you could buy them as young plants from garden centres.

Salad crops, including coloured-leaf lettuce, grow well in pots and window-boxes. They can also be used to edge paths and beds in the ornamental garden, together with a long row of parsley. Favourites include the frilly 'Lollo Rossa' and 'Red Salad Bowl', or you could try the new oakleaf lettuce 'Cerize' for purple-red pickings every week.

Other patio crops that perform well in large tubs are compact or trailing tomatoes, like 'Tumbler', bush varieties of marrow, like 'Tiger Cross', or courgettes, including 'Defender' and 'Burpee Golden Zucchini'. Patio crops need a warm, sheltered, sunny site, and must be watered daily during summer. Feed weekly with a liquid feed, such as a high potash tomato fertiliser.

Growing in beds

To maximise the crop returns from your vegetable plot, try making small beds, 90–120cm (3–4ft) wide. Ideally, each bed should be surrounded by a path to give you easy access to the centre. Instead of growing ordinary salad and vegetable crops, choose from the wide range of baby vegetables now being offered by seed companies. These vegetables can be picked small, when tender and full of flavour. The seeds can be sown closely, as all are compact growers, and the plants mature quickly for an early harvest, ensuring a regular crop of tasty young produce from every bed. The spacing between each row is about 15cm (6in), with the plants within each row sown just 2.5cm (1in) apart.

Crops to plant in your beds could include compact and quick-maturing varieties of spinach, carrot, turnip, leek, kohl rabi, lettuce, beetroot and Chinese cabbage, among many others. A good tip is to sow little and often because, by sowing a few seeds of different varieties every two or three weeks, you can ensure continuity of cropping. Vegetables should be picked regularly while young, and not left until they are too big, old and tough. Any spaces left from harvesting one crop can be filled quickly with a new sowing.

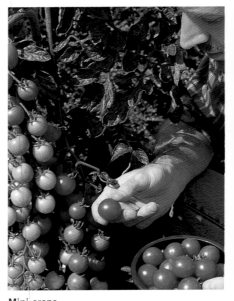

Mini crops
Even a single tomato plant will provide tasty pickings for several months from mid-summer.

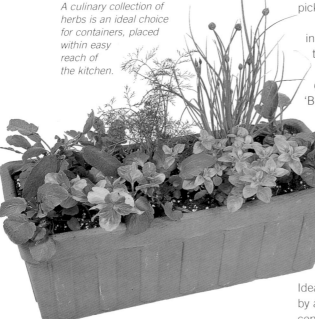

Herb box
A culinary collection of herbs is an ideal choice for containers, placed within easy reach of the kitchen.

Strawberry pots

Fresh strawberries provide a real taste of summer and by planting cold-stored runners, available from specialist fruit nurseries, you can harvest the fruit in just 60 days. Grown through the sides of a traditional terracotta strawberry pot, or in any large container, strawberries can be kept well watered and fed to maximise their yield, and can be easily netted to keep away hungry birds.

Fences for fruit

Many fruit trees will suit a small garden. Instead of being grown as traditional trees, they can be trained on walls or fences and pruned into forms known as espaliers, fans and cordons to restrict their size and spread. Pruning isn't complicated, and usually needs to be done once a year, in summer. Apples, pears, plums and cherries are all popular choices. If your local garden centre does not have a good range to choose from, try a specialist fruit nursery. While some fruit

trees need a compatible partner to ensure that their flowers pollinate one another and set a good crop, many varieties, like the majority of plums and cherries, are self-fertile and can be grown very successfully on their own.

There is also a wonderful range called Terrace Fruits. These naturally compact varieties are ideal for growing in patio containers. Peach, nectarines, apricots and pear are already available, and there are more fruits under trial for introduction in the near future.

Ornamental appeal

As a focal point on the patio, or as a centre-piece in a border, plant up a large terracotta pot with a standard bay tree. Provided it is carefully clipped, it will look striking and provide leaves for cooking as well. Compact fruit trees, like cherries, grow well in pots and can be moved within hand's reach of a

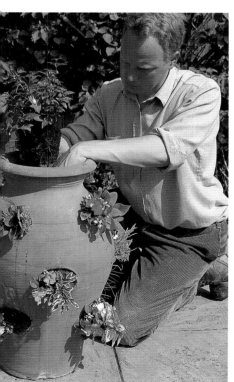

Left *Large terracotta pots with planting holes through their sides are perfect for strawberries, herbs, even trailing tomatoes.*

Cordons *Most apple varieties can be trained as upright columns, simply requiring an annual prune in early August to shorten sideshoots.*

seating area as their fruits ripen. Even a gooseberry bush can be trained as a standard to resemble a large lollipop on a stick. Choose a naturally disease-resistant variety, like 'Invicta' or 'Greenfinch', or, for a more painless picking experience, try the new, almost thornless 'Pax'.

You could include a few ornamental crops in your borders, too. Swiss and rhubarb chard, Florence fennel, beetroot, coloured-leaf lettuces and even bold, impressive artichokes would all look just as attractive and colourful as many flowering plants, with the added bonus that they are edible.

Instead of covering an arch with clematis and honeysuckle, you could turn to climbing marrows and squashes instead. Although their long stems will need some help to begin with, these plants will reward you with fruits for easy picking in late summer.

Potted fruits *Dwarf and compact peach and nectarine trees can be grown in large pots and kept in a sunny position to produce delicious fruits that can be picked from the comfort of a deck-chair.*

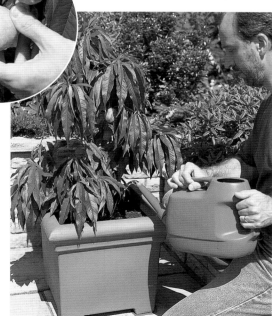

The story of
Gardeners' Question Time

Gardeners' Question Time **chairman ERIC ROBSON** traces the history of *GQT*, following its rise from a local radio programme to a national phenomenon.

Little did the BBC realise just what they were starting when, in 1947, the first episode of a new gardening series was broadcast with the aim of solving the nation's gardening problems.

More than 50 years later, *Gardeners' Question Time* goes from strength to strength, continuing to answer many of the niggling gardening queries that beset every gardener from time to time. Many of the programme's chairmen and contributors are now household names.

On April 9 1947, listeners to the BBC's Home Service in the north of England and Northern Ireland had a first-class evening's entertainment in store, and slipped into the schedules at 10.15pm there was a new programme. Called *How Does Your Garden Grow? A Gardener's Question Time*, it was a bold experiment. At a time when most factual programmes were heavily scripted, this one, recorded at a hotel in Ashton-under-Lyne, let people talk spontaneously. Members of the Smallshaw Garden and Allotment Association were able to put their gardening questions to a panel of experts. There was the

An early pioneer
Robert Stead was the man whose simple idea has now become a national institution.

head of Bolton Parks Department, a scientist from Manchester University and two real gardeners, FW Loads from Burnley and WE Sowerbutts from Ashton-under-Lyne.

In charge that night was Robert Stead, a talks producer from BBC North, who devised, chaired, produced and edited the programme. He'd already dabbled with public participation radio and felt that gardening was a suitable candidate for modernisation. The main gardening programme then was *In Your Garden*, which Bob Stead disliked because of what he considered its depressing tone. He set out to break the mould and almost broke his back in the process. The programme at Ashton was recorded on acetate discs, but each one only ran for just over five minutes and it took more than 50 discs to record that first edition.

The programme also had its chaotic moments. At one point during the evening

a chap who thought he had turned up for a recording of *Have a Go with Wilfred Pickles* insisted on playing his cornet.

Looking back through the programme files, what is perhaps most striking about those very early days is how the questions gardeners asked were so similar to the concerns that gardeners have today. In the second programme, one of the questioners was GC Moon, who wanted to know if vegetables grown with artificial manures were detrimental to the health of the consumer. One EJ Saint of Jubilee Cottage wanted to know the cause of clubroot in the cabbage family and an appropriate remedy. Sadly, only the questions have survived, while the answers have all been lost.

By April 1950, the show had settled down into an enjoyable routine that attracted tens of thousands of loyal listeners. That month, Doctor, later Professor, Alan Gemmell, a botanist from what was then called the University College of North Staffordshire, joined Fred Loads and Bill Sowerbutts in a radio partnership that was to last for more than 30 years. Bob Stead continued to chair the programme until 1952. He recalls

An enjoyable routine *By 1951, the programme had a loyal following and the team obviously enjoyed the relaxed format as much as the tens of thousands of listeners.*

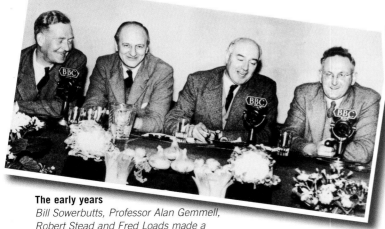

The early years
Bill Sowerbutts, Professor Alan Gemmell, Robert Stead and Fred Loads made a relaxed team in the 1950s.

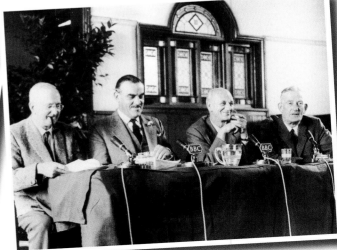

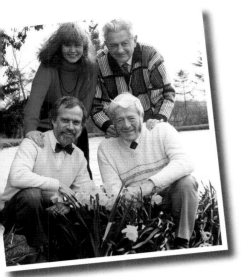

Well-known faces *The team in the 1980s included Stefan Buczacki and Fred Downham (seated), Daphne Ledward and Clay Jones.*

some memorable exchanges. Fred Loads was once asked why nobody had produced a yellow sweet pea. He flannelled for three minutes and then asked Bill Sowerbutts if he had anything to add. 'No Fred,' said Bill, enjoying himself, 'I don't know anything about it either.'

On another occasion a lady took Bill to task. 'I did just what you said I should to the plant,' she told him. When Bill asked what had happened, she replied that the plant had died. 'Funny, I thought it might,' was Bill's response.

Bob Stead also recollects the best pun of the early years coming from Alan Gemmell. Fred Loads had been banging on about the answer being in the soil when Alan sighed quietly to himself and said, 'As you see, all Loads lead to loam.'

Not everyone in the BBC hierarchy was as convinced of the success of *Gardeners' Question Time*. There are still memos on file from managers saying it would never be anything other than a regional programme. In 1957, the doubters were all overruled and *GQT* was launched on the national Home Service.

Freddy Grisewood had taken over as chairman of the programme in 1953 and continued to keep order until 1961, when he was succeeded by Franklin 'Jingles' Engelmann. Steve Race briefly held the job in 1972, the same year that Michael Barratt began his five-year term. Fred Loads died in 1981 and Alan Gemmell in 1986. Bill Sowerbutts retired in 1983 and died in 1990.

Ken Ford, who produced *GQT* for BBC Leeds for more than 20 years, chaired the programme from 1977 until 1985, when he was succeeded by Leslie Cottington and then by Clay Jones.

It was after Clay's retirement because of ill health that the fun and games started. Stories began to circulate that *GQT* was going to be modernised, that the programme was going to be aimed at a younger audience and include pop music, and that people ranging from Prince Charles to the Bishop of Durham and a bevy of children's BBC presenters were in the frame for the chairman's job.

What was happening was that the BBC had decided to have the programme produced by an independent company, the Taylor Made Group, run by Trevor Taylor. He had spent most of his working life with Radio 4 on programmes such as *Today*. Shortly afterwards he offered me the job. As only the eleventh chairman in the programme's long history, I found myself without a panel. Stefan Buczacki, Fred Downham, Sue Phillips and Daphne Ledward had set off for Classic FM, a channel where they really do play music alongside the gardening advice.

We had a bumpy week or two but this was not unique in over 50 years of broadcasting on the gentle hobby of gardening. Bill Sowerbutts had raised a bit of a storm when he left the programme and Alan Gemmell abandoned *GQT* for the dubious delights of television. The programme has changed over the decades and has continued to appeal to new listeners. If it hadn't, our audience would have gone in large measures to the compost heap in the sky. Each chairman has applied his own talents and eccentricities to the job. I hope that our present audience of over a million listeners a week will be as forgiving of me as they have been of all those who have gone before.

As the question papers have been passed from chairman to chairman over the years, I get the impression that we've all essentially

believed in the same thing, that the very simple idea that Bob Stead came up with is more important than any individual associated with it. What each one of us has tried to do is to cherish the idea, and leave it as strong at the end of our innings as it was at the beginning.

Down the years, *Gardeners' Question Time* has been a bit of a relay race, and the team holding the batten now is as rounded a bunch as the programme has ever had.

With a Yorkshire flourish, Geoffrey Smith transports us to the glorious hills of Tuscany, which can be useful when the rest of us are trying to identify some pest or disease that lurks in the corner of a polythene bag; Pippa Greenwood's grasp of plant pathology is unrivalled; no houseplant exists that Anne Swithinbank hasn't already grown; Bob Flowerdew espouses organic gardening with a passion; and Nigel Colborn combines the insight of a plantsman and writer with a down-to-earth delight in gardening.

An impressive team *The current panel of experts includes chairman Eric Robson, Anne Swithinbank, Bob Flowerdew, Nigel Colborn, Pippa Greenwood and Geoffrey Smith.*

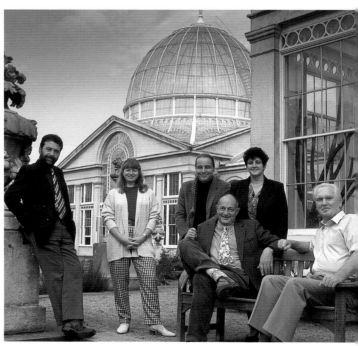

You can tune in to *Gardeners' Question Time* **every Sunday at 2.00pm on BBC Radio 4 (repeated Wednesday at 3.00pm). Eric Robson is the current chairman.**

Solutions to common gardening problems

Q Which bulbs can I plant to create colourful summer displays? I would also like some bulbs to grow in pots, and others to provide me with cut flowers.

A Once the last tulips and Dutch iris fade, you can look forward to glorious summer displays from alliums, camassias, summer hyacinth (galtonia), ornithogalum, crinum, canna and *Amaryllis belladonna*. Slightly more challenging is *Cardiocrinum giganteum*, which carries tall, bold heads of white trumpet flowers above beautiful glossy foliage.

Every bulb catalogue will be full of lilies, ranging from the dainty species to bright and gaudy hybrids. Lily bulbs are best planted from autumn to early spring and as soon as the bulbs can be purchased. Many lilies are ideal for growing in pots, with the new dwarf varieties being particularly suited to pot displays.

Some bulbs and dahlia tubers can be planted outside in early May to provide late summer and autumn cut flowers. But gladioli corms are best planted in groups

at two or three week intervals from mid-spring to early summer to produce a successional display, and all gladioli varieties make excellent cut flowers. Also look out for their relative called the watsonia.

An unusual patio display comes from a container filled with the pineapple flower, *Eucomis bicolor*. Start off in the greenhouse, bringing the container outside for the summer and autumn months. Provide frost protection during winter. These bulbs will then divide and multiply naturally.

Agapanthus also perform well in large containers, but in most parts of the country also need winter protection from cold and waterlogging. To round off the list of summer-flowering bulbs, take a look at tigridia, and for late colour do include colchicums, crocosmias, montbretia and nerine. For pots in the greenhouse, try begonias, sinningias, *Hymenocallis festalis* and scadoxus.

Q Can you recommend some grasses and dwarf bamboos suitable for growing in tubs?

A Bowles' golden sedge, if kept moist, *Arundinaria viridistriata*, a leafy, low, gold and green bamboo, and hakonechloa are all wonderful in pots. If you fancy growing dwarf bamboo, choose the *Pleioblastus pygmaeus*, which grows to just 15cm (6in).

But it's not only dwarf grasses and bamboos that look good in containers. Grow the taller kinds, such as *Arundo donax* 'Variegata', a reed grass which needs winter protection, *Arundinaria murieliae* and *Miscanthus sinensis* 'Zebrinus', all of which will make good backgrounds for groups of potted shrubs and flowers.

You could also try teaming up a potted bamboo with a Japanese maple in a separate container.

◁ **Lilies provide both flower and fragrance**

Q Can you recommend some fast-growing plants for a shady site that will smother the existing weeds?

A There are plenty of ground-cover plants for shade, such as *Alchemilla mollis* (lady's mantle) and bergenia.

Variegated plants are a great way to brighten up those shady areas. There are several good white or pewter-leaved forms of *Lamium maculatum*, such as 'White Nancy'.

The variegated Solomon's seal is beautiful and there are hundreds of variegated hostas. Variegated honesty is lovely, although the variegation only appears in the second season. Variegated periwinkle, a rampant spreader, will fill dark corners.

But no plant is good at smothering weeds. Plant them through sheets of slitted black polythene or woven landscaping fabric and cover this with a 2.5–5cm (1–2in) layer of chipped bark.

Q Why won't my wisteria flower? I've trained it for a number of years to the south-facing side of my house but it has never bloomed. What am I doing wrong?

A You certainly have the right spot as wisteria loves to grow in a sunny, sheltered site. A common cause of non-flowering is that the plant is seed-raised and therefore takes many years to bloom. When buying a wisteria, always look for plants that have been raised by grafting; the knobbly graft union is usually clearly visible near the base of the main stem. Also try to choose named varieties such as 'Issai', 'Black Dragon' and 'Purple Patches'.

However, this is little help in your present situation. Several things can be done to promote flowering. Training your plant to spread over the entire wall will ensure it receives maximum sunshine. The cheapest and most effective means of support is strong galvanised wire run through vine eyes. Twice-yearly pruning will develop the short lateral branches that

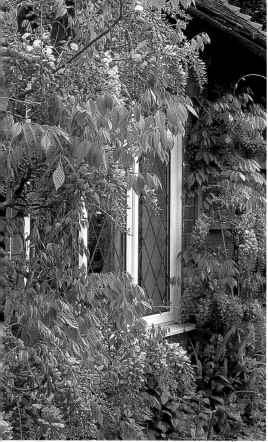

strongest-smelling varieties around.

Ten-week stocks can be treated as half-hardy annuals and sown in pots on a window-sill in late winter for spring flowers, or sown outside in April and May.

Sow biennials, such as *Hesperis matronalis*, in late spring to flower the next year. Other good biennials include honesty, wallflowers and sweet Williams. For climbers select *Lonicera periclymenum* 'Serotina' and 'Belgica', *L. caprifolium* with cream and pale pink flowers or *L. x americana* which has attractive yellow flowers.

Q We only have a small garden but would like to grow native wildflowers. Which flowers could we grow?

A If you want shade-tolerant wildflowers which can cope with neglect, then *Iris foetidissima* (stinking iris), *Convallaria majalis* (lily-of-the-valley) and *Lamium galeobdolon* (yellow archangel) are your best bets. Snowdrops and bluebells will provide lovely flowers in winter and spring.

If you're prepared to mulch and keep the soil moist, then all woodland flowers are suitable. *Digitalis purpurea* (foxgloves) and *Silene dioica* (red campion) are tall and tough. *Primula vulgaris* (primroses), *Viola riviniana* (dog violets) and *Galium odoratum* (sweet woodruff) are slightly more modest and require a little more care. In summer, *Lonicera periclymenum* (honeysuckle), will grow into the sun. The flowers attract moths and fill the balmy June evenings with perfume, while in autumn birds will feast on the berries.

Q Despite spraying, my roses always seem to succumb to the most common rose diseases of blackspot, mildew and rust. What

produce flowers so, in July or August, take the sideshoots back to 5–6 buds from the main stem. The following January, shorten these shoots even further, to 2–3 buds. Plants growing near walls may be short of nutrients, as the soil here is often poor quality and the shelter created by the wall also keeps off a fair amount of any rainwater. Tackle this by annual spring mulching with well-rotted compost or manure, watering during dry spells and applying a general fertiliser in spring. An application of sulphate of potash in late winter can also help to encourage flowering.

Q Having recently bought a house, my gardening budget is very tight. What scented plants could I grow that wouldn't cost much?

A Growing your own plants from seed is the most eonomical. Try hardy annuals uch as *Centaurea mosohata* (sweet sultan), *Lathyrus odoratus* (sweet peas), particularly the variety 'Snoopea' which needs very little support, as well as *Matthiola bicornis* (night-scented stock), *Reseda odorata* (mignonette) and zaluzianskya (night phlox). Use alyssum to create honey-scented edging. 'Sweet White' and 'Oriental Night' are two of the

can I do to control them and are there any resistant varieties I could choose?

A Prevention rather than cure is the key to controlling diseases, and a chemical control needs to start early, as soon as, or even before the disease becomes visible. For blackspot, spray as soon as possible after spring pruning to kill off any infection that may have survived the winter. Mildew and rust can be treated with a fungicide containing myclobutanil, as soon as the first signs appear. Keeping your plants fit and healthy goes a long way towards avoiding disease in the first place. Mulch the ground annually each spring with a soil conditioner like garden compost or well-rotted manure to help the soil retain water and nutrients. Feed regularly, ideally with a fertiliser that has been formulated especially for roses, and water during dry spells. In summer and autumn, gather up any diseased, fallen leaves so that any infections don't overwinter in the soil. Burn any diseased material or put it in the dustbin, not on the compost heap.

There are a number of varieties that have good, natural, disease resistance, and this really is something worth checking for when buying new roses. Good varieties to try include the hybrid tea 'Alexander', the ground-covering variety 'Flower Carpet', floribunda 'The Queen Elizabeth' or the climbing variety 'Aloha'.

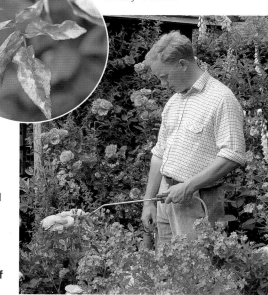

The kitchen garden

Q My runner beans produced plenty of brightly coloured flowers last summer but failed to crop well. Is there anything I can do to make sure that more beans form this year?

A Runner beans that flower but do not produce a good crop are invariably suffering from a shortage of water, although occasionally poor pollination may also be to blame. The old advice of incorporating loads of organic material deep under the site for runner beans may help, but it is far easier and more practical to give them a good soaking with a hosepipe, bans permitting, once a week from when the flowers first start to appear.

Often the first flush of flowers drops off because the plants know they are not yet strong enough to ripen them. If later flushes fail despite adequate water being provided, then it's probably due to poor pollination. Pollinators can be encouraged by syringing the flowers with a dilute sugar solution. Another simple method is to grow sweet peas with the beans; they flower earlier and attract the pollinators who are then already visiting when the beans start flowering.

For best results, sow plants outdoors at the start of May, then cover with bonded fleece until the threat of frost is past. Grow French beans, either dwarf varieties or climbers like 'Hunter', as these withstand hot conditions and crop reliably during summer.

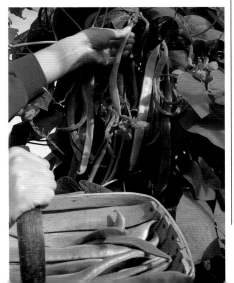

Q The leaves on my gooseberry bushes are being eaten away by something. What should I spray them with?

A If a gooseberry plant is being stripped of its foliage, the problem is almost invariably due to the gooseberry sawfly. It is quite a common pest and may produce three generations in one summer.

The larvae eat for about three weeks and can defoliate a bush, leaving just the leaf stalks. Eggs are usually laid at the centre of the bush, so damage is only noticed when it is already quite extensive.

The larvae then move into the soil to pupate. Try picking off the larvae and spray plants with an organic insecticide like liquid derris or a formulation containing permethrin, pirimiphos-methyl or bifenthrin. Make sure you observe the harvest interval.

Gooseberry mildew can also be a problem, but can be avoided by growing mildew-resistant varieties such as 'Invicta' and 'Greenfinch'.

Q Carrot is my favourite vegetable. By growing lots of different varieties and sowing in succession can I ensure a continuous harvest? How do I avoid carrot root fly?

A You can spread your carrot crop over quite a long season by using varieties that mature at different times, or sowing a variety of your choice every three to four weeks. Sow under glass in February, and outdoors from April to early June, then indoors in August and in September.

Protect your crop by dusting the drills with an insecticide such as Chlorophos, covering the rows

with fleece, or surrounding them with a 60cm (2ft) high barrier of polythene. Avoid thinning out, as the smell attracts the fly, and try to grow a variety like 'Flyaway' or 'Sytan', which claim some resistance to this pest.

Q I'm trying to cut back on chemical sprays in the garden, but do I have to keep up a regular preventive strategy against potato blight? Are there any resistant varieties?

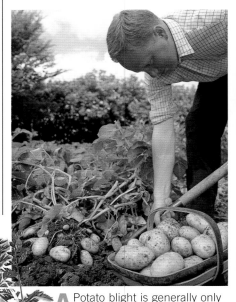

A Potato blight is generally only troublesome if conditions are moist and warm. You say that you want to cut down on spraying, so it is worth listening to farming programmes, which often draw attention to blight infection periods and advise when to spray.

For infection to take place, the blight fungus requires two consecutive 24-hour periods during which the minimum temperature is 10°C (50°F) and in each of which there are at least 11 hours when the relative humidity is 89 per cent or more. Preventive spraying at this stage when there is a risk will reduce the need to spray later.

Also bin or burn any infected material, don't risk composting any plant remains that have been infected. Good resistant varieties include 'Cara', 'Estima' and 'Wilja'.

Q I love fresh strawberries, but how can I grow them to provide pickings over the longest possible period?

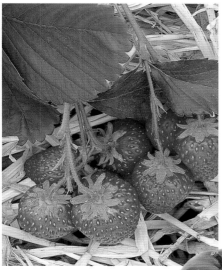

A Although strawberries aren't long-lived fruit plants, and are best replaced every three years or so, the way to extend the picking season is to choose different varieties, and use cloches to encourage plants to flower earlier.

Strawberries are classified as early, mid-season and late varieties, so selecting some from each group will provide the longest season of picking. For example, 'Honeoye' and 'Elvira' are good early varieties, while 'Elsanta', 'Hapil' and 'Eros' fruit mid-season, and 'Maxim' and 'Rhapsody' late season. Choosing varieties from each group should provide fruit for picking through the months of June and July. Covering plants with cloches from March will encourage earlier flowering and fruiting.

Some strawberries are classified as perpetual varieties, which means that they flower and fruit continuously throughout the season. 'Aromel', for example, provides useful pickings from August to October, while the new varieties

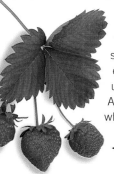

◁ **'Elvira'**

'Evita' and 'Marastil' both fruit over long periods.

To extend the season still further, pot up a few runners during the summer, leave the pots outside to receive a period of cold, and then move them to the greenhouse in late winter to encourage an early crop.

Alternatively, buy cold stored runners during spring and early summer. Plant them in containers or straight into the garden and they will flower and produce a small crop of fruit in about 60 days from planting.

Q I am planning to grow some apple trees. Could you recommend six varieties whose fruits are renowned for their good flavour?

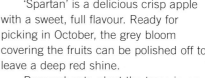

△ **'Redsleeves' apples**

A The following compatible selection will supply you with tasty apples from early autumn to late winter.

'Redsleeves' has medium-sized fruits flushed rosy red on a yellowish-green background. Ready from August to September, these apples are sweet, crisp and very juicy.

'Worcester Pearmain' is an old and reliable favourite which produces wonderful scarlet fruits in September and on into October.

'Elstar' is quite a weighty cropper. Its yellow fruits, flushed bright red, are ready for eating from October through to the end of January.

'Fiesta' offers good crops of large, red and yellow-flushed fruits from October through March and 'Kidd's Orange Red' spurs and fruits very freely. Its lemon-yellow fruits, with an orange-scarlet mottle, are ready from November through to January.

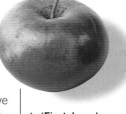

△ **'Fiesta' apples**

'Spartan' is a delicious crisp apple with a sweet, full flavour. Ready for picking in October, the grey bloom covering the fruits can be polished off to leave a deep red shine.

Remember to plant the trees in an airy but sheltered spot, in full sun, to attract pollinating insects and ensure a good fruit set.

Q I would like to have some autumn-fruiting raspberries next year. Could you recommend any particular varieties that I should look out for?

A The variety 'Autumn Bliss' is a deservedly popular one. It produces masses of lovely, large well-flavoured berries which ripen during late August, September and October.

'Galante' is a new variety from France, producing large fruits with an excellent flavour. And for something completely different, try 'Allgold', which crops at the same time as 'Autumn Bliss', but is yellow not pink.

Autumn raspberries are very easy to manage after fruiting because there are no stems to tie in. You simply cut them all down to ground level at the start of winter, and new ones will grow, flower and fruit in a single year.

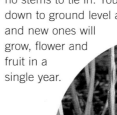
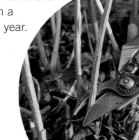

Pests and diseases

Q Lily beetles devastated my lilies a few years ago and, as a result, none of them came up afterwards. I really miss their scent in summer. Is it possible to keep this pest under control or grow resistant varieties?

A Until a few years ago, the lily beetle was limited to the Home Counties, but gradually, it has spread to other regions and promises to become an increasingly troublesome pest.

The beetle's scientific name is Lilioceris lilii. The adult insects are just under 1cm (½in) long with bright red bodies and black legs and heads. The larvae coat themselves with their own black, slimy excrement. Charming. Both larvae and adults attack the stems, buds, flowers and foliage, and can quickly do away with a patch of lilies. Adult beetles tend to fall to the ground and hide as soon as you go near. They can also fly.

They can be controlled by treatments containing malathion or permethrin. It is vital to take action as soon as the infestation is noticed since they are such fast workers. Follow the instructions on the insecticide packaging to the letter.

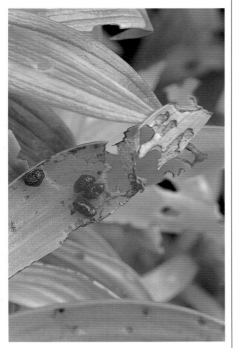

△ **Lily beetle larvae at work**

Q Every year, my ripening apples are eaten by a grub. I find one in each of the fruits and it devours the core. What is this creature and how can I control it?

A Codling moth is the culprit. Adults lay flat and translucent eggs singly on fruits and leaves. These will usually hatch within about 14 days.

The larva tunnels into the centre of the fruit, which it then eats. It remains within the core for about a month, before leaving it to overwinter under a flake of bark. It then emerges as a winged adult the following spring. Control it by spraying in mid-June with an insecticide based on pirimiphos-methyl, permethrin or fenitrothion. Repeat this process three weeks later.

Alternatively, hang a pheromone trap (*see inset*) in the tree in mid-May and replace it five weeks later. This releases simulated female sex attractants which lure the male pests to a sticky end. With no partners to mate with, the females cannot breed and so your apples are partially protected from attack.

Q The indoor cyclamen I bought last year has developed yellow leaves. Some are wilting as it starts to flower. I don't think I'm overwatering it, so what could be the problem?

A If you managed to care for the plant through last winter, rest it through summer and persuade it back into growth for another season, it seems unlikely that you have suddenly started to overwater. Cyclamen enjoy cool, light conditions, but could suffer on a cold window-sill.

Cyclamen are one of the favourite targets of vine weevil and it's likely a female beetle has laid her eggs in the pot. Nasty little pale-coloured C-shaped larvae will have hatched out and been feeding on the roots.

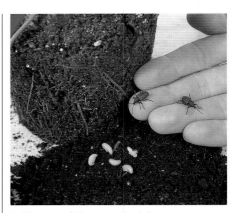

△ **Vine weevil larvae and adults**

Eventually, the plant will lose so many of its feeding roots that it won't be able to take up enough water or nutrients. Knock the plant out of its pot and inspect the roots. Squash all the larvae, repot the plant into fresh compost and with careful watering, it may yet survive.

If you think your plants are likely to be attacked by vine weevil, use a biological control. A solution containing millions of nematodes, which feed on the larvae, can be watered onto susceptible plants.

A new compost containing an insecticide that controls vine weevils and other pests is also worth considering. Called Plant Protection Compost, it can be used for ornamental but not edible crops.

Q My dahlias were magnificent last autumn, except that the first flowers had rough, ragged petals. Why?

A Earwigs may be to blame. They do most of their feeding at night and hide away in dark places during the day, so to find out if they are the culprits, you'll have to make some late-night expeditions into the garden with a torch.

You can use chemicals to control them. Try products based on pirimiphos-methyl, fenitrothion, bifenthrin or permethrin. To minimise the risk to pollinating and other beneficial insects, and to increase the chances of successful earwig control, spray after dusk.

You could also try trapping them.

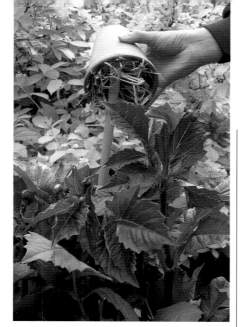

△ **Controlling earwigs**

Stuff flowerpots full of straw and invert onto bamboo canes in among the plants. If you remove the straw regularly, you will find earwigs hiding in it, which can then be killed.

Q All my lupins were decimated this year by a type of aphid. What can I do to ensure that they don't suffer the same fate again next year?

A Lupin aphids are remarkable as when they appear they are so big and always seem to be present in such large numbers. They demand extremely prompt action as they seem to be capable of sucking plants dry in a matter of hours.

Even if you managed to control them successfully last year, they may re-infest this year. So, your best course of action is to keep a very close watch on the plants and spray the aphids as soon as you see them with soft soap or an aphid-specific insecticide containing pirimicarb. This should control the pests while leaving the vast majority of beneficial insects unharmed. You may find that you need to spray the plant a few times, as the aphids could reinvade again later on in the summer.

Q My front and back gardens are being completely decimated by slugs. What steps can I take to control these pests?

A One of the most effective controls you can use is the nematode,

Phasmarhabditis hermaphrodita. Available by mail-order, this control is supplied as a powdered clay base. The nematodes are activated when water is added and the solution is then watered into the soil.

The nematodes enter the slug through a pore and once there, they release bacteria, multiply rapidly and poison the slug. Within a couple of days, the slug stops feeding and dies. As it breaks down, more nematodes move into the soil in search of more slugs.

This nematode will parasitise the most common slug species but does not harm earthworms and is killed off by the high temperatures of warm-blooded animals, including pets and humans.

Applied between March and October, the treatment will work for six weeks. However, it is expensive. Good garden hygiene and removing old leaves and plant debris help, and slug pellets based on methiocarb or metaldehyde are effective.

Q I suspect that a large crab apple tree in our garden has died from honey fungus as my neighbours said it had killed some plants in their own garden. What can I do to make certain it was honey fungus and have you any advice about future planting?

A Unfortunately, malus, in both its edible and ornamental forms, is rather prone to attack by honey fungus. However, you are right to check this is the culprit before assuming the worst.

Carefully remove some of the bark, either at the very base of the trunk or on

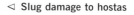

◁ **Slug damage to hostas**

some of the larger roots. If it is honey fungus, you will find the characteristic creamy white fungal sheet or mycelium sandwiched between the bark and the wood. Don't confuse this with harmless fungal growth that grows on the outside of the roots. The honey fungus mycelium also has a characteristic mushroomy smell. Another sign of honey fungus is honey-coloured toadstools which appear around the base of the trunk in late summer or autumn.

Dead trees and shrubs should be removed, preferably stump, roots and all, whether or not honey fungus is present. The greater the proportion of infected root you remove, the greater your chances of success in the future. When it comes to replanting, avoid using other trees or shrubs that are susceptible to this disease. These include roses, birch, hawthorn, forsythia, witch hazel, hydrangea, currant, rhododendron, lilac, wisteria, prunus, laburnum and paeony.

Fairly reliable subjects include abelia, actinidia, arundinaria, chaenomeles, cercis, aucuba, catalpa, cornus, cotinus, gleditsia, koelreuteria, pieris, parrotia, pittosporum, sarcococca, oak and beech.

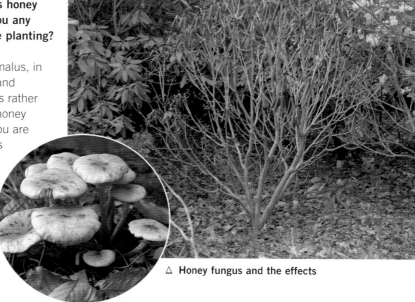

△ **Honey fungus and the effects**

The container garden

Q My hanging baskets are always rather boring. How can I ensure that they will be brimming over with colour this summer?

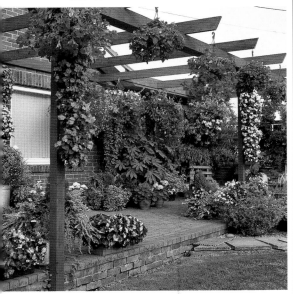

A The single most crucial factor with hanging baskets is water supply. In hot weather, you may have to water several times a day, so set your baskets up where they are easy to water. Automatic watering systems are great, too, but even these will need regular monitoring to make sure all is well and plants are sufficiently moist.

After water, feed is the next most important factor to consider. Summer displays must have regular feeding, about once a week in the growing season, using a dilute liquid feed. As for choice of plants, go for vigorous varieties, but be very careful with colour. There's a fashion, for instance, to plant mixed shades of lobelia, but many prefer the old-fashioned *Lobelia richardsonii*, the original trailing lobelia, because it is perennial and constantly produces flowers of a lovely mid-blue. With such a gentle colour, you could go for a strong, hot contrast, such as red ivy-leaved pelargoniums, or you could stay cool and gentle, bulking up the basket with trailing fuchsias.

Remember that foliage is as important as flower colour though, so try to include the variegated plectranthus or silver helichrysum.

Q How often should I feed my patio tubs during the summer months and what should I be using to feed them?

A The fertiliser in potting compost is only sufficient for the first few weeks, so additional feeding is vital to keep your plants performing really well. There are two options: regular applications of liquid fertiliser or a controlled release fertiliser added to the compost at planting time.

Liquid fertilisers need to be diluted in water and applied once or twice a week, usually by watering onto the roots, but they can be sprayed onto the leaves for an even faster response. Flowering plants benefit from being given a high-potash feed such as tomato fertiliser. In late summer, switch briefly to a high-nitrogen fertiliser to encourage a final burst of growth.

Controlled release fertiliser is a fairly new innovation and a real boon to busy gardeners. It takes the form of granules coated in a slow-dissolving resin which is temperature-sensitive, so nutrients are only released when it is warm enough for the plants to grow and need feeding. One application will last the whole of the season, although it is a good idea to top it up with a few liquid feeds towards the end of the summer.

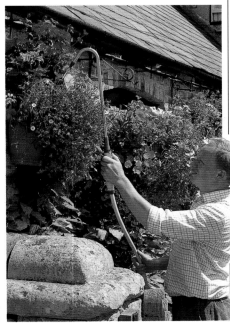

Q Can you explain how to make an alpine sink and suggest a selection of alpines I could plant in it to give some winter interest?

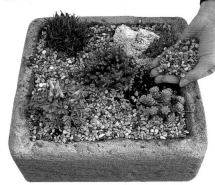

A The classic mixture for making hypertufa alpine sinks or troughs is two parts moistened, sieved moss peat, one part sharp sand or fine grit and one part cement. You can substitute sieved shredded composted bark for the peat with little difference.

The mixture can be stuck onto an old glazed sink, which needs a good roughening first, then covered with a suitable glue so that the hypertufa will stick.

Alternatively the mixture can be poured into a mould and allowed to set. Again, it will be made a lot stronger if wire chicken netting reinforcement is used throughout the walls and base of the container.

Many people like their alpine sinks to have an authentic aged look. To help speed up the greening process, paint on milk or live yoghurt once a week. This will encourage the growth of algae on the outside of the sink.

Surprisingly enough, there are quite a few plants to bring an extra sparkle to your sink in winter. *Hacquetia epipactis* is a low-growing herbaceous plant with yellow-green flowers. *Cyclamen coum*, in shades of magenta, pink and white, look splendid and have lovely attractive marbled leaves as an added bonus.

Don't forget to use evergreen plants like *Sempervivum* 'Mahogany' and *Saxifraga* 'Cloth of Gold', and bulbs like snowdrops need to be divided regularly to curb their spread.

The lawn

Q I have quite a passion for azaleas and camellias, but they simply turn yellow and die in my garden soil. Someone has suggested I try growing them in containers, but I would like to know which compost to use, and which varieties to grow?

A If your garden soil isn't naturally acidic, growing lime-haters in containers will be the ideal solution. Containers of 30–38cm (12–15in) diameter are suitable for dwarf rhododendrons and azaleas, but larger plants will need bigger pots. Use an ericaceous compost and feed every 10 days during the growing season with a general liquid feed. Also give one feed of sequestered iron each spring. Keep the compost constantly moist and protect pots from excess heat in summer.

Good cultivars include *Rhododendron yakushimanum* hybrids such as 'Grumpy' (pale yellow), and other dwarf rhododendrons like the Bow Bells Group (pink, dangling bell flowers), and tidy, compact Japanese azaleas such as 'Squirrel' (scarlet).

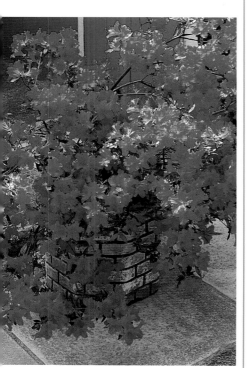

△ **Grow azaleas in an ericaceous compost**

Q My garden is on heavy clay and the lawn gets very waterlogged. What is the easiest way to improve drainage? I have tried forking over the surface but this hasn't helped.

A If you wanted to invest a lot of time and money, you could take up the lawn and install a drainage system. This gives the best results, but the easiest option is to hollow-tine aerate the whole area.

You can hire a hollow-tine aerator that removes plugs or cores of soil from the lawn. When you have finished hollow- tining, sweep up the cores and brush a very sandy top dressing mixture into the holes. The cores act as drainage channels, improving air circulation, which improves root growth of the turf grasses.

On a heavy soil you should do this every other year and, of course, avoid compacting the lawn any more than you have to. In particular, avoid walking on the lawn during wet weather.

Q Can you tell me if there is any permanent answer to controlling moss in lawns? I have tried using mosskillers in the past, but it just returns a few weeks later.

A The presence of moss in the lawn is a symptom of other problems, such as poor drainage, compaction, excessive shade or close mowing. Unless these are remedied, the moss will always return.

The warm, dry days of early September are an ideal time to apply lawn sand, which is the traditional control for moss. About two weeks after application, the moss turns black and can be raked out or scarified and bare patches reseeded. Other moss killers can be directly watered onto the lawn. After treatment, you should take immediate steps to rectify the actual cause of the problem.

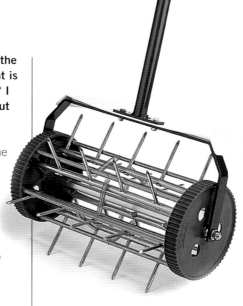

△ **Hollow-tined aerator**

Q My lawn contains a large number of broad-leaved weeds and is generally looking quite poorly. When is the best season to take some steps to improve it for next year?

A In early autumn months, eradicate weeds individually by spot treating them with a ready-to-use, spray-on herbicide. When the weeds are dead, rake over the surface of the lawn to remove any accumulated thatch. This will really help to improve aeration.

This is hard work, so if your lawn is large, it may be worth hiring or buying a powered scarifier.

Spike any compacted areas with a garden fork or lawn aerator and fill the holes with a mixture of equal parts of sharp sand and pulverised bark. Finish by feeding with a high potash/phosphate fertiliser plus moss killer, to strengthen the grass over the winter months. This should ensure plenty of lush new growth next spring.

◁ **Large, stubborn weeds can be spot-treated**

Problems with houseplants

Q I have tried growing just about every houseplant but they all seem to die in no time. Can you suggest some foolproof houseplants that I could try for a year-round display?

A As well as recommending some easy plants, do analyse your approach to their cultivation. The position you choose for your houseplants is vital to their survival. Most will thrive in good light away from radiators and fires during winter.

Getting the plants' watering regime right is the next challenge. Generally, plants need watering only when the compost surface has begun to dry out. Avoid frequent eggcupfuls of water: give them a soaking each time, so that all the roots benefit. If any water remains in the saucer after half an hour, empty it and allow the pot to drain.

Monstera deliciosa, the Swiss cheese plant, and *Dracaena* Deremensis Group can grow very large. If space is a problem, go for *Begonia rex*, chlorophytum, the spider plant, or *Asparagus densiflorus*

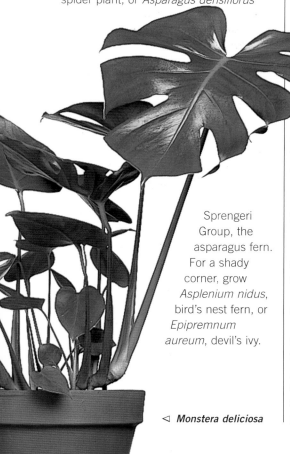

Sprengeri Group, the asparagus fern. For a shady corner, grow *Asplenium nidus*, bird's nest fern, or *Epipremnum aureum*, devil's ivy.

◁ *Monstera deliciosa*

Q My cymbidium orchid produced a lovely flower spike but the flowers then turned brown and dropped off. It is on a window-sill with good light and away from heat. What happened?

A Your cymbidium was either in a draught or experienced fluctuating temperatures by being close to the window. At night, there is quite a temperature drop around single glazed windows. The answer is to bring the orchid in from the window so it can benefit from direct light but has warmer air around it.

If you have tightly fitting windows, then the answer probably lies in watering. Too much or too little can result in flower buds dropping. Gauge its need for water by feeling the weight of the pot and empty excess from the saucer after an hour. However, it is also a mistake to leave the roots dry for too long.

Q Every year I am faced with red spider mite attack on my houseplants. What is the best way to control it, and are there any houseplants that are resistant to attack?

A The glasshouse red spider mite *Tetranychus urticae*, now more correctly known as two-spotted mite, seems to attack virtually all house-plants and biological control is the best solution. This means introducing another mite, in this case *Phytoseiulus persimilis*, to prey upon the red spider.

The predator feeds on adults, the young and even the eggs of the pest, so it is very efficient. *Phytoseiulus* is orange-red in colour with a rounder body than the greeny-yellow pest and, despite its portly appearance, rushes around the infested plant at great speed, catching and consuming its prey.

Provided you follow the instructions carefully and introduce the predators at the correct time, it works very well. In practice, this means introducing predators at the first signs of attack. Leave it too late and there may be too many red spider mites for the predators to cope with.

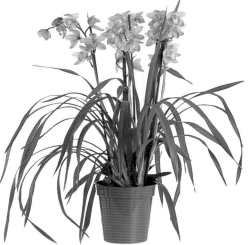

△ **Cymbidium orchid**

Introduce them too early and there will be insufficient prey for them to feed on, so they will die out quickly. You need a minimum daytime temperature of 21°C (70°F) if the predatory mites are to breed faster than the pest mites, so the method is generally most efficient from late spring until mid-autumn.

Before introducing the predators, check with the supplier that any chemicals used previously will not have remained on the plant as these could kill off the beneficial mites you introduce. Also check that any other chemicals used on or near your houseplants are not harmful to the *Phytoseiulus*.

All this may sound complicated but it really is easy, and usually far more effective than chemicals.

Q The surface of my houseplant compost is covered in tiny, black flies. What are they, will they do any damage and how should I control them?

A These are fungus gnats or sciarid flies, whose larvae feed on the organic matter present in the compost you are using. The adult flies are laying eggs into the compost surface, which hatch into tiny translucent maggots. You may have noticed them feeding on the remains of dead plants. Although generally said to cause no harm to healthy plants, they may feed on roots near to the surface and are certainly unsightly. Some houseplant insecticides will kill them, but try first to make their environment less welcoming. Leave the compost surface a little more time to dry out between waterings, or carefully remove the top 2.5cm (1in) or so and replace with small pebbles.

Problems with ponds

Q We didn't originally plan our pond as a wildlife haven, but it seems to attract all kinds of creatures, which we enjoy watching. What can we do to ensure that our pond is even more wildlife-friendly?

A Create a shallow area, lined with pebbles or gravel like a beach. The lack of depth enables hedgehogs to drink without falling into the water, and even if they do take a tumble, they'll be able to climb out again. A beach area also enables small frogs, toads and newts to find their way out. Partially submerged stones and logs provide basking areas for newts, but avoid large stones that overlap the pond as these make it difficult for pond life to get in and out.

Another way to attract wildlife is by introducing plenty of plants, especially oxygenators as these give tadpoles and insects somewhere to hide from newts and birds. Vertical plants, such as iris and grasses, are ideal for dragonfly nymphs to crawl onto before they hatch into adults.

Native plants can be vigorous, so choose carefully if you have a small pond. In particular, avoid duckweed. Never take plants from the wild.

If you want fish, avoid koi and goldfish varieties as they will uproot plants. There's no need to feed the fish as plants provide enough natural food. Any extra food only pollutes the water.

Q I own a tiny town garden and would love a small water feature. I saw one made out of a half-barrel. Is this easy to make and can you recommend any plants that would survive in such a confined space?

A It's very easy to make a water feature. First, you need a reservoir, in this case a half-barrel but you could also use glazed pots, urns, fibreglass containers and pebble pools. If using a barrel, make sure it's watertight. This may mean soaking it for the wood to swell; you can use a liner but it needs to be put in place well to look good.

If it's the sound of moving water you're after, a small pump is required. Raise the pump off the bottom of the barrel so you don't have to clean the filter too often.

If your moving water feature is just a small bubble of water, you can grow water lilies. Recommended varieties are *Nymphaea* 'Pygmaea Rubra', *N.* 'Pygmaea Helvola' and *N.* 'Pygmaea Alba'.

If you prefer more water disturbance, marginal plants are better. Those to choose from include *Caltha palustris* 'Pleno', *Houttuynia cordata* 'Flore Pleno' and Variegata Group, *Iris laevigata*, *Myosotis scorpioides* 'Mermaid', *Myriophyllum* 'Red Stem' and *Sagittaria sagittifolia* 'Flore Pleno'.

Recommended oxygenators are *Callitriche palustris, Hottonia palustris* and *Myriophyllum spicatum*.

Q Is there any way of making a pond safe for young children or can you suggest a safer water feature for the garden?

A For toddlers, it's best to remove the pond, and for older children, surround the pool with a childproof fence and lockable gate.

Complete safety with a pond and young children is impossible but there are ways of making it safer. One is to have a timber and plastic mesh grid lodged on the marginal shelf, just under the water's surface. The plants will grow through the mesh which, if it is black, will be hardly noticeable. Don't have steep slopes near a pool on which children can run down towards the water. Instead, plant the relevant pond side heavily with shrubs and marginals.

Water features that consist of a grid covering open water and supporting cobbles or pebbles are safe and attractive, especially with a wall spout or fountain.

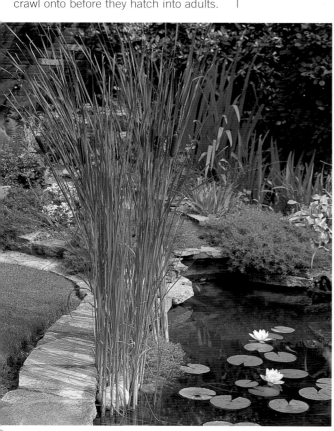

In search of
INSPIRATION

Kathryn Bradley-Hole

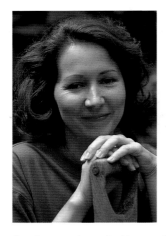

Some of the finest gardens in the world are to be found here in Britain. Whether they are large or small, visiting them is one of the great pleasures to be had in summer, or any other season. It has often been my good fortune to visit and write about gardens professionally for the past ten years, although I have toured them purely for pleasure for a good deal longer. My late mother was someone who enjoyed doing the rounds of stately homes, and I can remember, way back, being not greatly impressed by ornate plaster ceilings, portraits of swanky lords and ladies long gone, and dark wood carvings by Grinling Gibbons. As a child, I infinitely preferred wandering outdoors and nosing among the flowers, and that fascination has clearly withstood the test of time.

If the gardens featured here inspire you, too, you may wish to read *The Garden Lovers' Guide to Britain*, written in conjunction with *BBC Gardeners' World Magazine*. This gives a guided tour of more than 500 marvellous gardens and nurseries in the country, and is, I hope, a useful and entertaining book for anyone who loves plants and gardens.

Kathryn Bradley-Hole is a regular contributor to *BBC Gardeners' World Magazine*, *BBC Homes and Antiques* **and the** *Daily Telegraph*. **She is the author of** *The Garden Lovers' Guide to Britain* **(BBC Worldwide).**

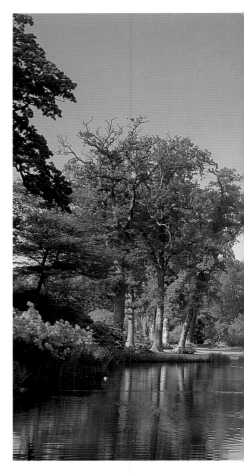

The Savill Garden, Berkshire

Only 35 of Windsor Great Park's 4,500 acres are taken up by this popular garden, which is one of my favourite springtime haunts. It is a woodland garden par excellence, with fine magnolias, rhododendrons, pieris and dogwoods filling out a middle layer under tree canopies of oaks and pines.

The garden also features a large collection of daffodil cultivars, individually grouped and well labelled, but even more attractive are the grassy slopes when covered with hoop-petticoat narcissi (*Narcissus bulbocodium*) and patches of the dainty *N. cyclamineus*. Informal gravel paths wind through the Dry Garden, where there are further colourful plantings of spring bulbs and Mediterranean plants. In the damper valleys, bright yellow kingcups and lysichitons line the bogs and streams among unfurling fronds of ferns. One of the garden's finest trees, an unusual Chilean *Podocarpus* in the herbaceous area, was quite unintended;

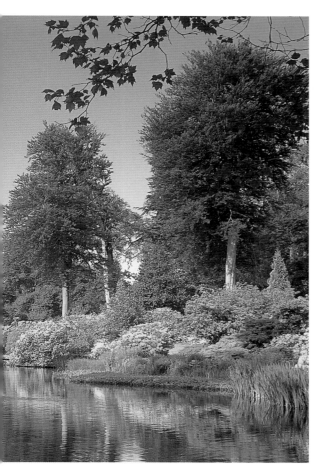

△ *The Savill Garden*

it was a discarded nursery seedling that took root here 60-odd years ago. A modern glasshouse was added in 1995 to house more tender rhododendrons and plants of the southern hemisphere.

Lyme Park, Cheshire

The grounds of Lyme Park are for ever etched in millions of viewers' minds as Pemberley, home of Mr Darcy in the BBC's popular adaptation of *Pride and Prejudice*. According to Vicky Dawson, the property manager, visitors of all nationalities want to know where Mr Darcy went for a dip, and whether they can see his wet shirt. Alas, we can't.

The property is one of the National Trust's most dazzling jewels, with a huge palladian mansion and 17 acres of fabulous gardens within a 1,400-acre landscaped park grazed by red and fallow deer. It also enjoys breathtaking views of

the Pennines and the lowland Cheshire plain. There is a formal, patterned Dutch garden with ivy-edged beds, infilled with bright spring and summer bedding. A sunken garden on the north side is more discreetly planted with trees and shrubs. An early 19th-century orangery houses a splendid fig tree and two enormous camellias, dating from Victorian times, plus a scattering of other fragrant and leafy conservatory stalwarts. Outside are terraced beds and a rose garden, leading on to less formal grounds with lawns and woodland. The lake and lime avenue are remnants of a 17th-century garden that has been absorbed into the gentler contours of the great 18th-century park.

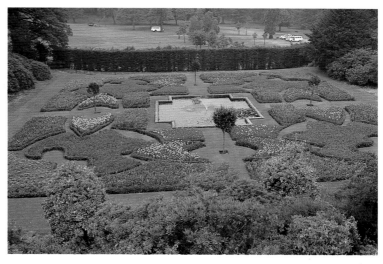

△ *Lyme Park*

Holker Hall, Cumbria

By any standards this unusual and spectacular garden is thrilling, because you are instantly aware of its high quality in design and maintenance. From a modest garden entrance at one side of the house, you come into the Elliptical Garden, a symmetrical, formal area laid out in 1993. Local materials such as slates and cobblestones from the nearby coast are used in the hard landscaping, and planting is of mixed shrubs and herbaceous perennials. There are ripples of blue catmint and fascinating delphinium 'cages' made yearly from hazel rods cut on the estate.

▽ *Holker Hall*

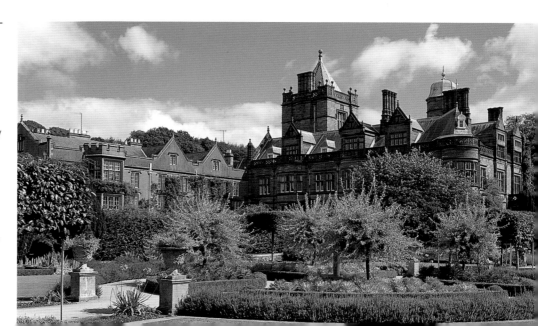

The Summer Garden beyond features a tunnel of Portuguese laurel casting shade along the central path, topiarised above clean stilt trunks. There are fragrant shrubs, lilies, roses and lavender, and the box-edged beds are filled with seasonal flowers. In contrast, the wildflower meadow beyond is home to 24 species of perennial native wildflowers, a glorious sight before hay cutting.

Long grasses and wildflowers are encouraged to great effect elsewhere in the gardens, among the numerous specimen trees that have been planted over the centuries. A fountain is surrounded by the lofty, twisted trunks of *Rhododendron arboreum*, hugely decorative when its deep pink petals carpet the ground, which was planted by Lord Burlington around 1840. A magnificent stepped water cascade, inspired by an ancient Indian water garden in Rajasthan, is a fairly recent addition. Across the lawns from the top of the cascade, you reach the small, intimate rose garden, a formal area with trellised gazebos supporting climbing varieties. Throughout the 25 acres there are many interesting, unusual trees and shrubs, making this a garden to return to, as new projects are continually executed.

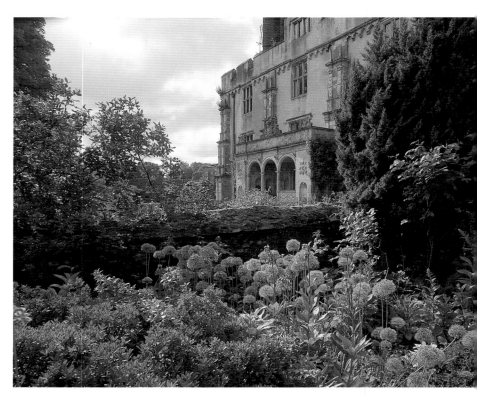

Coleton Fishacre, Devon

Sailing, sunshine and south Devon's fashionable resorts brought Rupert D'Oyly Carte, son and heir of the musical impresario partner to Gilbert and Sullivan, to this region. In 1925 he had a delightful house built of local stone, on an enchanting, south-facing valley. Around it the 22-acre garden is laid out in a series of beautifully planted terraces.

This garden offers a very satisfying blend of architectural and natural elements. There are dry-stone walls, circular water lily pools and a narrow water-rill near the house; but all of that soon gives way to a free-form, organic pattern of winding paths and shrubberies. Countless little streams feed luxuriant waterside plantings of irises, ferns and oriental primulas. Rhododendrons thrive, and the mild climate nurtures a huge collection of half-hardy plants from Australasia and South Africa. The Rill Garden is brilliant in high summer, with bright orange and scarlet-flowered cannas joined by salvias and assorted African daisies. Coleton Fishacre is tucked away down narrow lanes but is well worth seeking out for its beauty and tranquillity.

△ *Cranborne Manor*

Cranborne Manor Gardens and Garden Centre, Dorset

This is one of my all-time favourite gardens. It seems to have everything in perfect scale. The manor house is one of the prettiest in the country, being not too grand, and it is exquisitely proportioned. The original manor was built in 1207 as a hunting lodge for King John and was later remodelled during Tudor times. It subsequently passed to Robert Cecil, 1st Earl of Salisbury, in the early 17th century, and his descendants still live here.

A fine beech avenue runs down a gentle slope from the road to the twin pepperpot gate-houses. The house sits snugly in its 11-acre grounds, which were laid out in Robert Cecil's time under the instructions of John Tradescant the Elder, who brought back rare plants and bulbs from the European continent. A Jacobean mount, built for viewing the owner's rolling acres, and the walled and hedged enclosures reflect the intimate garden style prevailing at that time.

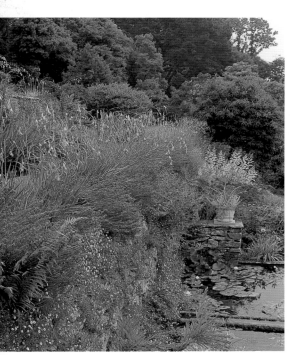

△ *Coleton Fishacre*

Broad stretches of grass, carpeting the ground beneath fruit and forest trees, are spangled with narcissi, cowslips, primroses, orchids and fritillaries in their thousands through spring. A rose- and wisteria-covered pergola runs beside the old kitchen garden. In addition, there are pleached limes, a garden of old roses and pale flowers and a herb garden with windows cut into an old yew hedge to give views of the countryside beyond.

The River Crane, from which Cranborne gets its name, runs along the northern edge of the garden. It is a winter bourne that dries out in summer. It is worthwhile pausing to admire the nearby ancient flint-and-cob walls.

Part of the old walled garden has been turned into a well-stocked garden centre, which is open all year round. It specialises in old-fashioned roses, herbs, fruit trees and garden ornaments.

Port Lympne, Kent

The county of Kent possesses an excessively generous helping of castles and historic houses set off by pleasing grounds. Port Lympne provides a fantastic cocktail of zoo, garden and eccentrically decorated house, adding up to a highly enjoyable outing for all ages and inclinations. From the garden visitor's point of view, it is certainly a novelty to walk through 100 yards of hydrangeas to the accompanying sound of baying wolves, or to hear the distant roar of rare Barbary lions while admiring the dahlia borders.

The 15 acres of gardens, within a 300-acre animal park, were originally designed by the wealthy art patron and political host Sir Philip Sassoon, and were laid out from 1919 onwards. From the hydrangea walk you reach the top of the 125-step Trojan stairs, offering wonderful views over Romney Marsh. The stairs lead down to a formal garden of roses, cotton lavender and Hupeh crab apples and further terraced gardens, divided by walls and hedging. Within the hedged compartments there are bedded-out areas, one in an intriguing chessboard design, another laid out with beds in

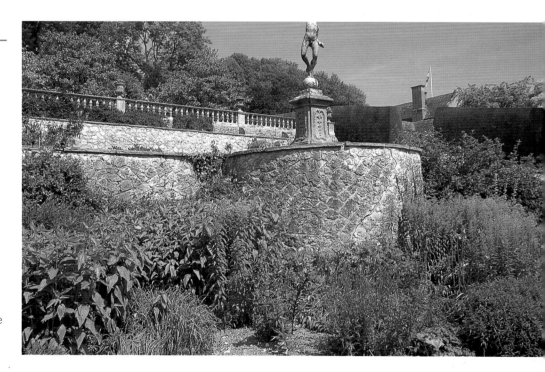

contrasting stripes. There is a terraced vineyard, a pair of long, mixed borders, a magnolia walk, rose terrace, dahlia terrace and a herbaceous border.

By the time you reach the end of the lower terraces, the animals are close at hand: lions, hyaenas, small cats, bison, gibbons and monkeys. It is also well worth

△ *Port Lympne*

your while looking inside the eccentrically decorated house, which has a delightful Moorish patio with a marble floor and five fountains. In addition, there is a tented room of exotic murals painted by the artist Rex Whistler.

Reads Nursery, Norfolk

There are three reasons to visit this nursery: fruit, interesting conservatory plants and the barn. Reads has been going for well over 100 years and it offers unrivalled selections of fruit, especially traditional varieties, available by mail as well as on-site. There are quinces and kiwi fruit, pineapple-guava and olives. There is also an extensive array of figs, with 34 different varieties, constituting the National Collection of these exquisite fruits.

Reads also specialises in citrus fruits, with oranges and lemons in variety, and limes, grapefruit, kumquats, limequats and tangelos – a cross between the grapefruit and mandarin, sometimes known as ugli fruit. The conservatory plants account for half of the nursery's catalogue, with more than 70 different varieties of bougainvillea alone, and the fragrant glasshouses are as thrilling as any you will see in a botanic garden, with the added piquancy that most of what you see is for sale.

Lastly, there is Hales Hall Barn. At 56m (184ft) long, with stepped gables and a wonderful ribcage of ancient

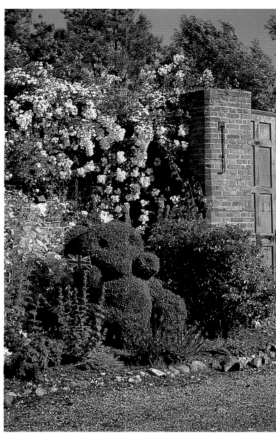

△ *Reads Nursery*

timbers supporting its newly thatched roof, it is one of the largest and most spectacular barns in the country, dating from around 1480. The one-and-a-quarter-acre nursery also offers topiary and hedging plants in box and yew.

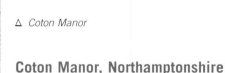

△ *Coton Manor*

Coton Manor, Northamptonshire

Coton Manor is a friendly farmhouse of local honey-coloured stone, with mullioned windows and a steeply pitched roof. The ten-acre gardens are among the most pleasing you will see anywhere, with exceptional ranges of plants and a high standard of upkeep. I bumped into one of the owners, Susie Pasley-Tyler, while she was immersed in a small sea of sisyrinchiums, her wheelbarrow on the turf path rapidly filling up with prunings and tidyings from one of the herbaceous borders. This is a hands-on family garden, as it has been for three generations.

Upon her mother-in-law's death in 1990, Susie and her husband, Ian, took over the manor and began some regenerative work in the garden. The results are very impressive. Roses and summer flowers billow around the footings of the manor and lady's mantle fills cracks in the stone paving. More roses and flower borders near the house are contained by yew hedges, with woodland and water gardens beyond. There are more borders in the lower gardens and grassy slopes leading to a five-acre bluebell wood, which is captivating in May. Beyond the recently made herb garden is a nursery. It is worth browsing here for interesting plants, while more are for sale beside the stable-yard café, where excellent home-made food is served.

CELEBRITY CHOICE

Geoffrey Smith, panellist of BBC Radio 4's *Gardeners' Question Time*

'I spend many a Sunday afternoon at Fountains Abbey, near Ripon in Yorkshire, because its landscape garden speaks of the tranquillity of centuries. Castle Howard is also magnificent – such an immense landscape. Its sheer extravagance is breathtaking.

'I also greatly admire the gorgeous herbaceous borders of Newby Hall and the way they sweep away from the house, down a gentle slope to the river. But the garden I love most is Parcevall, 305m (1,000ft) up in the Dales. It's a sublime place and not just because of the plants, although it has a fine collection, but also for the landscape around it. York Gate, at Adel, is second only to Parcevall; it's an intimate family garden, but full of good plantsmanship.'

Herterton House, Northumberland

It would be difficult to leave Herterton House without a boxful of souvenir plants, quaintly wrapped in newsprint, from the Lawleys' small but intriguing nursery, but there is more. The adjoining gardens, covering one acre around their farmhouse, are among the best to be seen in the country.

Facing the lane, in front of the low, Elizabethan farmhouse, the Lawleys, both of whom are artists, have planted a formal topiary garden of English evergreens, featuring ivy, box, yew and holly, and enlivened with golden-leaved and variegated forms. To one side, there is a fascinating cloistered herb garden displaying plants that were once greatly valued by medieval physicians and dyers. The plants include clary, a time-honoured remedy for eye complaints; betony, a cure-all since the days of antiquity; and periwinkle, sweet rocket, heartsease, gromwell and woad.

∇ *Herterton House*

Behind the house, full rein is given to colourful summer flowers, planted in graduated schemes of complementary tones. According to Frank Lawley, the scheme symbolises the passing of time, from 'pale colours in the morning (near the house), through the richest, brightest colours at midday (in mid-garden), to the deep reds and purples at the far end, signifying dusk and night-time'. The effect is captivating. The Lawleys are currently making another enclosed garden beyond: a box parterre, filled with bright annuals.

Felley Priory, Nottinghamshire

This three-acre garden has everything. It is of enormous interest to the plantsman, for there are many unusual trees, shrubs, bulbs and perennials, and the owner is a keen, hands-on gardener. A disciplined structure is provided by walls, mature yew hedges, topiarised with top-knots at regular intervals, and treillage enclosures. The borders are abundant and thoughtfully planted and the rose

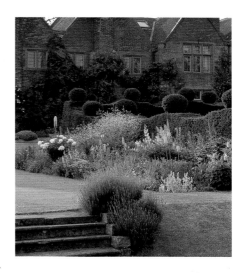

△ *Felley Priory*

garden is spectacular in summer, with late-flowering clematis providing colour once the roses have finished. The garden's layout is in sympathy with the priory house (not open), which has medieval origins, but it has a rewarding vigour and flair. The delightful lily pool has bog irises and shrub roses lighting up the banks.

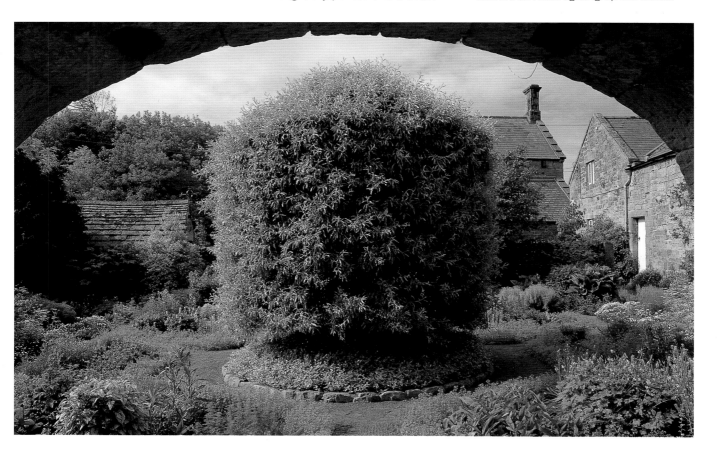

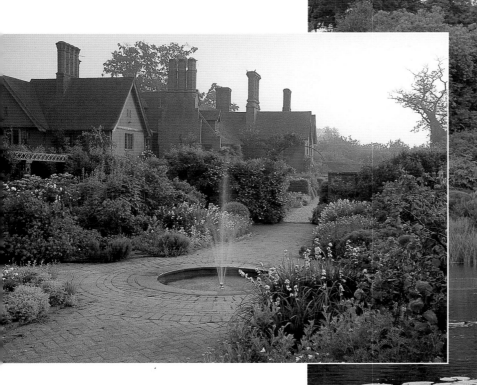

△ *Wyken Hall*

Wyken Hall, Suffolk

Wyken Hall, near Stanton, is an exquisite Elizabethan manor house, plastered and pargeted in the local vernacular style. It is painted the colour of raw salmon, a shade or two more daring than the average Suffolk pink. At the front of the house, several rocking chairs peer between espaliered apple trees on tall stems, in the manner usually employed for pleached limes. You know the garden will be interesting, for it has twists of originality while maintaining traditional form. Also at the front is a quincunx pattern of brick-and-flint circles with box hedging and seasonal infills of flowers.

Beyond, there is a small garden of edibles beside the house, leading to a border of hot colours: scarlet roses, geums and salvias among bronze-leaved impatiens and dahlias, for example. There are three small, linked gardens of traditional, formal design with box and yew hedging, herbs and a dining terrace, a rose garden with central fountain, a kitchen garden and orchard. A nuttery and dell have mown walks through long grasses and wildflowers leading to a young maze of copper-beech hedging. There are also fine old oaks in the grounds. From the wilder areas there are lovely views back to the house, which squats low and content in its wood-enshrouded gardens, while its ornate chimneys attempt to pierce the skyline.

Hodnet Hall, Shropshire

Two things about Hodnet Hall are etched for ever on my memory: the fantastic waterscape, created from a chain of big lakes, and the bizarre experience of taking tea with a snarling tiger, albeit a stuffed one, under the glassy gaze of hundreds of severed heads of assorted antelopes, buffaloes and

△ *Hodnet Hall*

rhinoceros. The late-Victorian hall sits on a plateau, looking down onto the main pool; half a dozen more lakes ascend the gentle valley to the west. Grassy banks on each side of the lakes are awash with daffodils, rhododendrons and cherry blossom through the spring, followed by astilbes and hydrangeas. There are acers in variety, with Japanese forms elegantly bowing to cast their reflections at the water's edge, and, with a variety of shrubs and trees, they bring a spectacular glow to autumn. Hodnet is a really splendid and unusual garden, laid out with imagination in the 1920s and well maintained today. If I lived nearby, its 60 acres would be a regular haunt.

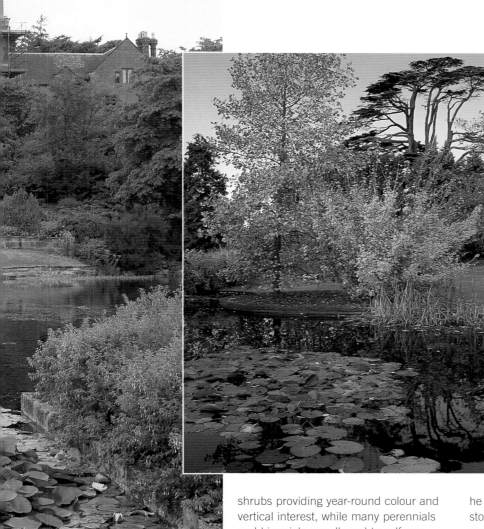

◁ *Denmans*

The Clock House, on the edge of the garden, and runs design courses from there. His style has blended well with the Robinsons'. The superb herb garden he made within the walled former kitchen garden is well known and much photographed. There is also a good nursery, offering many of the wonderful plants you see in the gardens, and the restaurant/tearoom serves good home-made fare in pleasant surroundings.

Iford Manor, Wiltshire

Several elements combine to make this a most pleasingly designed garden. The ancient manor itself (not open) is in a fabulous setting, perched above a picturesque meander of the River Frome. A wooded hill rises behind it, bearing traces of Roman settlements. When Harold Peto bought the property in 1899, he laid out a series of terraces linked by stone stairways, and added stone loggias and a colonnade to the grounds. Peto was influenced by Italian design. He made frequent excursions to Italy, in search of ancient artefacts and interesting

shrubs providing year-round colour and vertical interest, while many perennials and biennials are allowed to self-sow here and there, to enhance its informality.

Garden designer John Brookes arrived at Denmans in 1980. He lives in

Denmans, Sussex

Denmans was begun by the late Joyce Robinson, a great character who could often be met in her later years zooming about the garden in her powered wheelchair. She and her husband acquired the site in 1946 with 32 acres and a large house which they later sold, whereupon they moved into a cottage in the garden. The current three-and-a-half-acre garden is remarkable for Mrs Robinson's innovative design, with a 'dry river' of gravel running sinuously through it. The garden's original inspiration was a visit to the Greek island of Delos, in 1969, where Mrs Robinson saw that 'everything grew in hot, gravelly soil'. The style is relaxed, with mixed trees and

CELEBRITY CHOICE

Stephen Lacey, author, journalist and presenter of BBC2's *Gardeners' World*

'Powis Castle is practically on my doorstep, so I go there quite a lot at all times of the year and all times of the day. It's amazingly scenic and I love driving through the park. There is a lushness in the west of Britain, because of the rain, that you don't get in the east; Powis has a fertile feel to it with things growing buxomly. It is a rich source of planting ideas and the planting changes quite a lot from year to year. Colours in the planting are quite intense and the borders have helped me to develop a taste for strong colours, such as the scarlets and oranges of crocosmias. Unlike many gardens, this one gets better and better as the season progresses and it is particularly good in August, not only because of the flowers; you get other things, such as the great showers of rosehips from *Rosa glauca* and *R.* 'Highdownensis', and you will often see magnificent sunsets there.'

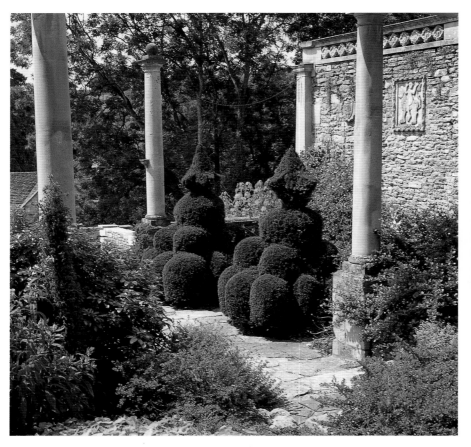

△ *Iford Manor*

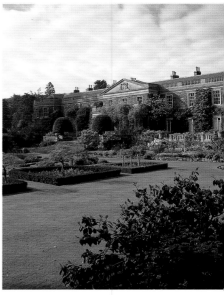

△ *Mount Stewart*

pieces of masonry, and his translation of the idiom into the Wiltshire landscape is deftly and sympathetically executed. A touch of the Riviera, where Peto also made gardens, is added by the planting, which includes wisterias, grapevines, irises, cypress trees and pines.

Peto admired the rigorous approach of Japanese design and added a small Japanese garden to Iford. There are also delightful streamside plantings and small, formal pools on this 15-acre site.

Mount Stewart, County Down

Some gardens are remarkable for their plant collections, some for their rigorous design and others are special for the particular atmosphere that has been imbued by their makers. Mount Stewart combines all of these three assets.

The 80-acre garden was chiefly laid out by Edith, Marchioness of Londonderry,

during the 1920s. Edith, known to her close friends as 'Circe, the Sorceress', was a remarkable woman by any standards. She was an influential political hostess, founding the Women's Legion in

1915, which helped to provide jobs for women while men were away fighting, and, as a result, greatly improved the status of women in the workplace. Following the First World War, Edith spent much of her time at Mount Stewart and refurbished the house interiors as well as giving ex-servicemen employment in laying out the formal gardens.

The Italian garden on the south front of the house comprises richly planted formal parterres, which are at their best

CELEBRITY CHOICE

Roy Lancaster, plant hunter, author and television presenter

'For me there are two great things in the world: mountains and the sea. Mountains are my favourite; you have to climb them, to explore them. And that is why I like Trebah. It's not mountainous, of course, but the depth of the valley is very much like a mountainside, and it has very good mountain flora, especially its Himalayan and Chinese content: the big rhododendrons, bamboos, a huge *Davidia involucrata*, one of my favourite trees. It's a primeval world. It is also about foliage and scale. To stand by the house at Trebah and look down the valley, glimpsing what appears to be the sea at the bottom, is very exciting. Then there is the huge gunnera grove in the valley. The path through it is very carefully cleaned up around the plants so you can see the huge rhizomes, and I love the lurid green light that shines through the gigantic leaves when you are standing under them. The plant content at Trebah takes in so many elements I've enjoyed in wild places. It's a rough, jagged garden, and one I love visiting.'

in summer, and are modelled on those of Dunrobin Castle in Sutherland, Edith's childhood home. Beyond is the Spanish garden, with rills and a formal pool, surrounded by impressive arcaded hedges of Leyland cypress. The sunk garden on the west side was laid out according to plans sent by post from Gertrude Jekyll, although its plantings of yellow and orange, blue and purple flowers and foliage are largely to Edith's own specification. Mount Stewart's gardens were deeply personal to Edith and are imbued with symbolism; its shamrock garden, enclosed by yew hedges, contains a topiarised Irish harp in yew and a ground pattern featuring the Red Hand of Ulster, planted seasonally with scarlet flowers. The Dodo terrace features cast concrete animals from The Ark, a dining club that was regularly hosted by Edith in London.

Mount Stewart's sheltered position, combined with dependable rainfall and lime-free soil, have all encouraged the rapid growth of rare and sub-tropical plants in the formal gardens and glorious rhododendrons and magnolias in the surrounding woodlands and lakeside.

Kellie Castle, Fife

A pretty, pleasing, utterly peaceful walled garden of one and a half acres, snuggling under the castle's massive bulk of buff-grey stone. My first impression upon entering the garden was of a distinctly feminine nature, and it is no surprise that the head gardener is a woman, Kathy Sayer, who has maintained the garden organically since arriving in 1990.

Knee-high box hedges line the gravelled paths which run around the garden's perimeter, dividing it into three main sections, with fruit tree-studded lawns filling the centre. The garden's chief function has always been to produce fruit, vegetables and flowers for the house. There are also many old roses, around 90 different varieties, and a pair of low hedges of the crimson-and-white striped *Rosa gallica* 'Versicolor', reputed to have been here for over 100 years. Poppies and paeonies, lupins, lavatera and dame's violet all contribute to the abundant beauty, and self-sown flowers are allowed to stay wherever possible. Kathy Sayer's hens are regularly allowed to roam the garden, assisting the organic slug-control.

A two-storey summerhouse in one corner of the garden was designed by the Arts and Crafts architect Sir Robert Lorimer. Kellie Castle was his family's summer home in the late 19th and early 20th century.

▽ *Kellie Castle*

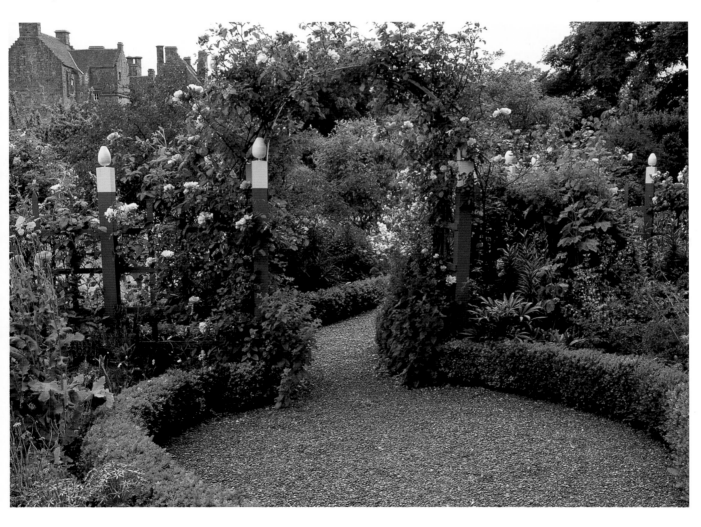

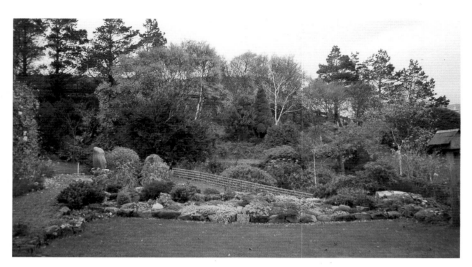

Glamaig Cottage, Isle of Skye

This is one of the most remote gardens I have ever visited. It is seven miles down a single-track road on Skye in the Western Isles, overlooking Loch Sligachan and the smaller islands of Raasay and Scalpay. It is an interesting two-acre plantsman's garden, made over the last 30 years by Richard and Ursula Townsend, who have fashioned it in a natural style befitting the steeply sloping site, which has a burn and waterfalls in its centre.

Spring and early summer see many rhododendrons in bloom, with waterside plantings of candelabra primulas and the bright crimson lanterns of *Crinodendron hookerianum*, which hails from Chile. There is a mini-pinetum, a wild heather bank, a productive kitchen garden, and a collection of exotic trees and shrubs around the burn. A lawn beside the house is surrounded by rock garden plants and summer-flowering perennials.

Plas Brondanw, Gwynedd

Formal gardens do not feature that strongly in Wales. The nation's gardeners have a tendency to respond to the mountainous topography and acid soils by taking a naturalistic approach. Not only is Plas Brondanw, situated in north-west Wales, a notable exception, but it is one of the most enchanting gardens you will see anywhere, although it is relatively little known.

The estate was given to the 25-year-old Clough Williams-Ellis in 1908 as a birthday present from his father. 'Nothing, just then, could possibly have been more ecstatically welcomed by me,' he recalled. A young architect with vision, and strongly imbued with the contemporary Arts and Crafts style, Williams-Ellis plotted the garden, a long, narrow strip of about two acres, dividing it into hedged rooms punctuated by slender columns of Italian cypress, which fare surprisingly well here.

This is an intimate, domestic and comfy garden, set against the awesome backdrop of the Snowdonia mountains. Its tiered yew topiaries are exceptionally fine, with deep crowns recalling traditional Welsh hats. The walls of local stone and slate shimmer in metallic mauves and browns in the rain, but transport the garden into dazzling Mediterranean mode when the sun shines.

Flowers do not feature strongly here, for this is chiefly a garden of green architecture and reflective pools, but with

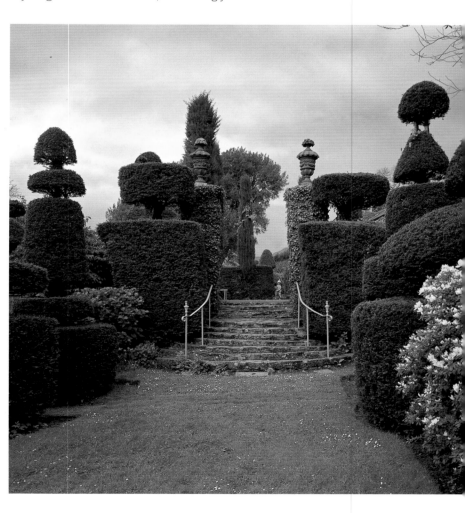

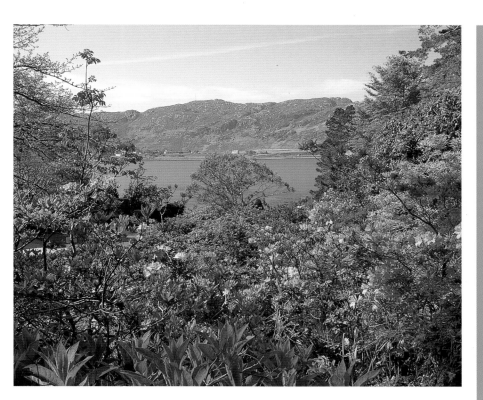

△ *Inverewe Garden*

its vistas directing your gaze to the summits of Moel Hebog and Cnicht in the distance, fancy blooms close to hand would seem an irrelevance.

There is a very pleasant walk, on the other side of the road, up a rather steep hill to a folly look-out. Williams-Ellis was serving in the Welsh Guards when he got married in 1915, but, always an individualist, he requested a ruin as a present from his fellow officers, instead of the usual silver salver. After the war he turned the gift of a pile of stones into the present viewing tower.

Inverewe Garden, Highlands

On my first visit to Inverewe in the Highlands of Scotland, I arrived at 8pm and had this fabulous garden all to myself, just me – and millions of midges. If you visit during the summer months, be sure to arrive liberally doused with repellent; the gardeners wear netted headgear on still summer days, when midges can be a serious problem.

Since a three-mile labyrinth of paths winds through the garden, you can lose yourself completely in the richly planted woodland featuring large collections of rhododendrons, eucalyptus, olearias and many other plants of the southern hemisphere, which thrive here due to the warming influence of the Gulf Stream. Among them are woodland perennials in variety, lily pools, bold drifts of candelabra primulas and shuttlecock ferns.

The front of the house is enlivened by a curved herbaceous border, which is spectacular from June to August, and below there is a rock garden sloping down to the shore. The sunny walled garden also faces the sea, and displays a sumptuous blend of herbaceous and annual flowers, vegetables, fruit and pergolas draped with climbing roses and clematis. The garden was made by Osgood Mackenzie in the latter half of the 19th century. Seeing all its rich variety, it is difficult to believe that when Mackenzie arrived the estate was a treeless wasteland. Positioned at 57.8°N, Inverewe Garden is, incredibly, closer to the Arctic Circle than St Petersburg and most of Labrador, and on one of the world's most windswept coastlines. The garden is also exceptionally well maintained.

Getting in touch

Barnsdale, Oakham, Rutland
Tel: 01572 813200

Castle Howard, York, Yorkshire
Tel: 01653 648333/648444

Coleton Fishacre, Kingswear, Devon
Tel: 01803 752466

Coton Manor, Guilsborough, Northamptonshire
Tel: 01604 740219

Cranborne Manor Gardens, Cranborne, Dorset
Tel: 01725 517248

Denmans, Fontwell, Sussex
Tel: 01243 542808

Felley Priory, Jacksdale, Nottinghamshire
Tel: 01773 810230

Fountains Abbey, Ripon, Yorkshire
Tel: 01765 608888

Glamaig Cottage, Portree, Isle of Skye
Tel: 01478 650226

Herterton House, Cambo, Northumberland
Tel: 01670 774278

Hodnet Hall, Hodnet, Shropshire
Tel: 01630 685202

Holker Hall, Grange-over-Sands, Cumbria
Tel: 01539 558328

Iford Manor, Bradford-on-Avon, Wiltshire
Tel: 01225 863146

Inverewe Garden, Wester Ross, Highlands
Tel: 01445 781200

Kellie Castle, Pittenweem, Fife
Tel: 01333 720271

Lyme Park, Stockport, Cheshire
Tel: 01663 762023

Mount Stewart, Newtownards, County Down
Tel: 01247 788387/788487

Newby Hall, Ripon, Yorkshire
Tel: 01423 322583

Parcevall Hall, Skipton, Yorkshire
Tel: 01756 720311

Plas Brondanw, Penrhyndeudraeth, Gwynedd
Tel: 01766 770484/770228

Port Lympne, Lympne, Kent
Tel: 01303 264647

Powis Castle, Welshpool, Powys
Tel: 01938 554338

Reads Nursery, Loddon, Norfolk
Tel: 01508 548395

The Savill Garden, Windsor Great Park, Berkshire
Tel: 01753 860222

Trebah Garden, Falmouth, Cornwall
Tel: 01326 250448

Wyken Hall, Stanton, Suffolk
Tel: 01359 250287

York Gate, Adel, Yorkshire
Tel: 01132 678240

What a blooming disaster

Judging by the happy smiles of the TV stars, you'd imagine that everything comes up roses in their gardens. Well, it doesn't. Like the rest of us, they have their disasters: the dog tramples the prize bedding, the fork impales their only champion-sized spud, or the lawnmower suddenly takes on a life of its own and scythes the herbaceous border. Here are a few, true, celebrity calamities.

Popular plantsman **Roy Lancaster** recalls the time he was leading a group of garden enthusiasts in Greece. Returning to the hotel after a day in the mountains, he discovered his woolly socks were covered with seeds. Instead of chucking the seeds away, he decided to sow them. Better still, why not sow the socks? On his return home, he 'planted' the socks in a seed tray, dreaming of discovering fantastic new flowers. Roy was so taken with his novel idea that he even wrote to a seed company to suggest his seed socks as a Father's Day present. The company responded enthusiastically and asked for photographs of the results. Roy waited with bated breath. The seeds germinated, and grew into a wonderfully lush crop of common weeds and grasses. He never did send those photos.

From the age of four, *Gardeners' World* regular **Pippa Greenwood** had her own little patch of garden and, when she grew up and left home, she added her treasures to her mother's garden. But there was something else she added, something she had lovingly purchased from a local fête with her hard-earned pocket money: a pot full of that rampant invader mind-your-own-business. It's now nearly 20 years since Pippa left home and she thinks her mother has only just succeeded in getting rid of it!

Perhaps actress **Susan Hampshire** could have helped. She loves weeding, but it reminds her of an early disaster. 'When I first started gardening, I pulled up hundreds of lily-of-the-valley thinking they were the dreaded ground elder.' She adds cheerfully, 'Thankfully, I've improved since then.'

Another type of planting disaster is recalled by celebrity hairdresser **Daniel Field**. He prides himself on his green fingers but was caught out when he and his wife, Julie, planted 30 rhododendrons last summer. Julie planted the first one and left him to plant the remaining 29. He woefully confesses, 'All my plants died while hers is thriving.'

Comedienne, actress and writer **Helen Lederer** probably hasn't got green fingers, judging from the day she helped out in her mother's garden. Noticing a tall, bracken-type thing in the centre of the lawn, she decided that it was spoiling the vista and 'had to go'. So, she promptly attacked it with the mower. On returning home, her mother peered at the lawn and asked, 'Where's my juniper plant?' 'Your what?' asked Helen, starting to feel rather cold. 'The juniper plant that was covering the drain in the middle of the lawn,' was the reply. Helen hasn't been asked to help out again.

Someone else who has learnt from his mistakes is *Gardeners' Question Time* panellist **Nigel Colborn**, who still has nightmares about his first pond. He borrowed a JCB to dig it out and got carried away. 'It was big enough to drown an elephant.' After partially filling it in, the levels were all wrong and a horrible wrinkled liner showed above the water line all down one side. In desperation, Nigel shovelled soil onto the edge and 'made the further mistake of planting vigorous British natives'. The resulting mat almost met in the middle of the pond. And

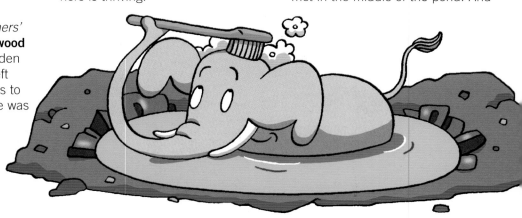

the final blow? 'My delinquent elder son accidentally speared the liner with a crow bar,' and the whole thing gradually emptied. Nigel filled it in, and planted grass and cowslips to mark the pond's grave. His second pond, he reports, looks fab.

Travel presenter **Anna Walker** wishes she had been a picky eater when she was young. She once made a 'pretend' tea from the garden, which included poisonous laburnum seeds. She ate them and had to be rushed to the hospital to have her stomach pumped!

A very different type of garden problem afflicted newsreader and presenter **Jill Dando**. Her new house sported a fine, green patch of astroturf, which she vowed to turf out. But four years later, the 'disastrous lawn' is still there. It turned out to be a blessing in disguise: 'It never needs mowing and the older it gets, the more it looks like the real thing.'

Television's **Sue Cook** certainly wouldn't want astroturf in her garden. She needs the grass to feed her pet disaster, her daughter's tortoise, Speedy. He's a picky eater, a good climber, but regularly falls off the garden wall and ends up on his back. 'I have to venture out on regular tortoise patrols to make sure he's upright and eating. The neighbours are treated to the daily sight of my bottom in the air as I search the undergrowth for him, calling out, "Speedy!". If only the blasted animal would learn to answer to his name!'

Leslie Ash, of *Men Behaving Badly* fame, had a startling and stomach-churning experience when she and her husband, footballer Lee Hurst, rented an old farmhouse in Italy.

Leslie was sure the garden was haunted, because every evening she could hear a spooky tapping noise that continued into the night. On their last night, they finally ventured into the garden and the ghostly tapping started up again. Leslie glanced in the direction of the sinister sound and, to her horror, saw what she thought was a ghostly robe floating through the air towards her. Needless to say, she was frightened out of her wits, but Lee, who hadn't seen the figure, bravely went to explore. Minutes later, he came back laughing. The spectre was nothing scarier than the spray from a garden sprinkler hidden in the grass. Just before they left the following day, they discovered that a kindly neighbour switched on the sprinklers every night!

Clare Bradley, the *Blue Peter* gardener, suffered a more natural disaster. One year the programme ran a giant pumpkin competition. Clare took part, sowing seed and tending her plant, but it took months for the first pumpkin to form. Back on air after the summer break, Clare had only four weeks to grow her tennis-ball-sized pumpkin into something more impressive. She tried every trick she could think of, including drip-feeding fertiliser directly into the stalk. But to her horror, it refused to grow larger than a football. On the big day, in rolled the viewers' winning pumpkins. They were so massive that they had to be manoeuvred into position with a forklift. Beside

them were placed glittering signs reading 'gigantic', 'massive', 'mega-huge' and 'enormous'. The cameras slowly panned along these monsters and eventually reached Clare's pumpkin. Plonked in front of it was a card saying, simply, 'puny'.

Take heart from Clare: when disaster strikes you in the garden, as it will from time to time, cheer yourself up with the thought that at least you don't have to share your plant howler with five million viewers.

Acknowledgements

The publisher would like to thank all those who have helped in so many ways to make this book possible. Everyone has given their help and support for free, from gardening experts and writers to illustrators, photographers and picture libraries. Without their enthusiasm, contributions and commitment this project would not have been possible.

Contributors

Stephen Anderton, Chris Baines, Clare Bradley, Steve Bradley, Kathryn Bradley-Hole, Nigel Colborn, Charlie Dimmock, Diarmuid Gavin, Pippa Greenwood, Ainsley Harriott, Carolyn Hutchinson, Richard Jackson, Roy Lancaster, Daphne Ledward, Anne McKevitt, Adam Pasco, Eric Robson, Peter Seabrook, Gay Search, Anne Swithinbank, Alan Titchmarsh, Tommy Walsh

Artwork

Vanessa Luff 42; Coral Mulla 58, 60, 61; Amanda Patton 45; Liz Pepperell 62, 63, 64, 67, Andrew Peters 94, 95

Photographers

A–Z Botanical: 25bc, Matt Johnson 17b, Malkolm Warrington 16br; **BBC**: Paul Bricknell/BBC 50, 51 all; Craig Easton/BBC 12b; Gus Filgate/BBC 55, 56; John Glover/BBC 12t, 13t, 57b; Tim Sandall/BBC 68 all, 69 all, 73c, 76l, 76r; William Shaw/BBC: 11t; *BBC Gardeners' World Magazine* 74tl, 78b; **Blakedown Nurseries** 25tc; **Bob Brown**: 27bc, **Jonathan Buckley**: 32, 33, 34, 35 (except portrait), 48 all, 49 all; *Country Life*: Felley Priory 87r; **Peter Durkes**: 74c; **Stephen Hamilton**: 73br, 74tr, 74bl, 75br, 77tl, 77tr 79; **Jerry Harpur**: 88l; **Derek Lomas**: 72; **Garden Picture Library**: David Askham/GPL 23br, 30bl, 31cl, Mark Bottom/GPL 26bl, back cover bottom, Lynne Brotchie/GPL back cover top; Chris Burrows/GPL 15tl, 22br; Brian Carter/GPL 26t, Kathy Charlton/GPL 91; Densey Clyne/GPL 31cr, 31b; Chrisopher Fairweather/GPL 30br; John Glover/GPL 23tc, 23tr, 25tr, 26c, 28tr, Sunniva Harte/GPL 24bl, Michael Howes/GPL 15tr, Clay Perry 85t, Howard Rice/GPL 6, 15bl, 25tl, 25bl; JS Sira/GPL 30tr; Steven Wooster/GPL 93; **Steve Gorton**: 19tr; **John Glover**: 9tb, 16tr, 19tl, 22t, 23c, 27c, 27tr, 27bl, 28bl, 29br, 39c, 39b, 44b, 73t, 82; **Julian Hawkins**: 41 all, 75tr, 75c, 76c, 80t; **Holt Studios International**: 14; **Anne Hyde**: 75tl, 75bl, 78l; **Andrew Lawson**: front cover top, 4, 8b, 16tl, 17t, 18l, 19br, 22bl, 25c, 25br, 27br, 38t, 44tr, 83b; Denmans Gardens, Sussex 89r; **National Trust Photographic Library**: Neil Campbell-Sharp 84b; Jerry Harpur 90r; **Clive Nichols Garden Pictures**: Emma Lush 54c; Garden Security and Lighting 57t; Herterton House 87l; Cotton Manor, Northants 86r; Clive Nichols 6, 15br, 20-21, 22c, 23tl, 23bl, 24t, 24c, 27t, 28c, 28br, 29tr, 29tc, 29tr, 29bl, 29bc, 30c, 31tl, 31tr, 36 all, 37 all, 38c, 38b, 39t, 47; **Photos Horticultural**: 2, 8t, 16bl, 19bl, 26b, 31c, 46 all, 54t, 54b, 57c, 58, 59 all, 61 all, 77bl, 77br, 79bl, 81 all, 83t, 89r, 90l, 93r; **TE Read**: 87l; **Mr and Mrs R Townsend**: 92l; **Jeremy Watson**: 85.

Also thanks to **Peter Anderson, George Brooks, Neil Campbell-Sharp, Steven Hamilton, Julian Hawkins, Richard Kendal, Gary Moyes, Tim Sandall** and **William Shaw** for their portrait photography.

Greenfingers Appeal Committee

Vicky Cooper, Jim Deen, Boyd Douglas-Davies, Mike Dunnett, Richard Jackson, Kevin Lannigan, Peter Marsh, Natalie McBride, Simon Richards, Alan Shaw, Dawn Smith, Jean Vernon and Chris Webb

Our thanks to the authors of the following books for allowing material to be taken from their work:

Anne Swithinbank's Container Gardening for All Seasons
Ainsley Harriott's Barbecue Bible
Ground Force Weekend Workbook by Alan Titchmarsh and Steve Bradley
The Garden Lovers' Guide to Britain by Kathryn Bradley-Hole

Material has also been taken from issues of *BBC Gardeners' World Magazine*.